INTRODUCTION TO Psychiatry

INTRODUCTION
TO
Psychiatry

O. SPURGEON ENGLISH, M.D.

PROFESSOR AND CHAIRMAN, DEPARTMENT OF PSYCHIA-
TRY, TEMPLE UNIVERSITY SCHOOL OF MEDICINE AND
HOSPITAL, PHILADELPHIA

and STUART M. FINCH, M.D.

PROFESSOR OF PSYCHIATRY, AND DIRECTOR OF THE
CHILDREN'S PSYCHIATRIC HOSPITAL, UNIVERSITY OF
MICHIGAN SCHOOL OF MEDICINE

W · W · NORTON & COMPANY · INC · *New York*

Library of Congress Catalog Card No. 64-11135

PRINTED IN THE UNITED STATES OF AMERICA
FOR THE PUBLISHERS BY THE VAIL-BALLOU PRESS, INC.
1 2 3 4 5 6 7 8 9

Contents

PART I   Concepts of Dynamic Psychiatry

PART IV   Personality Disorders

PART V   Psychophysiologic Disorders

PART VIII   Mental Retardation

PART IX   Therapy

Preface to the Third Edition

THE AUTHORS have felt considerable pride in the request for a third edition of this textbook—first because psychiatry has advanced sufficiently during the last few years to justify such an endeavor, and second because the textbook itself has been favorably received by students. Both authors have continued actively in the teaching of medical students and physicians and both have felt the need to try to keep such students abreast of newer advances in psychiatry. During the past few years the national interest in mental illness and mental retardation has increased remarkably. The Joint Commission Report "Action for Mental Health" has stimulated the public, the medical profession, and the various legislatures to turn more attention to this tremendous problem. Community psychiatry has now become almost a subspecialty of its own. Child psychiatry has attained official recognition as a subspecialty. Workers in many fields, both in and out of clinical medicine, have become increasingly involved in attempting to solve some of the problems of the psychiatric patient. The neurophysiologist, the endocrinologist, the geneticist, the biochemist, and others are providing us daily with new advances in our knowledge.

The authors still feel that the medical student and physician today should first understand the patient and his emotional adjustment. This is the essential cornerstone on which further knowledge about family interactions, parent-child relationships, community adjustments, and so forth are built. Essential to the understanding of the individual patient is a meaningful knowledge of psychoanalytic insights which, although refined and improved, remain basically the same as they were when the first edition of this book was published. We have attempted to bring up to date some of the areas in which the most noteworthy advances have been made. For example, the tranquilizers have made remarkable changes in the practice of psychiatry during the last few years and additional attention is therefore paid to this area. Community psychiatry has grown from its infancy to perhaps its adolescence. At the same time other areas have remained somewhat shrouded in mystery; an example is schizophrenia. When the last edition of the book was published the cause of schizophrenia was unknown. Today our knowledge is more sophisticated, but it still is true that we do not know what causes this group of disorders.

We have again decided in this edition to adhere in general to the official nomenclature of the American Psychiatric Association. While even the authors of this classification would be the first to admit that it has many weaknesses, it would also seem appropriate to follow the accepted, American Medical Association-approved, standardized method. The few departures we take from this nomenclature are explained in the text.

Acknowledgment is made to the many people who have helped us with this revision. We also wish to acknowledge the help of Dr. David Rubinstein in aiding with the discussion on family treatment. We are particularly indebted to Elizabeth Killins for her editorial assistance, and to Elizabeth Houston and Marion Mayer for invaluable help with proofreading and the preparation and typing of this manuscript.

O. S. E.
S. M. F.

Preface

THE DECISION to undertake the writing of this textbook of psychiatry was an outgrowth of the authors' teaching experiences at Temple University School of Medicine and Hospital. They have felt for some time that a textbook oriented along psychoanalytic lines was needed. The principles of dynamic psychiatry, as advanced by Sigmund Freud, have been mentioned and briefly explained in other texts, but often only in a fragmentary manner. Psychoanalytic thought has permeated both the practice and teaching of psychiatry to the point where there is a definite need for a book with this orientation.

Many new books are appearing in psychiatry, but unfortunately few of them are textbooks. Many of them deal with relatively limited aspects of psychiatry, such as treatment, psychophysiological conditions, or psychoneuroses. While a number of these books are brilliantly written, they have the disadvantage of covering only a limited sphere. Medical students, the authors feel, gain much of their initial acquaintance with psychiatry through the particular textbook which they use. It is important, therefore, that such a book be reasonably comprehensive and yet give the student a useful and practical view of personality formation and function.

The authors feel that a student can understand psychiatry only when he has mastered the concepts of dynamic personality formation and structure. Once these concepts are understood, the student may learn how such formation and structure may be distorted and disturbed. This is the same principle that in medical schools requires the student to become well grounded in anatomy and physiology before he attempts to learn the intricacies of pathology.

It will be noted that child psychiatry is given a new prominence consistent with its importance. It occupies an early and inclusive section of the book, rather than being put near the end in an isolated place. This is logical, since dynamic psychiatry stresses the importance of the childhood years in personality formation. The adult can only be completely understood if his childhood is taken into consideration.

In this book the authors have attempted to adhere as closely as possible to the new revision of nomenclature accepted by the Council of the American Psychiatric Association in the spring of 1952. It seemed most advantageous that the student and the resident adopt and conform to this nomenclature as closely as possible, even though it obviously does not represent the final answer to psychiatric diagnosis. The authors have accepted the fact that it was a difficult task to get a large committee to produce a nomenclature that would suit all groups and wish to commend the committee for the improvements in the new arrangement. There are, however, some diagnostic categories which overlap almost completely and others where subdivisions have been carried to a point of refinement that threatens to produce confusion rather than clarity for the student. Nevertheless, in the interest of consistency, the authors have tried to use the nomenclature as completely as possible.

Psychiatric and psychoanalytic knowledge has been applied in recent years to a progressively wider area of human endeavor. It has not only been found useful in other specialties of medicine, but also in law, religion, and other fields. It has not been feasible nor does it seem desirable in a textbook of this type to attempt adequate coverage of all of these applications of psychiatry. Reference is made to some of the books dealing with these subjects in the bibliography.

Acknowledgment is made to our colleague, Dr. Steven Hammerman, for reading the sections on organic and toxic brain disorders and making suggestions. Also, we are indebted to Dr. John M. Rhoads and Dr. H. Keith Fischer for supplying case material and to Dr. Francis H. Hoffman for material on tranquilizing drugs. Acknowledgment is made to Jeanne B. Speiser for her invaluable help with proofreading and her suggestions for clarity, readability, and arrangement of material.

For secretarial work and typing we are indebted to the conscientious and careful help of Dorothy K. Kallbach, Theresa Zubernis, and Nancy Snyder.

O. S. E.
S. M. F.

PART I

Concepts of Dynamic Psychiatry

CHAPTER I

The History of Psychiatry

MODERN psychiatry, with all its scientific concepts, is man's latest step in his age-long attempt to understand himself and his mental aberrations. Primitive man, ignorant of the phenomena about him, was both mystified and frightened by the appearance of mental disease, yet found a very simple explanation for it. He looked at the world about him, rather than within himself. He sought to find the reasons for mental illness in the various natural occurrences he saw. The sun, the moon, the wind, the rain, the lightning and thunder, all became repositories for his own inner "good" and "bad" urges; he could then blame these things for the strange diseases which befell him. Gradually, over a long period of time, many of these phenomena, as well as animals and objects, became deified and were assumed to exert mysterious forces. Slowly, from this early beginning, the idea of gods evolved and the belief arose that mental disease occurred whenever the gods took man's mind away.

Although some mention, and even description, of psychotic and epileptic syndromes is to be found in ancient writings of Western cultures, as well as in biblical writings, it remained for Hippocrates, the father of medicine, to make the first great contribution to psychiatry in the fourth century B.C. He removed mental disease from the realm of mysticism and put it into its proper place in medicine. In addition, this great Greek physician described many of the syndromes with which we are familiar today. Some of the understandable errors which he made, such as his theory of bile as a cause of mental disease, are comparatively insignificant in the light of the epochal strides which he made in bringing psychiatry into the realm

3

of medicine. Before Hippocrates' time the art of healing in Greece was primarily a religious one carried on in the temples of the god Aesculapius.

Aesculapius, according to legend, was the Roman god of healing who, along with his two sons, Machaon and Podalirius, was noted for his therapeutic ability, particularly along surgical lines. Temples were erected to him in many parts of Greece, near healing springs and high mountains. The practice of sleeping in these temples was common; it was believed that the god effected cures or prescribed remedies to the sick in dreams. The rites observed in these temples of Aesculapius were primarily religious in nature, so that Hippocrates' subsequent contributions seem even more remarkable in view of the then existing conditions. Notable was his challenge of the common belief of the time that epilepsy was a sacred disease and his statement that it originated from "natural cause," just as did many other diseases which he studied.

Hippocrates was an astute observer and described with accuracy the many syndromes which he noted. Among them were melancholia, *post partum* psychoses, and even various toxic deliria. While his understanding of the etiology of these syndromes was not accurate, his description of the various clinical pictures left little to be improved upon.

Plato, another great contributor of this same Grecian period, formulated a complex and rather confusing theory of psychopathology. He proposed a soul consisting of two parts, rational and irrational. His theories were a mixture of the theological past and the more advanced anatomical knowledge of his day. There was considerable disagreement among early medical writers and philosophers as to the body center of emotions and perceptions. Plato considered the brain to be such a center, while his famous pupil Aristotle located it in the heart. Both of these men played important roles in the beginning of our understanding of psychological functioning and the relationship between mind and body. Many areas of man's knowledge about himself and the world around him were enlarged during the period when Greece was the center of cultural learning. A great deal of mysticism and theology was mixed in with the medical and psychiatric thinking of the day. Plato's writings present a notable example of this mixture. Aristotle, on the other hand, was much more of an observant scientist, interested in describing the phenomena he saw and in forming deductions from his observations.

Another famous personality in the history of medical science is Asclepiades, who lived in the first century B.C. He was not only astute in his recognition of the role of emotions in the production of mental disease, but he also departed from some of the prevailing therapeutic views of the day. He prescribed a much more kindly treatment than had, up until then, been the vogue. Such things as music, gentle rocking, and pleasant conversations were among his recommendations for the treatment of mental disease. He opposed bleeding, which was widely advocated at that time.

Still another great physician from this early era who contributed much to the foundations of medicine was Galen. He lived in the second century A.D., and perhaps his greatest contribution was the gathering together of much of the knowledge which had accumulated during the height of the Greek and Roman cultures. He was essentially eclectic in his approach and his writings became a sort of a reference point for medicine throughout many centuries to come. Galen properly assigned psychic functions to the brain. However, in addition he proposed one irrational soul, ascribed to the liver, and a second ascribed to the heart. Some mental disease, he felt, stemmed directly from difficulties within the brain itself, although he also apparently accepted some of the humoral theories of Hippocrates.

Many of the scientific advances made during the Greco-Roman period fell into disuse and disrepute during the centuries following Galen. The rise of Christianity introduced many new theological ideas; among them were concepts regarding mental illness. Many of the psychotics, then as now, suffered from delusions and hallucinations with religious content and this fact led to the assumption that there was a supernatural quality to mental illness. As the Dark Ages closed in there were a few bright spots in psychological thinking, but for the most part, scientific progress in psychiatry was slowed and most of the past advances were eradicated. The devil was felt to be the primary cause of mental disease and thus it was eliminated from the realm of medicine.

In 1494, two monks wrote a book which solidified, outlined, and clearly defined much of the thinking of the day concerning mental illness. This book dealt with the problems of witches and was called the *Malleus Maleficarum,* or "witches' hammer." It has been described as "the most authoritative and horrible document of that age," and inseparably linked mental disease and witchcraft for many centuries. It is truly difficult for modern man to conceive of the conditions which existed during the Dark Ages, particularly in regard to mental illness. The Church played a prominent role in state affairs and both Church and state accepted demonology. A person who became hallucinated or delusional was considered to be afflicted with the devil and to be a witch.

It was during the fifteenth and sixteenth centuries that some voices began to be raised against the prevailing demonic theory of mental illness. Juan Vives, a Spanish scholar, was a pioneer in the trend toward more humanistic and scientific thinking. He spoke out in his belief that emotions were important in the understanding of personality problems. He agreed to the existence of a soul in man which was within the realm of theology, but he also felt that many of the workings of man's mind were subject to scientific study and therefore to greater understanding. Vives was not a physician, but a Swiss contemporary of his, Paracelsus, who shared the same views, was a medical man. Paracelsus was an individualist who was considered to be a heretic by many of his contemporaries. He often criticized existing medical beliefs and demanded an end to the idea that demons were responsible for mental illness. Another famous physician of the period was Cornelius Agrippa. He, like Paracelsus, was ridiculed and maligned for his radical ideas, but he too spoke out clearly against demonology. Johann Weyer, a student of Agrippa, was the first "psychiatrist" in that he was primarily interested in mental illness. He left a wealth of descriptive material covering a variety of clinical entities and, in so doing, furthered the separation of psychology from theology and thus helped to bring mental illness back into the realm of medicine.

As more enlightened attitudes gained ground in medical as well as psychological areas, a school of organicists arose during the seventeenth century who looked for the answer to mental disease in anatomical studies. At the same time, the humanistic school of psychological thought was occupied with attempts to correct legal and social problems of the day as they related to the treatment of the mentally disturbed. During this period the insane were housed in poorhouses, almshouses, and in a few scattered mental hospitals. The latter hardly deserved the name of hospital, since patients received abominable care, often being chained for years in dark and filthy dungeons. Bethlehem, or as it was properly called, Bedlam, in London, had been in operation since the thirteenth century. The Bicêtre, in Paris, was another example of the "mental hospital."

It was during the eighteenth century that Philippe Pinel came to the Bicêtre and upset the traditions of his day by removing the chains from patients and treating them as human beings. This drastic step took great courage and daring and Pinel was subjected to severe criticism. During the latter part of this same century York Retreat was founded in England by William Tuke, a layman who was horrified by the poor treatment afforded mental patients. This institution, along with the Bicêtre, pioneered in more freedom for patients and the removal of chains.

Another milestone in psychiatric history occurred during the latter part of the eighteenth century with the meteoric rise of Anton Mesmer. This histrionic performer originated, or at least popularized, hypnotism, which was also known as mesmerism. He gave demonstrations and produced widespread interest in this phenomenon, which he attributed to "animal magnetism." An interesting sidelight to this development was the spread of mesmerism to the United States where a local watchmaker, P. P. Quimby, was stirred to an interest in faith healing and successfully rid Mary Baker Eddy of a hysterical paralysis. The most important result of Mesmer's somewhat theatrical career was the interest stirred up in the medical profession by his techniques. This led to the use of hypnosis as an anesthetic agent and also to experimentation with it as a means of treatment of emotional disorders. Jean Martin Charcot, a famous French physician, and another contemporary, H. Bernheim, became the centers of study groups who investigated neuroses, often using hypnosis. One of Charcot's pupils, a neurologist named Sigmund Freud, was to make epochal contributions to the field of psychiatry.

Psychiatry officially began in the United States in 1751, when the Pennsylvania Hospital was founded in Philadelphia. It was the first hospital in the Colonies to care exclusively for the sick, and provisions were made for the care of mentally ill patients. Benjamin Rush, one of the signers of the Declaration of Independence, was an early American physician who, along with his many other achievements, helped psychiatry get its beginnings in this country. In 1844, thirteen physicians gathered in Philadelphia for the first meeting of the Association of Medical Superintendents of American Institutions of the Insane (later to become the American Psychiatric Association). At that time there were very few mental hospitals in the States and the tendency was to follow the prevalent European theories and practices. It was in 1841 that Dorothea Dix, a school teacher, began her forty-year crusade for improved institutional care of the mentally ill. In 1908, Clifford Beers[1] wrote a book entitled *A Mind That Found Itself*. It was an account of the author's nervous breakdown which had resulted in his spending several years in various mental institutions. The book stirred wide interest and Beers became instrumental in the founding of the National Committee for Mental Hygiene, now the National Association for Mental Health. He remained the secretary of this organization for thirty years.

Classification of mental disease had, from early and slow beginnings, become increasingly common during the nineteenth century. Unfortunately, while many syndromes were described, there was little real system to the many classifications. Emil Kraepelin (1862–1915) introduced the first really comprehensive organization in the classification of mental diseases. His elucidation of the varieties of dementia praecox and manic depressive psychosis had a beneficial, stabilizing effect on the psychiatric thinking of the time. Although this vastly improved classification had many merits and represented a great stride forward, it nevertheless had one disadvantage. This was that the nosological approach put the emphasis on symptom patterns rather than on a better understanding of the underlying reasons for symptoms. Soon after the turn of the century, Eugen

[1] Beers, Clifford. *A Mind That Found Itself*. New York, Doubleday, Doran and Co., 1936.

Bleuler introduced the term *schizophrenia* to replace the older term *dementia praecox*. In his writings he stressed the fact that schizophrenia was not a single disease entity, and pointed out the inner origins of autistic thinking. Such contributions were important in stressing a better understanding of mechanisms beyond the area of pure classification.

Near the end of the last century, Sigmund Freud turned his attention from organic neurological problems to emotional disorders. After his work with hypnosis he gradually evolved his theories of dynamic personality function and gave the name *psychoanalysis* to his therapeutic procedure. His was a dynamic orientation based upon gaining insight into the underlying reasons for neurotic disturbances. Freud's early theories of the unconscious and of the importance of sexual material led to a great deal of opposition in both medical and lay groups. He gathered about himself a small group of workers, some physicians and some laymen, and so was born the new science of psychoanalysis. It has grown in spite of many vicissitudes until at the present time psychoanalytic concepts have diffused throughout the entire field of psychiatry, with applications in the field of many of the social sciences and education as well.

Soon after the turn of the century, a few of the early Freudian group split off to pursue their own divergent views as to the causation of neurosis. C. G. Jung, a brilliant psychiatrist, became more and more convinced of the existence and importance of what he called a "racial unconscious," that is, fantasies and emotional trends inherited from ancestors. Jung formed his own group to pursue this orientation and his work showed an increasing emphasis on the creative impulse in man. Alfred Adler, another of the early workers, founded his school of individual psychology based upon what he considered to be man's all-important striving for power. Otto Rank, another of the early group who went on to form his own school, stressed the importance of anxiety experienced at birth as a prototype of much future anxiety in the life of an individual. Wilhelm Stekel stressed skill in dream interpretation and the importance of homosexuality in the production of psychopathology. He, like the others, formed a group of his own. While there are still practicing therapists of all these smaller groups, the majority of psychoanalysts adhere to Freudian concepts.

James J. Putnam and A. A. Brill are the two men who were responsible for the introduction of psychoanalysis into the United States and its integration into medical and psychiatric thinking. Brill translated many of Freud's basic works into English for publication in this country and in 1911 he founded the New York Psychoanalytic Society. Two other vigorous supporters and exponents of psychoanalysis in psychiatry were Smith Ely Jelliffe and William Alanson White. Both men were prominent psychiatrists, coedited psychiatric and psychoanalytic journals, and lent much prestige to the early analytic movement.

One of the most important figures in American psychiatry was Adolf Meyer, who, in 1910, became Professor of Psychiatry at Johns Hopkins. He was a contemporary of Freud, and the views of the two men had some similarities. Both regarded mental illness, in the main, as a personality reaction rather than a disease. Both felt that the life history and the vicissitudes of the individual were important etiological factors. They differed in that Meyer did not accept the concept of the unconscious or the importance of infantile sexuality. Meyer did not evolve as definite a technique of therapy as did Freud. Yet both these two great scientists contributed immensely to the wider acceptance of a concept of mental disease seen as a result of the individual's difficulty in adapting to his environment.

Meyer has been properly called the "dean of American psychiatry." Basically, as we have mentioned, he looked upon emotional and mental disorders not as disease entities but as reaction types. He called his school of thought *psychobiology* and to him the total man was to be considered in the light of all aspects, including organic, cultural, sociological, and psychological ones. His was a "common-sense approach," based on all factors involved. His students were many; psychobiology became a prominent orientation in American psychiatry. Meyer's lack of acceptance of psychoanalysis was unfortunate, since it hampered the relationships between the two schools of thought and produced, at times, an intraspecialty conflict which interfered with efficient co-operation. However, it may be said that at the present time most psychiatrists accept and utilize at least some of the basic theories of psychoanalysis and that the conflict between the psychoanalyst and the nonpsychoanalyst is not nearly as sharp as it has been in the past.

Psychoanalysis, although originally intended by Freud to be a specific technique for treatment of the psychoneuroses, has been applied to other conditions, such as psychoses, children's disorders, and psychophysiologic conditions. With some modifications, its basic principles have proven useful in furthering our understanding of disorders in fields other than psychoneurosis and have improved treatment procedures. Consequently, while the authors freely and gratefully acknowledge the important contributions of other psychodynamic systems, they feel that the time has come when, for simplicity and cohesion, a psychiatric textbook should be written which adheres primarily to the application of Freudian principles. They believe that the future of psychiatry seems likely to be further organized around Freudian psychology because it is the most comprehensive. Freudian psychology considers the interaction of life processes with environmental events from the very beginning of existence. It presents a dynamic psychology that is inextricably interlocked with body physiology. This fact alone makes it the ideal physician's psychology. It seems important, therefore, to focus attention on a system of thought which is so far-reaching and which has been subjecting itself to experimental work and scientific validation along with other scientific medical disciplines.

The growth of psychiatry during the past fifty years has been phenomenal. It has assumed an increasingly important position in the curricula of medical schools. Many new mental hospitals have been built, and the public has become increasingly aware of the importance of mental and emotional disorders. Psychiatrists are more numerous (the American Psychiatric Association now has more than 12,000 members); preventive psychiatry is making rapid strides; and increasing attention is being given to emotional disorders in children. It has been estimated that one of every ten persons in the U.S. is now suffering from some form of mental illness. Approximately 10 per cent of all public-school children are sufficiently disturbed to need help. Over one-half of the hospital beds are occupied by mental patients—this is more than all the hospitalized patients with heart disease, cancer, polio, tuberculosis, and all other diseases combined. Over one-half million new juvenile delinquents are seen by courts each year. The divorce rate continues to grow. These are only a few indications of the magnitude of the problem.

Action for Mental Health,[2] the report by the Joint Commission, points out the need for drastically increased services for the mentally ill. Community psychiatry as a new approach is rapidly gaining impetus. Certainly we cannot spread the principles of mental hygiene unless we ourselves are initially well-grounded in them. And, as physicians, we cannot covet the right to care for the mentally and emotionally disturbed unless we assume the obligation of learning the basic principles of psychiatric thought.

[2] Joint Commission on Mental Illness and Health. *Action for Mental Health*. New York, Basic Books, 1961.

CHAPTER 2

The Development and Structure of the Personality

PSYCHIATRY is that branch of medicine which deals with the human psyche and its various disturbances. Like other branches of medicine, it deals with human beings who are ill. It cannot treat directly a disturbance of the psyche, but must rather treat a person who has a pathological emotional process. The internist does not see an ulcer, but a man who has an ulcer, and so it is with the psychiatrist. He does not see a conversion reaction, but an individual whose emotional dysfunction falls within the group of patients utilizing conversion patterns. After all, man is a unit and one cannot consider the psyche without the soma, nor the soma without the psyche. Psychiatry, even more than any other branch of medicine, considers not only the total man, but also the environment from which he comes. It is man's psyche which interprets his environment and which is constantly trying to adjust him to that environment.

A basic principle of living organisms is the attempt to adjust to the environment. In its simplest form this is seen in the phenomenon of the reflex arc, a matter of a stimulus calling for a response, where the principle of irritability applies. As man has progressed up the phylogenetic scale and successfully crammed more and more brain tissue into his cranium, he has complicated many of the basic principles of simpler animal life. For example, he has added the all-important function of reason to his armamentarium. Yet, since he is still a living organism, he is not entirely different from the simpler forms of life. The principle of homeostasis propounded by Cannon [1] is an example. This principle postulates the tendency of all living matter to attempt to return to a resting state. Equilibrium is constantly being disturbed by various stimuli from the environment, and the organism is equally constant in its attempts to re-establish its initial equilibrium.

The environment continuously makes demands upon the psyche from the outside, and, at the same time, organic demands press on it from within. The forces and counterforces which are engendered produce a complicated but nevertheless understandable pattern of attempts of the individual to adjust to the environment and to achieve a satisfactory state of existence.

As the five special senses bring to the brain a constant stream of impressions from the outer world, they indicate the dangers and demands, pleasures and satisfactions, of the environment. At the same time, from within the body, there are the urges of those organically based drives which are called the instincts, and which have their origin within the somatic processes of the body. Basically there is a tendency to attempt to satisfy these inner urges immediately, but various complicating factors are at work. Previous experience, training, and the environmental situations very often make control and postponement of these inner urges necessary. It is with such processes and their vicissitudes that psychiatry deals.

Instincts are the somatically based urges arising within the body and seeking as their aim gratification through some object, the object often being a person. The term *instinct* is commonly used to indicate stereotyped patterns of behavior as seen in other species, and one must be certain not to confuse this with the term as used in psychiatry. Man, as a matter of fact, would appear to have relatively few instincts of this stereotyped nature. Examples of the common usage are such things as the migratory habits of birds and the spawning habits of certain fish.

It must be borne in mind also that psychiatrists and particularly psychoanalysts use the word *sexual* in a different and much broader sense than a purely genital one. The term as Freud used it indicates

[1] Cannon, W. B. *The Wisdom of the Body.* Revised edition. New York, W. W. Norton & Company, 1939.

anything pleasurable. He broadened the traditional concept of sexuality to include "love" in a limitless sense, embodying positive creative forces which he saw as the core of man's instinctual life. This means of course that adult genital union is only part of the sexual picture. The infant who derives pleasure from sucking is getting sexual pleasure in the psychoanalytic sense. The same holds true for the toddler who is getting pleasure from his excretory functions.

It is with the instincts as psychiatry defines them that the very close connection between psyche and soma is best illustrated. It is here that body and mind have a relationship which as yet is not fully understood, but which we know is of great importance in maintaining an organically and psychically healthy state. It would certainly appear that pathological processes in either the psyche or the soma are capable of upsetting each other's operations. Modern medicine is paying progressively greater attention to this all-important link between mind and body in its attempts to view man as a whole operating unit.

Attempts to describe the human personality can proceed from two directions—developmental and structural. But because *personality* is a term that will be used often in this book it should now be defined. Specifically, personality is the sum total of experience, in that everything which has happened to an individual from birth onward has produced some effect on him. The infant is born with certain constitutional endowments, and the eventual form which his personality takes will depend both upon this original endowment and how the environment acts on it. The personality will also include the sum total of the ways in which he has gradually learned to deal with his inner needs (instincts) in relation to the outer world.

It is possible to describe the structure of an adult personality as it exists at a given moment. However, using this method alone has certain disadvantages in that it may deceive the student into adopting a sort of static concept of a rigid personality structure, almost in the anatomical sense. On the other hand, it is possible to describe this same personality in terms of its various formative stages. Combining the two has the advantage of giving the student a more dynamic understanding of the various processes at work within the human personality.

PERSONALITY DEVELOPMENT

One of the main contributions of psychoanalysis to modern dynamic psychiatry has been the delineation of various steps in the development of personality from infancy to maturity. It may be said that the human infant is born without a personality, but with certain potentials for forming one. It has been determined through extensive and intensive study that in the process of maturing each individual passes through certain definite levels of personality formation. These particular levels of psychosexual development are dictated primarily by a combination of the individual's ability to relate to his environment and the variations in his instinctual needs. The phases are not sharply differentiated from each other, and it is perfectly normal to see evidences of more than one phase in an individual child at one time. However, in the normal developing youngster, one particular phase is seen as being in ascendancy, while others at that time appear less noticeable. It is of some importance for the student to master a general knowledge of the demands and behavior of each particular phase, since only through such knowledge can he accurately evaluate the status of a personality, either in an adult or in a child. Another aspect of the same problem of maturation is the progression from the pleasure principle of infancy to the reality principle of adult life. The pleasure principle indicates behavior on an "I want what I want when I want it and I don't want to postpone my wants for anything or anyone" level. Infants function on this principle and are unwilling, and to a degree unable, to postpone gratification of their instinctual demands for any period of time. The reality principle refers to a more adult kind of adjustment, namely the ability to set up long-range goals and undergo temporary frustration and difficulties to attain these goals. The healthy adult will be able to withstand tensions from ungratified instincts if he is able to progress steadily toward his eventual and larger goals.

ORAL PERIOD

At the time of birth and for some time thereafter the human infant is totally dependent upon the adults who surround him. Without them existence would be impossible. To this first period of life, extending through the initial year, Freud gave the name *oral period*. This name was chosen because of the importance of the oral mechanism in the infant's relationship to the world about him. Most basic is the fact, of course, that his nutritional needs are met through the use of the mouth. The inner hunger tensions which develop are relieved through this route and the experience is a pleasurable one. The satiation of hunger brings with it, both during and following the process, a sense of pleasure and contentment and security. Mounting hunger tensions are painful and the extremely immature ego of the infant is unable to master or postpone such tensions, which therefore become increasingly unpleasant.

There exists during this first period of life an extremely close relationship between mother and child. The mother supplies both nutritional and emotional essentials to the child. It is during this period of life that certain basic attitudes are formed as a result of the degree of security provided by the environment. The infant whose mother is able to provide warmth, love, and the necessary comforts develops an inner feeling of security. It is from such security that the adult personality derives many of its desirable features, such as friendliness, optimism, and the proper ability to give and take in relationships with people. If, however, the infant's mother is incapable, perhaps because of her own emotional deficiencies, of providing these necessary ingredients for the baby, personality formation does not progress satisfactorily. The infant is constantly threatened by painful tensions which he is unable to master. His mother becomes for him a source of frustration, rather than a source of gratification. He comes to not expect satisfaction from the environment. His growing personality will have at its core a basically distrustful and pessimistic concept of the world about him. He will have difficulty progressing through later levels of psychosexual development because of the large elements of early unsatisfied dependency. Evidences of residual oral traits which are often seen in adults include such things as alcoholism, excessive smoking, excessive gum chewing, an unduly demanding attitude, and overeating. Such individuals have an attitude that the world owes them not only a living but princely rewards as well. They are basically anxious, insecure people who are quite sensitive to rejection, but at the same time quite demanding.

The oral period is considered to extend through the first year. However, evidences of orality are quite normally seen throughout much of childhood. They are pathological only when they persist to a degree that prevents a smooth continuous development through the following psychosexual phases.

ANAL PERIOD

The *anal period* is that phase of personality development extending from approximately the end of the first year to about the fourth year. It derives its name from the fact that during this time the functions of elimination have a position of great importance in the child's life. During the oral phase, the infant is totally dependent upon his environment and cannot be expected to give to those around him. However, following the end of the first year, demands are made upon him toward learning conformity. One of the most important areas in which these demands are made is in that of learning to control his excretions. Both the retention and finally the expulsion of urine and feces become pleasurable acts to the child. The youngster's willingness to bring his functions of elimination under control depends primarily upon his relationship with his mother and the methods by which she attempts to achieve her goal. The child during the anal period has certain personality characteristics which are normal at this particular time, and which have to be taken into consideration by those who would help him learn to conform. Obstinacy, parsimony, ambivalence, and sadism are all characteristics of this particular phase. *Ambivalence* is a term indicating the simultaneous existence of both love and hate impulses toward an individual. Whereas a mature individual is capable of loving others, the ambivalent person automatically loves as he hates and hates as he loves. This state of affairs exists as a normal condition only during the anal phase.

The greatest single motivating factor stimulating the child to learn to conform is the high value he puts on the love from his parents. He gradually becomes willing to renounce his infantile pleasures and to adopt more mature ways of behavior in order to continue to receive his parents' love. However, these renunciations are no easy task for the very small child, and therefore the demands which are made upon him must be very gradual and supported by ample quantities of approval. Excessive parental demands or insufficient parental love bring about a state of conflict between parent and child and lead to a perpetuation of various anal characteristics in the personality.

Residual anal characteristics in the adult are apt to manifest themselves in one of two ways. They may, for instance, be expressed in their true form, as in sadism or stubbornness. However, the individual may have tried to prevent the emergence of such characteristics by adopting exactly the opposite characteristics in an attempt to compensate. It is during the anal period that the growing personality has its first experiences with authority. If this authority, usually in the maternal demands, is considerate, just, and kind, the child's later ability to both give and take authority will be good. If, on the other hand, the early authority is inconsiderate, inconsistent, and harsh, the youngster's future reactions to authority will undoubtedly be distorted; his reactions to authority will be hate or fear or both.

It is during the anal period that the youngster absorbs many of his feelings of shame, disgust, and inferiority as a result of the methods utilized by his parents in dealing with his anal drives and in helping him bring them under control. It is difficult to convey to the student of psychiatry the importance of these earliest years in the formation of personality. One is prone to look at a one-, two-, or three-year-old child and feel that he is too young to be completely aware of all the emotional attitudes of his parents. But when one realizes that to the three-year-old child the major part of the world is populated by his parents and immediate family, such an awareness is not too difficult to understand. He is actually more sensitive to the emotional atmosphere created within the home than is the adult. His personality is in a very formative stage and as such is markedly influenced by emotional tones even without words. A generally inhibited home, even though it is not actually a punitive home, will convey to the child the dangerousness of emotional expression. An overprotective, ever-watchful mother will convey to the child a sense of wariness about the expression of his own individual impulses.

In contrast to this, the more wholesome, healthy, relaxed home, which tolerates instinctual and emotional gratification within limits, is much more apt to produce a relaxed and contented youngster, who is then willing gradually to bring under control his more infantile instinctual energies.

Examples of home attitudes are easily seen in the important matter of toilet training. Parents who are themselves filled with shame and disgust about matters of excretion cannot help but pass this attitude on to their youngsters as they attempt to train them to conformity. Even if parents "follow the book" and begin toilet training at the proper time, their own emotional reaction to the problem will be conveyed to the child and he will sense in it an over-demanding attitude. Obviously, this will call forth rebellion in him. Because of their own particular emotional constellations, many parents have great difficulty with their children during the anal period. They are capable of understanding and tolerating the dependent oral period, but rebel at the signs of obstinacy, stubbornness, and "dirtiness" which they see in the ordinary anal period. They become anxious to suppress, repress, or otherwise do away with all signs of anality, and set forth with grim purpose to stamp out all evidences of this perfectly normal phase in far too short a time. The result is either a child who is extremely rebellious and refuses to go along, or a child who is forced too suddenly into a passive pattern.

The student should note that observations on infants show differences in reactions to light, sounds, heat, and cold, and varying tolerances to discomfort generally. These early differences in response seem to be constitutional. In some children there is a more prominent oral phase; in others, a more highly emotionally toned anal phase, with such traits as stubbornness predominating. The problem of parents is that of helping the youngster toward a more normal range, rather than forcing him into a fixed and rigid pattern which he obviously cannot fit without more stress than is healthy for his age level.

GENITAL PERIOD

Between approximately four and six years, the child passes through a fairly well-delineated phase. By this time he has theoretically overcome many of his oral and anal characteristics. It is at this time that he becomes more interested in the differences between the sexes. The boy comes now to recognize more clearly that he is a boy—the girl that she is a girl—and that the other belongs to a different sex. He now recognizes particularly that his mother and father are of different sexes, and his curiosity begins to awaken. He asks questions of his parents about the difference between men and women and boys and girls. Much of the natural curiosity we see in youngsters of this age is stimulated by the desire to learn the answer to the great riddles of why there are two sexes and where babies come from. At the same time that he is attempting to gain more information about sexuality, the youngster passes through a particular emotional constellation called the oedipus complex.

Oedipus Complex

"Oedipus complex" was the name adopted by Freud for a particular psychological occurrence which takes place during the genital period, during which the child becomes more attached to the parent of the opposite sex and begins to struggle with some negative feelings toward the parent of the same sex.

It is during the genital phase that we find heightened the pleasurable sensations arising from stimulation of the genitalia. As will be remembered, during the oral phase the mucous membrane of the mouth is particularly capable of giving pleasure. During the ensuing anal phase, the child derives the same pleasure from the act of defecation and stimulation of the mucous membrane of the rectum and anal area. During the genital phase, there is heightened excitation of the genitalia and stimulation of the genitalia gives considerable pleasure. Whereas masturbation is a frequent, if not universal, occurrence during the first two phases of life, it does not have the organized directiveness that is seen during the genital period.

Coincidental with this rise in genital erotization, there occurs the psychological complement of increased feelings of attraction to the parent of the opposite sex. Many theories have been advanced to explain the existence of the oedipus complex, but none has seemed completely satisfactory. However, it has been determined through psychoanalysis of both children and adults that such a complex is universal. It exists whether the child has one or both parents, or whether he must seek in his environment parental substitutes, as is often the case in orphanages or foundling homes.

If we consider the small boy during the period of the oedipus complex, we find that he has now begun to look at his mother somewhat differently than he did before. She now becomes an individual of the opposite sex to whom he is attracted because of her difference in sexuality. He now, for the first time, recognizes himself as a boy and her as a woman. While it is true that his attraction to her does not bear the marks of adult mature sexuality, certainly it develops the prototypes of this same sort of attraction. She is no longer merely the provider of things or the giver of orders; there now appears a new sort of relationship. He begins to want her for his own. He begins to picture himself as her little man and in his small ways to attempt to fill this role.

Obviously, however, as his attraction to her in this direction develops, his father becomes a threat. He recognizes daily that his father has a preferred relationship with his mother, much of which excludes him. He sees clearly that he cannot have his mother for his own as long as his father has this preferential relationship with her, and this stimulates within him certain jealous and negative feelings toward his father. However, it must be stressed that the ordinary boy also has many warm friendly feelings toward his father, who provides him with many other gratifications. The situation gives rise to a difficult problem with which the boy must struggle for some time in his attempts to find a solution. While he is attracted in a sexual way by his mother and so seeks her exclusive attention, this, of course, would require the absence of his father; and yet he may be firmly attached to his father.

As the boy gradually works his way through the oedipus complex, the normal child reaches the conclusion that he may not have his mother in the way that he has desired, and that he must give her up as a sexual object and retain only a tender feeling toward her. In addition to this he comes to the conclusion that, instead of opposing his father, he must grow up to be like his father, a process called *identification,* and eventually marry a woman like his mother. It has often been said by psychoanalysts that the solution or failure of solution of the oedipus complex is the point upon which future neurosis or psychosis depends. We must bear in mind that the nature of the personality with which the child faces the oedipus complex is important. If his earlier oral and anal phases have been completed satisfactorily, he comes into the oedipal phase with much more strength for solving it than if the earlier phases have been full of deprivation or overindulgence.

Obviously, however, a certain amount of his success in the oedipal phase depends upon the personalities of his parents. For instance, the small boy who has a dominating and rejecting kind of mother will have great difficulty in focusing his positive oedipal attachment upon her. Similarly, the young girl whose father is too busy or too frequently absent will have great difficulty in working through this particular phase. Conversely, the boy whose father is punitive, dangerous, and distant will build up much more fear of his father than will the normal boy, and consequently will stand much less chance of making a successful solution to his oedipal problem. To make the examples complete, if a young girl has a mother who bitterly resents any attentions that the father may pay to the girl because the mother feels that they detract from her own wifely position, the girl will have a great deal of difficulty in reaching a complete and satisfactory solution to this phase of her personality growth.

If the child is not able to reach a successful conclusion of the oedipal phase, he is most apt to bury the whole complex within his unconscious, where it continues to operate for the rest of his life. On the other hand, it is equally possible that such a youngster may literally retreat from the oedipal phase back to one of his earlier and more comfortable phases in an attempt to escape from an insoluble problem. Many adult neurotics have never solved their oedipal problem, either because they have repressed it completely, or because they have retreated from it and taken up an earlier anal or oral orientation which has persisted into adult life.

Castration Complex

The important subject of the castration complex now arises. Because of the increased erotization of the genitals, the small boy feels during the oedipal phase that the punishment which he deserves from his father for his guilt-laden desires toward his mother would be directed toward his genitalia. Masturbation has ordinarily increased during this particular phase and is unfortunately often met with parental threats which, of course, increase the boy's fear of harm to his genitalia. After all, if his main source of pleasure during this particular phase is his penis, he obviously expects retribution to be directed toward this object. It is not too far in the distant past that the small boy has become really aware that there are people in the world who do not possess penises. At this stage of experience and knowledge he cannot but postulate the possibility that they have been born with penises, but that the organs have been taken away for reasons of punishment. This knowledge of the difference between the sexes is apt to heighten the boy's castration fears. It is partly because of castration fear that the boy goes on to his normal solution of the oedipus complex, that is, giving up sexual feelings toward the mother and retaining tender feelings toward her.

The little girl faces a somewhat different problem. She becomes attached during the oedipal phase to her father. Part of her attachment is due to a disappointment in her mother because she has discovered that her mother, who has always been her provider, has failed to give her the anatomical equipment which is possessed by the male part of the family. In her disappointment, she turns to the father. If, in her attempts to gain his affection, she finds that she is successful, she is more than apt to become satisfied with her own sexuality. If, however, she is met by rejection or withdrawal, she is apt to continue with her envy of those who possess more anatomical detail than she feels she does. The continued existence of *penis envy* in girls through adult life is by no means uncommon, as is evidenced by the mannish characteristics adopted by certain women. The normal little girl, like her male counterpart, eventually recognizes the hopelessness of competition with her mother for her father. She gradually gives up her father as a love object and proceeds to identify herself with her mother in the hope of growing up to be able to marry a man like her father. The final reason for the collapse of the oedipus complex in boys is the castration fear, and this may take place quickly within a few weeks or months. In girls, however, the dissolution of the oedipus complex is much more gradual, since the little girl does not face the immediate threat of castration.

LATENCY PERIOD

The latency period covers the ages between seven and eleven or whenever puberty appears. It was given this particular name because the outward evidence of psychological changes did not seem to be as pronounced as in previous phases. However, the name is in some ways misleading. Before the latency period, the youngster, if normal, has solved the oedipus complex, and between that time and puberty devotes many of his energies to broadening his horizons. It is during this time that his learning capacity is quite large, which is, incidentally, why educators have found that schooling should begin during early latency. As noted in our discussion of the oedipal phase, the child has identified himself with the parent of the same sex. This particular mechanism of identification plays a prominent role during the latency period. It is at this time that the youngster tries to adopt the characteristics of those he admires—often heroes of history, religion, sport, and public life. His personal heroes can range from George Washington to the most recent rock-and-roll idol. He patterns himself after his older brother and his male teacher. All these individuals contribute a certain amount to his personality formation through his identification with them. Now that the oedipal problem is solved and the genital excitation has subsided, much of his ego energy is freed for consolidation and learning. Part of his earlier sexual curiosity has been sublimated into learning, thereby supplementing his energies in this direction.

During this time, his horizons widen immensely. He learns about many things past and present which have influenced adults, and thinks about them. Psychologically, he is essentially a homosexual, since he has little interest in the opposite sex. Boys during this time play with boys and girls with girls and the two rarely mix.

It is during this phase that the boy begins to develop many of the traits and characteristics which he admires in older people. It is a phase of fairly rapid development, of increase of knowledge, and of ego strength. The main neurotic mechanisms and symptoms which are seen during this period are remnants of an inability to solve the problems associated with one of the earlier phases.

PUBERTY AND ADOLESCENCE

Puberty is that phenomenon characterized by the increase in biological and psychological sexuality with its concomitant development of secondary sexual characteristics. Adolescence is the period which follows puberty and exists until physical maturity is attained, usually toward the end of the teen-age period. Puberty is the phase during which the individual begins to change from being a child to being an adult—a stormy period characterized by wide swings and variations in moods and interests. It is ushered in by the increase in biological and psychological sexual drives. Puberty occurs at different ages, depending on race and environment, and follows the relatively quiescent period of latency. There are also so-called prepubertal phases during which actual preparation for puberty is begun. It is important to bear in mind that both physically and psychologically adolescence represents the transition between childhood and adulthood. The two factors, physical and psychological, interact upon each other markedly during this particular period of personality development. The child, previously dependent and immature from a psychological standpoint and impotent from a reproductive standpoint, is during this time to become mature, potent, and capable of parenthood.

The groundwork for puberty has been laid in previous years. In progressing through the earlier phases with more or less success, the youth has developed a personality which will be tested at the onset of puberty and throughout adolescence. If this personality has been constructed well, it is able to withstand the onslaughts of a marked increase of instinctual urges and to master and control them. If, however, it has been built on a rigid, inflexible basis, it is liable to crack and crumble and begin to show evidence of psychosis or neurosis. Inevitably, while attempting to master these newly risen instinctual and biological urges, the personality is put to great test and even the most healthy personality will show wide variations and swings in its functioning. Adolescence is one period of life during which it is extremely difficult to form a concept of "normal." More so-called pathological processes and symptoms are considered to be within the range of normality in adolescence than at any other period of life.

There are four prime achievements to be accomplished during adolescence. They are: (1) emancipation from parents, (2) choice of a vocation, (3) acceptance of heterosexual goals, and (4) integration of the personality in the direction of altruistic goals. The success or failure of the adolescent in achieving these four goals will determine in the main his future adjustments. Again it cannot be overemphasized that his ability to achieve these points depends in the main upon the personality which he has formed in his earlier years. If, for instance, his early oral traits have been continued within his personality, it will be extremely difficult for him to achieve an independent relationship to his environment. On the other hand, if he had difficulty during the anal phase with authority and learning to conform, this again will crop up during his adolescent phase and cause him great difficulty. Normal parental identification may also pose problems in this period.

If work, as far as his father is concerned, has always been a drudge, a misery, and a duty, rather than having been combined with pleasure, the youngster is more than apt to have difficulty choosing a vocation. If he has never been given the idea of the pleasure of work and the pleasures of accomplishment, he will find himself without a great deal of interest during this particular phase and will be unwilling or unable to make any choice of a vocation. It is equally true that if his father has forced him into a vocation for which he does not have enough interest or aptitude, he will again find a problem facing him.

With the male there is usually only the vocational problem, while with the female there is the more difficult task of choosing (1) marriage and home-making, (2) a career, or (3) a combination of both. Each of the first two have their attractive features, and if a girl feels she must choose between them she can fall into considerable conflict. The combination of both is entirely possible but it takes careful planning and co-operation from the environment. A woman has to have education and training for a career, the moral support of husband and family, a job that can allow time off for childbearing, and a community that contains the kind of home help that can act as substitute for the mother if she continues her career during her child-rearing years. It takes a careful and conscientious division of labor to satisfy the demands of a job and a family.

In regard to his adjustment to sexuality, the individual's progress during adolescence will depend in great measure upon his success in having completed the oedipal phase. If he still retains, usually unconsciously, a sexual attachment to his mother, it will be very difficult for him to adjust to the other sex because of the incestuous taboo which will remain. If, on the other hand, he is still concerned, even though unconsciously, with a castration threat from his father, it will be equally difficult for him to adjust to women. If his family have been extremely inhibited in their view of sexuality, it again will be a difficult job for him to admit to himself his own inner sexual urges. If, however, his family has been more relaxed and comfortable about such things, he will not find his own inner sexual instinctual energies so difficult to manage and face. He will join in the social life and engage in the harmless and conventional love play of this age, and think more or less clearly of the time when he will repeat the pattern of marriage and family that he sees around him. The female is subject to similar psychological paths. She may be crippled by a strong emotional tie to the father or fear of harm by the mother. Moreover, she carried a great general burden of moral and aesthetic taboos laid down by society. Therefore she has more difficulty in freeing herself for an uncomplicated sexual adjustment than the male. Fearing sexuality and love too much, she may also take little enjoyment in motherhood.

The integration of the individual's entire personality will depend first of all upon the successful accomplishment of the first three of the responsibilities of adolescence and also upon a certain ability to develop a pleasant, altruistic, co-operative spirit toward his fellow man. This last point again depends in great measure upon the earlier emotional atmosphere of his home. If it was filled with co-operation, pleasantness, kindness, and industry, he is more than apt to find his way in the world as a friendly place. If, on the other hand, it was fraught with conflict, punitiveness, and inconsistency, he is more than apt to look upon the world as a distrustful and hostile place and fight against it rather than co-operate with it.

The biological changes of puberty and adolescence occur with or without the adolescent's acquiescence. Either his personality is capable of tolerating and handling the increased inner sexual urges, or it falls by the wayside into neurosis, psychosis, or personality disturbance. This, of course, depends in great measure upon the type of earlier emotional environment in which he has lived.

The average adolescent's attempts to handle and control his increased sexual urges and his needs for independence often lead him to a wide variety of temporary personality patterns and behavior. As a means of making peace with his superego—that is, his conscience—about his sexual urges, he may attempt to renounce them completely for a period of time. He may adopt an ascetic approach to life and picture himself as completely removed from all aspects of sexuality. However, it is fairly characteristic that within a short period he has forgotten all about his temporary attitude and is swinging toward the other side of the scale, where many of his interests, feelings, and thoughts are directed toward the opposite sex. Eventually, out of all these wide swings through the teen-age years should come a more mature and stable personality.

Similar conflicts occur within the adolescent in regard to independence. He has still not inwardly renounced all of his childhood dependency on his parents and other adults. However, during the phase of adolescence, he begins to strive for a more independent adjustment. He tries to hide from himself and his contemporaries any evidence of childish dependency. When and if his parents attempt to exercise their previous authority over him, he is apt to rebel, not because he completely disagrees with their orders, but merely because to obey would indicate a childish dependent relationship to them. Obviously, such a situation makes parenthood as well as adolescence a state requiring flexibility.

As the foregoing would indicate, the adolescent literally must grow up during the teen-age years and can do so only if given a certain amount of responsibility in increasing doses. Continued parental authority exercised as it was in childhood prevents the adolescent from learning to handle his own inner needs and from meeting reality. Adolescence is a phase that cannot be gone through in a short period of time, and during this phase a wide variety of experiences are good for the healthy adolescent.

ADULT PERIOD

The adult phase of life is that period between the end of adolescence and the onset of senility. Theoretically, it is the phase at which the individual is at his peak of efficiency and maturity. Unfortunately, however, not every person achieves either of these goals to an optimum degree. Maturity, from a psychological standpoint, can be said to have been achieved when certain conditions are present. They are: (1) freedom from neurotic symptoms, (2) satisfactory heterosexual adjustment, (3) an adequate working capacity, and (4) freedom from emotional conflict. It is often asked whether the psychiatrist feels that anyone has really attained complete maturity. This is a rather hypothetical question, since our means for measurement of maturity are somewhat gross in nature. Certainly it can be said without fear of contradiction that far too many people are unable to meet the criteria noted above for maturity. Every day we can see all around us ample indications of widespread emotional problems in our society. Tranquilizers are being gobbled up at a prodigious rate by the many who would seek relief from chronic, recurrent anxiety. Divorce rates continue to climb as more and more people are unable to choose marital partners wisely or to work out reasonable marital adjustments. Juvenile delinquency is a major national problem and many thousands of young people drop out of school prematurely. Their adjustments are usually marginal and they often have poorly integrated personalities. Other examples are seen in those adults who still have many childish and unmet emotional needs and who overeat or who drink too much in attempts to satiate these needs. Still another example is the homosexual segment of society. Some of these individuals have achieved a reasonable adjustment in many areas of their lives but are still hampered by an inability to love someone of the opposite sex. The mature individual is an effective person, able to work productively and love satisfactorily. He enjoys his life and contributes to the society in which he lives. Too many of our citizens fail to achieve this level of adjustment.

The adult period can best be examined by dividing it into two phases—the early adult phase and the middle life phase. During the twenties and early thirties, the initial adult phase, there are many major adjustments to be made in life. Two of the most important are the beginning of a vocation and entering into marriage. Both of these experiences involve the assumption of major responsibility, and both, to be performed adequately, require a flexible and stable personality. Unfortunately, the present divorce rate in our country reveals that far too few individuals have reached the state of maturity which enables them to choose proper partners and to live harmoniously with them for life.

The personality which the individual developed up through childhood and adolescence is of major importance in determining how wisely he will choose his vocation and his marital partner. Residual neurotic conflicts or personality disturbances can influence the choice in such a way as to make failure much more probable. An individual with a psychologically healthy background and a mature personality looks forward to work and marriage with the recognition of the responsibilities they will demand from him, but also with the knowledge that they will give him certain pleasures. It is also during this time that an individual ordinarily becomes a contributing member of the community in which he lives.

The next phase, or middle life, extends from about thirty-five years of age to the climacterium. It is ordinarily the period of life during which the individual has achieved some stability in his occupational endeavors; his children are beginning to grow up and in some ways to become less dependent upon him. He has become more firmly established in the community in which he lives. By this time he should have achieved at least some of the goals he originally set for himself.

However, middle age may well be a time of difficulty for those whose lives are fraught with emotional problems. One of the most common of these is the recognition that many of the goals which were originally set earlier have not been achieved. There is along with this the realization that the passage of time has made their ultimate achievement impossible. All of this may lead to a growing dissatisfaction with the individual's present situation in terms of his job, his marriage, and his children. It may lead to an increased sense of frustration and restlessness, or to irritability. It is also during this age period that there may be a gradual onset of physical problems and limitations which the individual, if he is struggling with emotional problems, may not be able to accept with equanimity. He is no longer able to think in terms of adventure, romance, and excitement, as he may have done in the past. It is difficult for him to accept the ordinary pleasures of his family and working life and to feel satisfied. Although he admits they are good, his behavior would seem to indicate they are not enough.

LATER-LIFE PERIOD

It is difficult to separate the later-life period from the preceding phase with any degree of accuracy, at least in the normal individual. The mature person continues to develop his personality resources with advancing age until the onset of organic changes of deterioration. However, in many less mature individuals, there may be noted the onset of a downhill psychological change beginning somewhere in the fifties or early sixties. In these individuals there seems to be recognition of advancing age, which carries with it morbid omens. Whereas they have proceeded previously in a semisatisfied state, they have always been able to hope that they would achieve more in the future. Now they begin to recognize that their goals probably cannot be achieved if they have not even been begun as yet, and with this recognition comes a tendency to give up. The accompanying sense of frustration and futility can be painful if not actually incapacitating.

Aside from organic factors, there is no reason why the personality should not continue to show ego growth far into this later-life phase. New experiences and interests should always contribute to ego strengths, and in the mature individual, the ego never stops developing.

PERSONALITY STRUCTURE

Personality cannot be said to have a structure in the anatomical sense, although to simplify understanding, it is divisible into certain areas or parts. Such division is permissible only with the recognition that the dynamic orientation of personality function must be recalled. There is a constant interplay of forces without static or rigid separation of one part from the others. Somatic processes of the body which give rise to the instinctual urges are responsible for the inner pressures upon the personality. From the environment come forces which necessitate postponement, variation, or suppression of gratification of certain of these instinctual urges. Each individual gradually develops his own characteristic patterns of dealing with these inner needs in his attempts to adjust to his environment.

The first important division of personality from a dynamic standpoint concerns the quality of mental activity. Not all of the mental processes at a given time are within an individual's awareness, and only a small portion of them are what we know as conscious. A much larger area of mental activity lies beneath this and is only under certain circumstances capable of rising to the level of consciousness. It is to this last large area that we give the name *unconscious*. For the sake of completeness the term *preconscious* should be mentioned. It is possible to be conscious of only a small amount of material at one particular moment, yet there is a sizable body of material which can become conscious if the individual calls it into his awareness. This latter material is called preconscious. In other words, preconscious material is available to consciousness with voluntary effort while unconscious material is not, except under special circumstances to be elucidated later.

CONSCIOUS AND UNCONSCIOUS

It is to Freud that we owe our basic understanding of the remarkably influential area of the personality called the unconscious. His initial postulates regarding its existence and strong influence over the personality function called forth considerable resistance from both scientists and laymen of fifty years ago. It is not difficult to understand why this concept resulted in such vigorous denial.

Basically it indicated that a man was not really as much his own master as he had considered himself. It indicated also that many of the forces motivating him originated and operated in a manner of which he had little direct control or knowledge. To accept such a concept was, at least at that time, a painful blow to the self-esteem of the average person. For essentially the same reason it is not always easy to impress the student of modern psychiatry with the tremendous importance of the unconscious.

There are additional reasons why an understanding of the unconscious is so difficult. There are forces operating within the psyche which maintain a constant vigilance to prevent unconscious material from entering into the conscious. The mental qualities of the conscious and the unconscious also reveal markedly different principles of operation. For instance, man has laboriously built his ability to think logically and places great value upon this proclivity. However, in the unconscious, logic does not hold sway over the mental activities. Urges contrary to each other and striving in opposite directions can coexist in a way that would be thoroughly unacceptable to the conscious mind. Another point of interest is time. Ordinarily the passage of time gradually diminishes the importance and clarity of events. In the unconscious, however, time does not exist, so that repressed memories can retain their original strength for years.

One of the more dramatic and convincing evidences of the existence of the unconscious is hypnosis. This is a strong form of suggestion which is sometimes histrionic in its effect. It was with hypnosis, or mesmerism as it was called at that time, that Freud began his investigation into the neuroses. It is possible to implant into the mind of a hypnotized subject ideas which will remain beneath his awareness in the waking state and yet be capable of exerting influence. To give an example, the hypnotist may tell the subject who is in a trance that within a few minutes after awakening he will have a desire to sing, but will not know why. Soon after he is wakened, he begins to show obvious signs of discomfort and embarrassment. When questioned about it, he is apt to say that he feels an urge to sing but he also is embarrassed because it would obviously be inappropriate to do so. He is unable to explain this urge and questioning only brings forth weak excuses. If he is allowed and encouraged to sing he will subsequently feel relieved of this tension. If, however, he is not allowed to do so the tension will continue and he will probably break into song as soon as he is alone. The explanation for this phenomenon lies in the fact that the hypnotist has implanted in the unconscious of the subject the urge to sing. There it remains pressing for discharge and producing tension as long as it is ungratified.

A somewhat more ubiquitous if not as startling demonstration of the unconscious is found in what Freud has called the "psychopathology of everyday life." He showed that such occurrences as slips of the tongue, forgetting of names and dates, and certain erroneously carried-out actions can really be understood on the basis of the unconscious. Such slips are brought about by the existence of unrecognized feelings in the deeper layers of the mind which are pressing for discharge. These feelings, although not sufficiently strong to overcome resistance and reach consciousness, are capable of changing a word or a phrase so as to alter its entire meaning, or to prevent conscious recall of the name or date. For instance, a patient who had been describing to the interviewer his fondness for his wife said, "You know, I really love my mother very much." When the slip was called to his attention he emphatically denied that he had said "mother" instead of "wife." In this particular instance the patient had a strong attachment to his mother and was really, in his marriage, unconsciously seeking the same protecting maternal attitude from his wife which he had had from his mother. To recognize this consciously would have been painful for him, but his unconscious managed to express his underlying feeling by merely changing a word in the sentence.

Freud conceived of the mental structure of the personality as being divided into three parts. It is necessary to superimpose these upon the concept of the mental qualities of conscious and unconscious. At the same time it is essential to retain the concept of dynamic personality function involving a constant interchange between all areas and portions. The three divisions are the id, ego, and superego.

THE ID

The id, which is unconscious, contains all the basic instinctual drives. It is the oldest of the three portions and as Freud says, "It contains everything that is inherited, that is present at birth and was fixed in the constitution—above all therefore, the instincts which originate in the somatic organization which find their first mental expression in the id in forms unknown to us." Throughout life the id remains the reservoir of instincts. It is the original undifferentiated portion of the psyche from which develop the other two portions.

THE EGO

The ego is a more specialized area of the personality, which develops originally out of the id and acts as an intermediary between the id and the outer world. The ego is the seat of consciousness and tester of reality. To it come the stimuli from the special senses which establish contact with the environment. Also to it come the stimuli from within the body. The task of the ego is to synthesize and integrate these factors and initiate appropriate reponses. To the ego is relegated the control of voluntary movement. It stores up stimuli from external events and thus is also the center of memory. From the stimuli reaching it from the inner instinctual activity, the ego must decide which urges are to be allowed satisfaction and which are to be suppressed or postponed.

At birth nothing exists of the psychic structure except the id. Gradually over the first few months of life there begins to separate from this undifferentiated id the more specialized ego structure. The latter gradually assumes control of voluntary musculature. In the beginning its very existence is tenuous. It is not ready at that time to take over the duties for which it is intended.

In the early months of life, excessive instinctual frustration leads to tensions which an immature ego cannot possibly handle. For this reason modern psychiatric teaching stresses the importance of maternal support for the struggling, and as yet very weak, ego during these crucial early months. The older person, by virtue of his more mature ego strength, is capable of controlling and postponing his instinctual gratification. The infant, on the other hand, because his ego is just beginning to form, finds it impossible to accomplish this task and his ego is often overwhelmed if his instincts are left ungratified for any length of time. In the healthy individual the ego continues to grow throughout life. New experiences constantly modify, change, and enlarge the area of the ego. In the emotionally disturbed person, either psychoneurotic or with a marked personality disorder, the ego is limited in its strength and hampered in its activity by the presence of conflictual material.

The ego, even in the mature individual, has a difficult task. It must mediate between the demands of the instincts and the reality of the environment, and at the same time not transgress the codes of the superego. The ego of the immature and disturbed individual is put under a doubly difficult burden. Since its growth and maturation have been hampered by the pathological environment, it must expend a great deal of its limited energy to keep infantile conflicts within the unconscious. The basic orientation of dynamic psychotherapy is to bring within the realm of the ego material which has previously been in the unconscious, thus allowing a more satisfactory and realistic solution of various conflicts.

THE SUPEREGO

The third division of the personality, the superego, is really a special portion of the ego which contains the individual's censorship mechanisms regarding right and wrong, good and evil. The very small child has little real concept of social mores and what is considered correct and incorrect. For the first few years of his life the moral codes of society are gradually impressed upon him, particularly by his parents. By the time the child passes his sixth birthday he has begun to develop a fairly well-organized superego. The basis of this portion of the personality is really the child's concept of his parents which he has internalized and therefore uses as a guide to his own behavior. It is of importance to note that we have said the child's own impression of his parents rather than, necessarily, his parents as they actually are.

In ordinary discussions the word *conscience* is often used as synonymous with superego. However, it would be more correct to utilize *conscience* to indicate the conscious portion of the superego, since the latter has many unconscious elements. Lest this statement appear confusing, some clarification is advisable. The conscience, as the word is ordinarily used, indicates that portion of the superego of which the individual is aware. For instance, he cannot steal or cheat because he knows it is wrong and knows he would feel guilty. The large and psychopathologically more important area of the superego is unconscious and deals with conflicts which are unconscious. This, then, is the area of true neurotic conflict. One woman whenever castigated by her critical mother would hurt herself, sometime within the next few hours, in some type of minor "accident." It developed that when criticized by her mother she resented it but felt that anger at her loved mother was wrong so she did not express it or even become clearly conscious of it. Yet her superego, through its ability to see the unconscious anger, threatened to cause guilt unless punishment were arranged. The latter was "arranged" through an inadvertent "accident."

It is extremely important to realize that the transgression of superego dictates produces guilt and that this is a feeling (an emotion) which is extremely uncomfortable. As a result the individual will go to many lengths, both consciously and unconsciously, to avoid this painful state. Whenever possible the person avoids such acts as would produce guilt, or utilizes mechanisms of ego defense to escape it. Rationalization is an excellent example of such utilization. If, however, certain unconscious and forbidden impulses exist and are expressed, even if in a disguised manner, guilt is forthcoming and efforts are expended to assuage the guilt. Punishment is the "neutralizer" of guilt, so the individual often unconsciously seeks punishment. The best example is found in the neurotic type of criminal who must act out his emotional drives yet does it in such a way as to be caught and punished. Were his superego not active he would use his intelligence more efficiently and lessen his chances of capture. The person who has a chronic, unsolved, unconscious problem is constantly struggling with inner unconscious guilt which leads him to seek punishment in various disguised ways. The unconscious conflict is a steady source of guilt and guilt constantly requires punishment. Since he hasn't access to his unconscious conflict it continues the endless cycle of guilt and punishment.

As the child begins school and his horizons widen he begins gradually to add to his superego formations his concept of various teachers, heroes, historical and fictional figures, thus building his own inner set of rules and regulations by which he must thereafter live. That part of the superego which deals with higher ethical concepts as opposed to the prohibition "thou shalt not" is sometimes called the *ego ideal*. The strength and rigidity of the superego obviously depends in great measure first upon the parental personalities, and second upon the other training requirements to which the child has been subjected. It is possible for the superego to be very underdeveloped and exercise little control over instinctual gratification, thus allowing the individual to live on the pleasure principle without regard to the rights and privileges of others. On the other hand, it is possible for the superego to be so rigid and severe as to hamper gratification of almost any sexual or aggressive instinct, regardless of situation or appropriateness.

The most healthy superego is one which fits well within the demands of society and of reality and yet allows adequate instinctual gratification under appropriate conditions. From time to time one finds an individual whose superego is very rigid and strict in certain areas and yet extremely lax in others. It is necessary to understand that only a certain portion of this part of the personality is within the realm of consciousness and that much of it operates beneath the level of awareness.

SUMMARY

Growth of the personality proceeds in an orderly fashion beginning with events which surround the nursing experience, the toilet-training experience, and the response to increasing awareness of genital tension. This is followed by the learning experiences of the grade-school years, puberty and adolescent emancipation experiences, choosing and preparing for vocation, and learning adaptation to the opposite sex. We have seen that the ego must serve as the outlet for instinctual urges, must meet the demands of reality, and must meet the demands of the superego. Instinctual demands tend to remain more or less constant throughout life, with the exception of the periods of puberty and the menopausal age. During these times we find an increase in the pressure of instinctual demands. From the standpoint of external pressures one can readily see how a marked increase of restriction of environmental pressure is capable of placing an increased load upon the ego. The most obvious illustration is that of wartime combat, where constant severe environmental pressure forces a breakdown of ego function in many soldiers.

It is also easy to see how the superego, if its demands are rigid and unrealistic, will place the individual under a severe burden. The chief mechanism by which the superego enforces its demands upon the ego is the production of guilt—the painful feeling from which the ego tries to escape.

To recapitulate what has been said about personality structure and mental qualities, we have noted first the mental qualities of conscious and unconscious, with the latter producing by far the larger portion of mental activities. Beneath the level of awareness are found not only the instinctual impulses as they arise from the somatic processes within the body but also the past, buried environmental experiences which have conditioned him to expect certain reactions from those about him.

From the standpoint of the psychic apparatus we have discussed the id, the ego, and the superego.

The id, of course, is the reservoir of all instinctual impulses, that portion of the personality which is present at birth.

The ego is the conscious portion of the personality which has separated slowly from the id and which thereafter contains the controls for motility and receives sensations from the environment. Its chief functions revolve around attempting to keep harmony between the demands of the id, the demands of the superego, and the demands of reality.

The superego is the inner censorship mechanism regulating rights and wrongs, and may vary widely in strength from near nonexistence to dominance—an extremely severe and punitive portion of the personality.

The goal of psychotherapy is to enhance the function of the ego and to bring into ego control the material which has hitherto been inefficiently dealt with in the unconscious. It also attempts to change the superego by strengthening or lessening its controls, depending upon whether the original structure is inadequate or excessively demanding.

It is well to stress again the fact that personality function is dynamic and that there can be no rigid separation of either the mental qualities of conscious from unconscious or among the various portions of the psychic apparatus. The instinctual stimuli are constantly arising within the unconscious and pressing for discharge through the ego. The ego also is constantly receiving impressions from the environment as well as strictures from the superego and is striving to bring harmony into the entire structure. The ego's chief ways of dealing with conflict are the various mechanisms of defense—the means by which the personality attempts to achieve adjustment between the inner self and the outer world.

CHAPTER 3

The Development of Mental and Emotional Disorders

PSYCHIATRY, as a branch of medical science, is concerned particularly with disorders and diseases of the psyche, and is therefore interested in any etiological factor capable of producing them. Some of these factors are similar to those with which various other branches of medicine are concerned, such as tumors, infections, blood dyscrasias, endocrine disorders, vitamin deficiencies, tissue degeneration, and so forth. As these various etiological agents or physical symptoms have been discovered, it was found in many instances that they were capable of producing mental disorders. For instance, a brain tumor can so disturb central nervous system function as to produce a psychosis. Degeneration of tissues may result in the psychoses seen in senility and arteriosclerosis. Infection such as the spirochete of syphilis may invade the brain and cause tissue changes which give rise to general paresis. Various toxins are capable of upsetting the central nervous system physiology and producing psychoses. Bromide and alcohol intoxication are examples of this.

However, there is still left a large segment of mental disease for which no demonstrable tissue pathology or physiological malfunction has been found. Therefore, it has been necessary to acknowledge, and in some cases reluctantly, another etiological factor for mental diseases—that of becoming ill from disturbed human relationships. When integrative disturbances in the body produce mental disease, we refer to these disturbances as *physiogenic*. When inte-

42

grative disturbances arise from inner emotional maladjustment (aided perhaps by environmental pressures), we refer to these disturbances as *psychogenic*. In psychogenic illness, the structural, biochemical, and physiological changes are absent, or, if present, are secondary to the emotional factors.

GENERAL CATEGORIES OF MENTAL DISEASES

Prior to proceeding with a more complete discussion of the various etiological factors of emotional and mental diseases, it is necessary to describe first the general categories into which these conditions may be divided. Broadly speaking, mental disorders express themselves in terms of psychoses, psychoneuroses, personality disorders, and psychophysiologic disorders. The dividing lines between these divisions is not sharp and clear, and many individuals present evidences of more than one.

PSYCHOTIC DISORDERS

A psychosis is a severe form of mental disease characterized by an extensive disorganization of the personality function. In the typical psychosis the individual has lost contact with reality and reveals severe disturbances in all areas of his life. The psychotic reaction is a much more thoroughly and severely abnormal one than is the psychoneurosis. Psychosis may be precipitated by organic, toxic, or psychological factors. The psychotic individual, as his personality disorganization progresses, becomes incapable of making an adequate social adjustment. He has lost his reality-testing functions and often must be hospitalized. As the ego of the psychotic breaks down, previously unconscious material is allowed expression in its raw form, and its expression is bizarre, confusing, and difficult to understand. *Reality testing* means the individual's ability to perceive and evaluate accurately events and situations in the world about him. Messages are brought to the ego through the five special senses, which are then weighed in terms of past experience through memory, and a judgment made. The loss of reality testing indicates an impairment in the ego's ability to perceive, integrate, and act realistically upon events taking place in the world. Misinterpretations are made because the presence of strong conflict within the psyche has shattered the ego functions.

PSYCHONEUROTIC DISORDERS

In the psychoneurotic there is a less severe personality disturbance in which the individual is able to retain at least some measure of social adjustment. His ego, although warped and distorted, retains its reality-testing functions. Whereas the psychoneurotic may well warp his concept of reality, he does not lose it entirely, as does the typical psychotic. The entire psychoneurosis is an attempt on the part of the individual's ego to find some solution to its unconscious problems. Psychoneuroses have a basic psychological etiology, although it is possible for organic and toxic factors to contribute to the condition. The psychoneurotic individual retains at least some measure of his ability to relate to those about him, whereas this is lost in the psychotic.

PSYCHOPHYSIOLOGIC AUTONOMIC AND VISCERAL DISORDERS

Psychophysiologic disorders or psychosomatic disorders, as they are commonly called, are physiologic conditions resulting from chronic emotional states of one type or another. These particular pathological states become chronic when the personality is unable to deal satisfactorily with the environment. The individual, for instance, who remains chronically angry for one reason or another, but unable to deal adequately with this hostility, may well develop hypertension. The personality of the psychophysiologically ill individual often does not reveal overt symptoms of emotional maladjustment. This would seem to be primarily because the chronically stimulated emotional reaction is drained off in the form of autonomic hyperactivity in a particular area. The dependency of the ulcer patient may not be obvious in his ordinary relationships, but its constant existence stimulates autonomic activity which eventually leads to ulcer formation. It has often been found that where, for one reason or another, the psychophysiologic symptom is removed without adequate psychological insight, the patient becomes psychotic. There are some observers who feel that psychophysiologic disorders replace or prevent psychoses.

PERSONALITY DISORDERS

Personality disorders are conditions in which the individual acts out his various conflicts through noticeably aberrant behavior. To take a simple example: If an individual is full of an inner resentment, he may do one of three things with this anger. He may form defenses in order to prevent its expression, in which case he is apt to fall within the category of a psychoneurotic and behave as if the anger were not there. He may develop a psychosomatic disorder. If, however, it is possible for him to react in a hostile, aggressive way toward everyone in his environment, he falls within the group of personality disorders.

The same sort of thing is true of inner or unconscious strivings toward homosexuality. If the individual forms defenses against the homosexual impulse, he may appear on the surface to be heterosexual, but reveal neurotic symptoms, or even become paranoid to a psychotic degree. On the other hand, these homosexual impulses may be carried out in action, in which case the individual has a personality disorder of the homosexual type. The question of whether an individual defends himself against his inner impulses, finding them unacceptable, or gives free expression to them depends upon the experiences of his early formative years and particularly upon the strength of his superego in relation to these particular impulses. If the impulses are of a socially unacceptable type and have not been channeled into other conventional behavior, then they either must be defended against or be given free expression.

HEREDITY

The role of heredity in mental and emotional disorders has undoubtedly been both over- and underestimated by investigators at various times, although there is no doubt that each individual comes into the world endowed differently from others, from the standpoint of innate strengths and weaknesses. As knowledge about mental disease advances, there is probably less and less importance attributed to heredity. While it cannot be completely ignored, its importance as an etiological factor has diminished over the years.

From a psychological standpoint, certain hereditary factors are of importance. The potential intelligence or I.Q. is determined at birth, although its development is influenced by environmental factors. The various strengths and weaknesses of physiological systems are present at birth. There is a constitutional predisposition toward a certain degree of motor activity. Some children are more aggressively active from birth onward than others, without a demonstrable reason to be found in the environment. The various levels of psychosexual development seem inherently varied. Where one child may show a prolonged and intensified oral period, the next may show an exaggerated anal period, again without any demonstrable environmental reason. It is well to bear in mind, however, that the environment is the first and most obvious place to look for the reason for such exaggerations. Certain children seem to be born with poorly integrated faculties and have great difficulty, literally, in grasping life. Their success or failure depends in great measure upon the environment meeting their needs.

Certainly, while heredity may play a role, there is little if anything that can be done about it from a practical standpoint. The most important thing is how the environment through various stresses and strains takes full advantage of strong points and strengthens weakened points in the heredity scale.

ORGANIC AND TOXIC FACTORS

Herein we would group all the various organic and toxic etiological factors which are capable of producing mental disorders—in general, anything which is capable of upsetting the body physiology or destroying tissue. Central nervous-system tissue cannot be regenerated and once destroyed remains inoperative although other areas may partially compensate for the loss.

The developing fetus is influenced by the maternal organism and if, during pregnancy, the mother's health is in some way deleteriously influenced, the growing fetus may be affected and result in an infant whose endowments are limited. It is not within the scope of this book to go into the various maternal disorders which are capable of influencing fetal growth, but certainly they are important in the growth of the future central nervous system. In addition there are innumerable problems associated with the act of birth itself which are capable of influencing, from a toxic or organic standpoint, the infant's central nervous system development. During the first year of life especially, such things as contagious diseases, particularly if accompanied by a high fever, are capable of producing irreversible damage.

PSYCHOGENIC FACTORS

As psychiatry has developed its knowledge of dynamic personality function, the importance of psychogenic factors in the etiology of emotional and mental disorders has become progressively more apparent. While it is true that various organic, toxic, and even constitutional factors are capable of producing disorders, there still remains a large percentage of disturbance which is in great measure produced by psychogenic factors.

Chapter 2 traces the progress of the child from infancy onward through the various levels of psychosexual development. We have shown that at each of these particular levels definite inherent psychological characteristics are found. During the oral phase, for instance, dependency is the dominant psychological factor. During the anal period the youngster relates in an ambivalent way to all the people in his environment and obstinacy, parsimoniousness, and sadomasochism are prominent in his growing personality structure. During the genital period of psychosexual development the child becomes involved with the problem of the differences between the sexes and becomes enmeshed in the all-important oedipus complex. It has been pointed out how the various mental institutions—id, ego, and superego—are gradually differentiated. Throughout the discussion the importance of environmental factors upon personality development and therefore the future intrapsychic relationships as well as relationships with others has been noted.

To the child of five years or under, his parents or the members of his immediate family are by far the most important individuals in his environment. At this early age the four walls of his house essentially are the boundaries of his world. Most of his earliest personality formation is a response to the emotional atmosphere which is created within the home by the various family members, particularly the parents. Obviously in the earliest year or two of life the maternal personality is the most important. Recent research has thrown more and more light on this so-called *primary unit,* the mother-child unit. It has become increasingly evident through this research that the maternal personality creates the emotional atmosphere on which the very young infant depends for its earliest ego formation. While it is true that the umbilical cord is separated at birth, which places the infant physiologically on his own, there is no similar sudden severance of the "psychic umbilical cord." In these earliest months of life, the infant continues to introject "emotional nutrition" from the mother. Her ability to provide a warm, loving, secure atmosphere is of great importance in the formation of the basic layers of the personality, particularly in regard to ego development. Extremely rigid mothers, narcissistic mothers, prepsychotic or psychotic mothers are incapable of creating such a healthy atmosphere and the obvious result is inadequate and slow ego development.

As the work of René Spitz [1] has shown, the absence of a constant maternal figure, even in the presence of all other requirements of food, clothing, and shelter, will leave an infant unable to develop along his normal physiological or psychological channels. Such infants remain on an extremely immature level. The best examples of such infants other than those seen in Dr. Spitz's work are found in the so-called *autistic* children, whose mothers have been severely lacking in the healthy maternal qualities. These youngsters do not develop a normal ego. They have great difficulty in distinguishing between themselves and others. They have not learned to relate to other people and literally remain in a world of their own very similar to that of earliest infancy or that of the psychotic individual.

The attainment of psychological maturity requires the successful passage through each level of psychosexual development. The neurotic or psychotic individual is one who has retained typical characteristics of an earlier level of psychosexual development and has

[1] Spitz, René. "Hospitalism, An Inquiry into the Genesis of Psychiatric Conditions in Early Childhood," in *The Psychoanalytic Study of the Child*, Vol. I. New York, International Universities Press, 1945.

in many ways left part of his personality in that particular level. Generally speaking, two possible environmental (parental) attitudes are capable of arresting a portion of the child's psychological development in one or another of these phases. The first and perhaps most common is that of deprivation. If the child is deprived of normal outlets for his needs during a particular phase of psychosexual development, he will literally leave part of his personality there, as if in an attempt to fulfill these needs eventually; as if he has not finished with this particular phase and therefore cannot move on to the next. On the other hand, overindulgence can have the same result as deprivation. If the parents make one phase particularly attractive, and especially if they make the next phase very difficult for the child, he may well remain in or regress to the earlier phase.

It should be mentioned here that it is difficult if not impossible to overindulge the child during the oral phase, but this phase can be prolonged far beyond the normal. It is possible to make the anal phase, including the requirements for conformity, so difficult that the child reverts to the earlier oral phase. Also of importance is the fact that the child attempts to deal with each succeeding level of psychosexual development on the basis of, and utilizing, the personality that he has formed during the earlier phases. If this has been inadequate or faulty, he is that much less able to deal with the new problems that are presented to him.

During the oedipal period either one or both parents may make it difficult and sometimes impossible for the child to resolve this conflict. Seductiveness or rejection on the part of parents as well as excessive punitiveness are potential factors in hindering the child's ability here. The youngster may develop excessive anxiety if the parent of the opposite sex is more seductive than is advisable. On the other hand, the youngster may be led to bitterness, disappointment, and frustration if the parent of the opposite sex is withdrawn, cold, or punitive. The parent of the same sex may arouse the child's incipient oedipal resentment by being excessively punitive or dangerous to the child. It is possible for the parent of the same sex to be so "good" that the child is unable to find any reason at all to vent any of the built-up oedipal hostility that he has slowly accumulated. All of these situations are capable of reducing the youngster's ability to solve his oedipus complex and move on to the next phase.

Essentially what is needed in each level of adjustment is a mature, warm, loving, understanding attitude that is capable of sensing and meeting the child's various needs. The mature mother understands that her infant during the first year requires a great deal of intense care, love, and attention, and she meets these demands without requiring the infant to give her anything in return. During the anal phase, she intuitively understands the necessity for training her child to some degree of conformity, and yet at the same time is willing to go at it slowly and easily and with a great deal of reassurance and love. Both parents, if mature, understand the necessity of presenting to their children an example of a happily married couple in a congenial, friendly home.

It is of importance to remember that the child must mold his personality to fit into the particular environment in which he finds himself. At an early age he has little basis for judgment, since his past experience is minimal. He can only do what to him at this particular stage of events seems to be best. This may or may not be the most advantageous solution, but nevertheless the child chooses it and it remains with him throughout the rest of his personality development. The process of maturation is never easy and comfortable even in the best circumstances. The most normal children have occasional phases of seemingly distorted behavior. Yet if the environment is consistent and healthy, the inherent urges toward maturation will overcome these temporary difficulties and allow personality development to proceed in a mature direction. If, however, the environment is pathological, these minor distortions become crystallized and exaggerated and result in neurotic or personality disturbance patterns or possibly even psychoses.

NARCISSISM AND ANXIETY

Because of their close relationship these two particular topics will be discussed together. The term *narcissism* indicates basically the quality of self-love, and it is derived from the mythological tale of Narcissus, who fell in love with his own image as he gazed at himself in a pool. To a degree this narcissism or self-love is present in every human being. It is normally most pronounced in infancy when, in the child of a few months of age, it is essentially 100 per-cent present. Gradually as the youngster matures and passes through the various levels of psychosexual development, part of this narcissis-tic self-love becomes available for so-called *object love*. The latter refers to the ability of the individual to love someone other than himself. There should be, by the time maturity is attained, a correct balance between object love and self-love or narcissism. If, as is most often the case in pathological personalities, the narcissism remains too great, object relationships are bound to suffer because of an in-sufficient amount of libido available for them. The ego itself is the reservoir of this libido and in the process of its development even-tually reaches a level where a certain amount of its love is given to others in the environment and a certain amount remains vested in itself.

It is chiefly through early family relationships of a warm, mature, loving nature that the child learns to invest a portion of his love in those about him. In the absence of this mature type of love from those within the family, the child will remain in the infantile state, loving himself to the exclusion of others and also having great and insatiable desires for love from others without feeling the need or ability to give love to them. Whereas it is possible in infancy to have great narcissistic needs met by the mother, it becomes a very diffi-cult, if not impossible, task to have such infantile narcissistic needs met when one is an adult.

Anxiety refers to that very common syndrome resembling fear, but differing from actual fear in that there is no external object of which the individual is afraid. Anxiety in a sense is the ego's warning mechanism that something is awry within the personality. The ego itself uses anxiety to indicate that either something within the id or something within the superego threatens the ego.

Here it is necessary to tie in our earlier description of narcissism. The ego, being the reservoir of narcissism or self-love, attempts to escape any situation which would threaten its sense of well-being and integrity. Such threats may come from instinctual urges which are not acceptable and cannot be discharged, or from threats of superego reprisal in the form of guilt. The individual may use anxiety as it should be used, namely, as a warning device, and may therefore seek a more satisfactory solution. Or the ego may at times be overwhelmed by anxiety and go into a panic, which, incidentally, is one of the most painful situations to which the human being is heir. Patients who suffer extreme anxiety would cheerfully trade this state of events for the most severe organic pain.

All human beings, because of this inherent degree of narcissism, try to protect themselves from any insult or injury to their self-evaluation. It is with such attempts and vicissitudes that the personality is constantly enmeshed and from them that it may develop various emotional problems.

MECHANISMS OF EGO DEFENSE

The ego, as explained in Chapter 2, begins in earliest infancy to differentiate itself out of the amorphous id and to become a more or less separate portion of the personality. It is to the ego that all instincts must make their bid for gratification, for it is only through ego-initiated activity that such gratification can occur. In its early immature childhood stages, the ego is hard put to exercise an inhibiting effect upon instincts and is frequently threatened by them in their search for discharge. Throughout childhood the ego builds up a series of so-called *mechanisms of defense,* by which it attempts to deal with instincts whose gratification would be dangerous or painful for one reason or another. When a forbidden urge for instinctual gratification threatens to seek expression, anxiety appears, and anxiety is a very painful affect. Mechanisms of defense attempt to avoid the sensation of anxiety. Ordinarily we find that out of the possible mechanisms, perhaps slightly over a dozen, each individual tends to use a particular few to deal with the majority of his instinctual urges. These mechanisms become more or less characteristic of him, and while he may use others at times, these are the ones with which we expect him to try to meet the majority of his conflicts.

The concept of the mechanisms of ego defense was introduced by Freud [2] in 1894 in his paper entitled "The Defense in Neuropsy-

[2] Freud, Sigmund. "The Defense in Neuropsychoses," in *Selected Papers on Hysteria.* Nervous and Mental Disease Monograph Series, No. 4. New York and Washington.

choses." In that publication he described the mechanism which we now call repression. Other mechanisms have since been added to the list, and unfortunately in some instances two names have been given to one particular type of mechanism, thus introducing a certain amount of confusion. It is not always easy to draw a clear, distinct line between the various mechanisms of defense, since certain ones are similar to others and can only be differentiated at minor points. To complicate the picture still further, one usually sees a combination of perhaps three or four mechanisms utilized by an individual in dealing with his conflicts.

It is important to realize that all of these defense mechanisms operate at an unconscious and more or less automatic level, so that the individual is unaware of their existence or scope. While the motivation for the ego's mechanisms of defense has been subdivided into three types, it remains that in the last analysis the basic underlying motivation is that of the necessity of preventing clear recognizable gratification of an instinctual urge because of possible untoward effects.

Perhaps the simplest as well as the earliest motivation for the ego to utilize defenses is the threat it feels at the possibility of being overwhelmed by instinctual pressure. This undoubtedly plays a particularly large role in the earliest years, when the ego structure is as yet immature and unable to cope with the powerful instinctual urges.

There are other times in life when this fear of being overpowered by instinctual pressure is found. At puberty, when the biological upsurge of sexual instinctual energy occurs, we find the ego having to protect itself against this increased pressure. There is also evidence that a similar type of difficulty often occurs at the menopausal period. Another situation of this same type is found in the incipient stages of a psychosis where the ego is gradually disintegrating and falling prey to the ever-present instinctual pressures. The anxiety in these various situations causes the ego to increase its activities in terms of defense mechanisms. A second possible source of difficulty from unimpeded instinctual gratification is that arising in the environment. The ego may recognize that a particular instinct, if gratified, will result in environmental retaliation which will be dangerous to the individual. For instance, the little boy who becomes angry with his father may clearly recognize that if he openly expresses this anger with motor activity his father may retaliate.

Finally, the third area which the ego must take into account prior to giving instinctual gratification is the superego. This mental institution stands ready to punish the ego with its weapon of guilt, should the latter allow instinctual expression which is contrary to the superego's dictates. In summary, therefore, we see that the ego must constantly watch both the environment and the superego, as well as the instinctual impulses, as it makes its decisions regarding which instincts may be gratified. Wherever gratification is potentially dangerous or painful to the ego, the ego tends to utilize any one or a combination of its mechanisms of defense.

SUBLIMATION

Only one defense can be considered well within the limits of normality, and that is called *sublimation*. This particular mechanism requires a change in either the aim or object of an instinct and then subsequent gratification. Whereas the other mechanisms of defense meet the instinct head on and prevent its discharge, in sublimation the instinct is turned into a new but useful and more acceptable channel, which may then be allowed expression. An important feature of this mechanism is, of course, that the ego does not have to maintain a constant energy output equal to that of the instinctual urge in order to prevent its discharge.

Examples

Examples of sublimation are numerous. Generally speaking, the early infantile instinctual urges are the ones which may be dealt with by sublimation. The child has a tendency, for instance, toward destructiveness, which in its pure form later becomes unacceptable in an adult. Another such inner urge seen in children is that of intense sexual curiosity or a desire to know more about sexuality. The early destructive element might eventually be sublimated into the necessary and useful occupation of building-wrecking. The infantile curiosity may eventually be used to strengthen the researcher's acumen and drive in unexplored fields. A childish desire to exhibit oneself, which is ubiquitous in youngsters, may be sublimated subsequently into a theatrical career which proves enjoyable to everyone. In all of these examples it may be clearly seen that the ego is merely changing the aim or object of the infantile urge. It does not need to erect rigid and energy-consuming defenses in order to prevent the instinctual discharge. Such a mechanism, of course, leaves the ego free to grow and expand and makes the individual a more useful and contributing member of society.

The remainder of ego defenses, although found to some degree in everyone, can properly be labeled "pathological." In spite of their widespread occurrence, they cannot be considered perfectly normal because of the inefficient way in which they operate. The ego is forced to allot a certain amount of energy in order to maintain these defenses in effect, which is therefore not available for other more constructive uses. Certain of these mechanisms are more or less characteristic of definite clinical entities and are ordinarily associated with them. For instance, when we see a patient with a conversion reaction, we know immediately, through experience, that he makes great use of the mechanism of repression. On the other hand, we know that the obsessive compulsive patient utilizes isolation in its typical form. The paranoid schizophrenic attempts to deal with many of his conflicts by projection. As already mentioned, it is rare to find only one mechanism operating in an individual. Instead we find that each person develops a tendency from childhood onward to use two or three particular defenses more than any others and that these become characteristic of him. He is apt to deal with new conflict situations by using this particular combination of defenses.

We will discuss individually these various mechanisms, citing examples of each.

REPRESSION

Repression is an unconsciously purposeful forgetting of either internal urgings or external events which if they were to become conscious would be painful. It is interesting to note that this defense was the first one described by Freud, who became aware of it in his work with hysterical patients. It formed the cornerstone of some of his early theories of psychoanalysis. Simply put, the ego exerts sufficient energy against the objectionable memory, or affect, or instinct, to prevent its reaching consciousness. This energy on the part of the ego obviously must be equal in amount to that exerted by the objectionable material. The latter is relegated to the unconscious lest it disturb psychic equilibrium by becoming conscious. Since the pressure from beneath is constant, the ego must maintain constant vigilance. There is always the danger that thoughts or affects too closely related to the dangerous one will reach consciousness and possibly be followed by the objectionable material. Therefore an increasingly wide repressive process often occurs, in the way a wave expands after a rock is thrown in the water. The efficiency of this mechanism is questionable, since it requires this increasing expenditure of ego energy to achieve its success.

It is a psychoanalytic contention that early infantile sexuality through the oedipal period is subject to a mass repression which obliterates most if not all of the memories of the first six years of life. This is the reason, of course, that most individuals cannot remember much of anything prior to their fifth year. The child during this time becomes enmeshed in the oedipal conflict with all its unacceptable incestuous strivings. In the neurotic individual particularly, who cannot find a satisfactory solution to his oedipal problems, the mass repression of literally all memories occurs. This, as we would expect, is most evident in individuals with conversion symptoms, where this particular mechanism plays an important role.

Examples

1. Probably the simplest examples of repression are in the situations described by Freud [3] in his *Psychopathology of Everyday Life,* where the forgetting of names and dates is discussed. The common phrase, "It's on the tip of my tongue," may cover a minor and temporary repression. It may be that the name in question is that of an individual who is disliked, or it may merely mean that there is some particular type of association between that name and an objectionable affect or idea.

2. A more complicated example of this particular type of mechanism is to be found in circumscribed amnesia, where an incident or series of incidents covering a period of time is completely "forgotten." Again we are apt to find this particular type of phenomenon in a dissociative reac-

[3] Freud, Sigmund. *The Psychopathology of Everyday Life,* in *The Basic Writings of Sigmund Freud.* Edited by A. A. Brill. New York. The Modern Library, 1938.

tion following some painful or traumatic experience which results in a subsequent repression of the entire period of time.

PROJECTION

Projection is a mechanism whereby painful or objectionable affects or ideas are projected outward upon persons or things in the environment and felt by the individual as belonging outside of himself. This is one of the most primitive types of mechanism, presumably dating from early infancy. At this time there is a tendency to consider all "good" or pleasurable things as part of the self and all "bad" or painful things as part of the outside world. The infant literally projects everything that is unpleasant or painful to the outer world and retains as part of himself only what is pleasant. It is the type of defense that cannot ordinarily be used to any great extent as long as the ego's reality-testing functions are preserved. However, it is still surprising the degree to which this mechanism can occur in neurotic individuals. In its simplest form, projection is merely the denial by an individual of certain unacceptable things within himself and the attribution of them to something outside himself.

Examples

1. A very common occurrence of this type of mechanism is to be found in the woman who unconsciously feels herself inadequate as a woman, mother, and wife, and who accuses her husband of possessing all of the same inadequacies which she unconsciously feels she has. Consciously she behaves as if she considers herself to be a good example of a woman, wife, and mother and is thoroughly unaware of her own unconscious insecurity and feelings of inadequacy.

2. A more complex and much more serious example of projection is seen in the paranoid schizophrenic, in the form of hallucinations. His loss of reality-testing function allows him to project to the degree that he literally hears voices coming from the environment which accuse him of various things which are present only in his unconscious. For example, he says, "They say I'm a fairy and I'm no good. They call me a lousy bum and say that I can't do anything right." The basic motivation for the paranoid's having to defend himself against unconscious homosexual impulses is the fear of superego retaliation. His superego would find such impulses thoroughly untenable and he would be punished by

overwhelming guilt. It is quite clear that the ego's reality-testing function is seriously disturbed, otherwise the projection to the point of hallucinations could not possibly occur.

DENIAL

Denial is a mechanism of defense whereby obvious reality factors are treated by the individual as if they did not exist. For one reason or another the patient finds certain of these factors painful or unpleasant and he literally denies that they are present. This mechanism, similar to projection, while quite common, is representative of a psychotic state if it is used excessively in adults. It is seen most frequently in children where play itself often represents a denial of reality. Healthy children, while capable of denying reality by "playing house" with all the authority of mother and father, are capable of returning to reality on quick notice if called from their play. In the world of children, with so many things unknown and potentially dangerous, denial is almost an essential to help them master some of the anxieties they would otherwise develop. As an individual grows older, however, he is expected to face reality and to learn to cope with it. Almost everyone has some fantasy life which is a form of denial, but which is relatively harmless if it does not interfere with the individual's tasks in the real world. However, if the person continues to live in a world of his own making through fantasy and continues to deny things as they are, he is psychotic. It should be stressed here that the mechanism of denial operates on an unconscious, or at best preconscious, level and it should not be confused with the conscious process of deliberate prevarication.

Examples

1. A simple and very common example of denial is the frequent refusal we find in a person to "read the handwriting on the wall." For instance, consider the boy of military age who continues to rule out any possibility of being called into the service through the draft, in spite of the fact that such an occurrence is a strong probability. It may be evident that all such young men in his particular condition are rapidly being drafted into military service, and yet he continues to act as if this could not possibly happen to him. The more normal boy in this situation would at least make some tentative plans regarding his education, his

courtship, and his family. He would not dwell incessantly upon the prospect of being called into the service, but certainly would treat it as a very realistic possibility. Denial reaches even larger proportions in our population in times of growing world tension with such remarks as "We can't go to war; we wouldn't go to war; there won't be any war." Such statements as these may be much more comfortable than they are realistic. They certainly are not a very accurate appraisal of the environmental situation.

2. A more complex and pathological example of denial is seen in the schizophrenic, who amid the noise and turmoil of the disturbed ward in a mental hospital proclaims himself to be a free man who may come and go as he pleases. He completely ignores the fact that he must remain in the institution, and that he is ill, but rather sees only the more pleasant self-made pictures that he chooses to see. It is obvious that such a patient has lost his sense of reality testing, or he would not be able to use this mechanism to such a degree. The normal individual, while he may use denial on certain occasions, is not able to maintain it with the steadfastness that we see in psychotics. If reality is presented to him in convincing doses, he finally must accept it.

INTROJECTION

Introjection is a mechanism by which a person incorporates into himself a certain human characteristic, trait, or force. This characteristic, trait, or force may be incorporated for the purpose of using it or of destroying it. In many ways introjection is the opposite of projection, and both are very primitive in their origins. Like projection, introjection relates back to the infantile feeling that everything "good" belongs to the self and everything "bad" or painful is of the outer world. Originally the infant finds that the incorporation of food is pleasurable, but as he gradually grows older, he also learns that destruction follows the ingestion of something. Introjection has about it therefore an aura of orality. We find that introjection may be used by the individual either to acquire some trait or characteristic or force which is considered advantageous, or to destroy something which is considered dangerous. Something which is "good" or pleasurable may be introjected for positive reasons. On the other hand, something which is potentially dangerous may be introjected for the purpose of destroying it. Once again it must be stressed that, as with all defense mechanisms, this process occurs unconsciously.

However, examples of conscious introjection may be found in primitive societies where, for instance, it is believed that if portions of the powerful but defeated enemy are eaten by the victors, the strength and skill of the dead warrior will be gained by those who partake of the feast.

Examples

1. A common example of introjection is found in children who "ingest" the standards and mores of their parents to form the nucleus of their superego. The rules and regulations which they have taken within themselves then become a part of their developing personality rather than having to be received from parents constantly as was the case earlier in childhood. It is as if the child figuratively swallows these regulations which have surrounded him and makes them a part of his growing personality.

2. A more pathological example of this particular mechanism is to be found in the depressed patient. This individual has powerful undercurrents of hate in his relationships to loved persons. When one of these loved persons rejects him, the depressed patient literally "introjects" him, hate, love, and all, and then becomes the recipient himself of all the hate which he has previously had toward the other individual. He is full of self-recriminations and self-accusations which unconsciously he always harbored for the "loved one," but which he now turns against himself.

REACTION FORMATION

Reaction formation is a defense mechanism which involves the setting up of a more or less rigid attitude or character trait which will serve as a means of preventing the emergence of a painful or undesirable attitude or trait, usually of the opposite type. Reaction formation produces a noticeable change in the character or demeanor of an individual. Such a mechanism, however, usually involves an excess, seems to be static, rigid, and unrealistic. Since unconscious pressure for the discharge of the objectionable trait remains constant, the reaction formation must remain constant, regardless of the usefulness or suitableness that it seems to have on the surface. This type of defense is actually very close to, if not the same as, overcompensation.

Examples

1. A common example of reaction formation is the too-agreeable, anxious-to-please person who never shows hostility or disagreement. His demeanor, while pleasant for a time, soon strikes one as artificial. This person could not possibly agree with everything and everyone and still be human, and yet he seems to do it. Actually his manner is really a reaction formation to cover underlying hostility and prevent its expression. He must constantly maintain this attitude, since it is by then ingrained into his personality thoroughly and operates on an automatic basis. He is unaware of his underlying resentment and truly feels himself a totally "agreeable" person.

2. Another typical reaction formation is seen in the obsessive-compulsive patient, who has numerous compulsive rituals through which he must go. For instance, he may have an elaborate set of ritualistic actions through which he must go prior to starting a car. If these actions are performed according to his inner dictates, he feels that the drive that he is about to take will be safe. However, if they are not performed, he finds himself in constant fear lest he run over someone with the automobile. Actually his meaningless and ritualistic behavior is a method of attempting to control and keep unconscious his hostility and sadistic urges. It is as if he feels that by the magical gestures he can keep such unconscious material from emerging into awareness.

UNDOING

Undoing is a mechanism in which the individual does one thing for the purpose of "undoing" or neutralizing something which in his imagination or in reality was done before, and which he feels was objectionable. It is a sort of expiation mechanism. As we have already mentioned and as we will see here, it is not always easy to differentiate between the various mechanisms of defense, and there are no distinct boundaries limiting one from the other. Some are related quite closely to each other, as are reaction formation and undoing. In general, in the latter there is a definite act or thought initiated which is the direct counterpart of the initial and unacceptable one. In reaction formation, however, there is an underlying attitude against which an opposite attitude is constantly maintained.

Examples

1. Most of the clear examples of undoing are to be found in certain compulsive acts or obsessive thoughts. For instance, the man who would occasionally be disturbed by thoughts that his father might suffer from some incurable disease would immediately "undo" this with the thought that his father is the most healthy man in the world. Obviously his first thoughts arose from his unrecognized and unconscious hostility toward his father, which slipped out as an idea that his father might have cancer or become a victim of it in the future. Lest the "magic" of this thought produce paternal cancer, it was immediately counteracted by the equally "magic" thought of the remarkable health possessed by his father.

2. Since the gas jets are common focal points for excessive worries, an example concerning them is useful here. A patient, for instance, must first turn the gas jets on and then turn them off, thus undoing the original harmful act. Here again the obsession that the jets are on is accompanied by the fear that the whole household might be asphyxiated and stems from unconscious hostility. Turning the jets off after turning them on symbolically "undoes" the damage and makes things all right again.

ISOLATION

Isolation is a mechanism where the original memory and its affect are separated and the affect remains unconscious, while the idea is allowed access to consciousness. This mechanism, like undoing, is typical of obsessive-compulsive neurotics. It is one of the reasons why a compulsive patient is often able to relate what must have obviously been a highly charged incident and yet do it without a trace of emotion. He seems not to be able to recapture any of the original feeling associated with the incident. This mechanism incidentally allows these patients to remember much farther into their childhood than can the average conversion or dissociative type of person who has repressed both ideas and affects.

Examples

1. One of the examples of isolation most frequently seen is that of the man who isolates physical sexuality from its ordinary emotional component. Such a man can have sexual relations only with women for whom he feels no tenderness or warmth. On the other hand, he cannot

have sexual relations with a woman for whom he does have these warm emotions. This is often referred to as a "madonna-prostitute complex." Women belong, as far as such men are concerned, either to one class or the other and become therefore either sexual objects or the recipient of positive love feelings, but never both.

2. Another example is found in a patient who was able to describe accurately and vividly a scene where his sister had been run over by a truck and horribly mutilated when he was five years of age and she three-and-a-half. As he described the various gruesome details, one was struck by the obvious lack of emotion. At the time of the incident he felt a great deal, but the affect and memory had become separated and the affect had remained unconscious. While it is true that the passage of time ordinarily diminishes to some degree the affect associated with an incident, we ordinarily find at least a reasonable proportion of the affect retained with the memory and recurring at the time of relating the incident, even though it may be years later. At times this mechanism of isolation works in such a way that the affect is allowed to become conscious, but only when attached to some unrelated and trivial incident which has nothing to do with the original incident. At such times of course the affect seems somewhat incongruous in its improper setting.

REGRESSION

Regression is a mechanism of defense by which the ego abandons a level of psychosexual adjustment which it has achieved and returns to an earlier and more infantile level. Generally speaking there are three possible motivating factors for the use of the regressive phenomenon of returning to an earlier level. In the first place, we must consider the possibility of a constitutionally enhanced level of psychosexual development. Some children seem to be endowed from birth onward with an exaggerated oral, anal, or genital period of psychosexual development. Certain children, for instance, present obvious signs or symptoms of a prolonged oral phase. They require the bottle for longer than is ordinarily seen. They may well have much more difficulty going through the teething process. They generally seem to have greater problems obtaining freedom from the oral dependent period. Other youngsters may reveal increased anal signs in terms of obstinacy, ambivalence, aggression, and so forth. In many such youngsters, we find no obvious reasons in terms of family environment for this difficulty and have to attribute it to constitutional endowment.

The second possible reason for difficulty in overcoming and out-growing a level of psychosexual development lies in parental over-indulgence. If the mother and father make a particular phase of psychosexual development especially easy and comfortable for a youngster and subsequently make the next phase very difficult, it stands to reason that the child will attempt to maintain the earlier phase. For instance, in certain families, we find the beginning anal phase very difficult to tolerate and children tend to rebel against learn-ing the conformity that goes with this particular period. The previous oral phase holds much greater promise of gratification and the new and oncoming phase means only frustration to the children.

The third possible reason for regression in a child's personality lies in deprivation during a particular phase. If a youngster, to take the same example, is deprived severely during the oral phase, his needs and gratifications remain unmet and he tends to retain the particular urges that are characteristic of the early phase, perhaps in the vain hope of satisfying them prior to moving on to the next phase. He has literally never been able to outgrow completely the previous phase because the needs of that phase have never been met. He may be said to be fixated in the oral phase. He will probably continue to some extent to mature emotionally, but there will re-main a basic tendency to orality which, especially under periods of stress, will become more evident. In other words, when an individual regresses under pressure, he will regress to his level of fixation.

Examples

1. Perhaps the commonest and simplest example of regression is that seen in a child at the birth of a younger sibling. For instance, the boy who has reached the age of four-and-a-half and has satisfactorily de-veloped through the oral phase to the anal phase is apt to have difficulty at the birth of a younger sister. When presented with this new family member, his sense of security is threatened and he will attempt to regain what he considers to be lost in security and love by means of regression. This regression may go all the way back to the oral period and result in infantile habits which he has long since given up. On the other hand, he may again revive some of the anal characteristics which he had previously conquered. He may begin to suck his thumb or demand to be

rocked like his younger sister; or, on the other hand, he may begin to wet and soil. His regression is an attempt to regain an earlier period where his security seemed more in evidence to him.

2. The most pathological regression we know is that seen in the schizophrenic patient. There we find the typical example of the catatonic schizophrenic who regresses to an extremely infantile level. Bowel and bladder training are completely lost and ego functions disintegrate to that early formative state before the ego had a chance to become an operating portion of the mind. An individual with this disorder may assume fetal positions and display other marked characteristics of the very young infant. This type of regression includes giving up reality-testing functions.

RATIONALIZATION

Rationalization is a mechanism of defense in which the ego substitutes an acceptable reason for an unacceptable one in order to explain a given action or attitude. This is carried on primarily to delude the superego into accepting something which might otherwise result in guilt. We all prefer to feel ourselves capable of acting in a reasonable, logical, and realistic way. If our inner urges of a more infantile nature attempt to push us into action in some other direction, we are apt to substitute "better" if not truer reasons for the action which we have taken, or will take. This mechanism of defense is one of the most common of all and is utilized to a certain degree by almost everyone. However, it is easy to see how, if used to excess, it can become quite pathological and disturbing. It allows expression of unacceptable urges which are based on inner instinctual drives of a childish nature and yet deludes the individual into believing that he is behaving on a mature level.

Examples

1. The student who has an examination on the following day and as yet has not studied the material should obviously spend some time in reviewing his lecture notes and consolidating them in his mind. However, since this is not always a pleasant task, and since the neighborhood theater may be showing a movie he would really like to see, there ensues a conflict within him. For him to admit that he would really prefer the movies to studying would engender considerable guilt within him, and

if he went to the show under these circumstances, he would not be able to enjoy it because of guilt. Therefore, there comes to his mind all that he has heard about the need to relax before an examination and the uselessness of "cramming." After all, he says to himself, it would be harmful to strain his eyes on lecture notes and to lose sleep worrying about learning them. He begins to think that he would be in a much better position to do well on the examination the following day if he were to spend time relaxing. Thus, he eventually goes to the theater without guilt and for "good" reasons and enjoys the movie.

2. Rationalization is common and most students have used it to one degree or another. However, when it reaches a chronic and constant level it is dangerous. The student who finds school much more difficult than he had anticipated and cannot form any good study habits may see failure coming. He may then quit studying completely and fail, but rationalize himself out of the guilt by claiming that he could have passed had he studied, but that he really didn't try very hard. The basic idea is to tell himself that he is intelligent enough and capable enough to pass the medical-school curriculum had he wished to do so but that he really did not care or try. This person is apt to use this mechanism elsewhere also. Perhaps he cannot get along with people or make friends. Rather than admit this painful thought, he rationalizes by saying that he prefers to be alone and does not like "lots of noisy people." Such a state of affairs can cover a multitude of difficulties so that he does not recognize what they really are.

DISPLACEMENT

Displacement is a mechanism of defense by which an affect which was originally attached to one object is displaced to another. As with other mechanisms of defense, displacement has as its purpose the preventing of distress from developing within the ego. The affect is ordinarily displaced onto a more innocuous object which has access to consciousness and the original memory is relegated to the unconscious.

Examples

1. A simple and unfortunately common example of displacement occurs in many American homes. The husband is berated during the day by his boss for some error that he has made. He cannot, for obvious reasons, vent the anger which is stimulated in him immediately in the

office. However, when he arrives home to find dinner is five minutes late, he becomes unreasonably angry with his wife. Actually, of course, his anger was mainly directed towards his boss, but circumstances which have prevented its expression lead the way for displacement onto another object which is "safer," namely his wife.

2. A more pathological example of displacement is seen in phobias. These are fears of animals, places, or objects which do not seem to have a rational basis. The little boy who in the height of his oedipal period is struggling with negative feelings toward his father fears retaliation from his father. Such fears make living with his father difficult and the whole situation becomes a problem to him. Therefore, he is apt to displace his fear of the father onto an animal. Then the animal can be avoided and the father can be tolerated. Obviously this is a more convenient solution than attempting to suppress and control the whole complex.

SUMMARY

Thus it can be seen that the ego is quite busy with its various mechanisms of defense. We may reasonably ask why the ego needs these particular mechanisms and why it should be so fearful of painful problems developing. The answer lies in the narcissism of the human being, or, in other words, his self-love. We all need to feel a certain amount of lovableness. The ego of the personality has great need for approval. If during childhood the youngster is made secure by the basic conclusion that he is loved, it is of great help to him in going on further in personality development. If, on the other hand, he is made unhappy by teasing, neglect, or punishment, there comes an inner and unconscious conclusion that no one could possibly love him. This inner conclusion, whether it be that of lovableness or unlovableness, tends to remain basic within the personality as chronological growth continues. The mature and secure person develops an inner core of his personality during childhood which gives him the feeling that he is potentially lovable. The immature, neurotic, or psychotic individual has an inner insecure core built out of a feeling that he could not possibly be loved by anyone and in addition in many ways is unable to love himself.

This last statement needs certain qualifications, in that the neurotic or psychotic individual also has the opposite feeling, namely an enhanced self-love; but this is not enough to convince himself of his own worth-whileness. The mature person feels himself relatively capable and useful in his environment, while the immature individual is constantly beset by feelings of insecurity or is busily engaged in over-compensating them to the point of appearing to be markedly ego-centric. True humility is seen only in persons whose egos have been well filled with early childhood love and warmth and who are confident of themselves and secure in their abilities. They feel that their impulses are acceptable, their intentions good, and they proceed to do the best that they are able. They therefore need few if any mechanisms of defense, since they are unafraid of fantasied attack from the environment or from those whom they knew long ago and who now exist within them as a conscience.

Unfortunately the average person uses many defenses in his attempts to deal with his instincts and the environment. When such defenses are exaggerated, we call that individual "defensive." Generally speaking, he may either retire shyly from the environment or meet it in an exaggerated pseudo-aggressive way. We soon sense that there is an obvious artificiality in his demeanor. Keeping such defenses in operation requires a considerable amount of psychic energy to meet the environment. The defensive person is less flexible, interesting, and likable than a mature person. Much of psychotherapy consists of studying the defenses with which the patient tries unrealistically and inefficiently to deal with the environment or with his own instinctual impulses or rigid superego demands.

CHAPTER 4

History Taking, Examination, and Diagnosis

THE WISE physician considers an evaluation of the mental and emotional factors an integral part of every examination which he performs, no matter what the presenting symptoms have been. However, it is an unfortunately common attitude of many medical students and physicians that such an evaluation is an undertaking completely alien to ordinary medical practice. They feel that this procedure requires an extensive amount of specific psychiatric knowledge, possessed, as far as they are concerned, only by psychiatrists. Such medical students and physicians may be quite capable of tracing down an organic complaint to its minutest components and yet seem painfully unable to form any useful impression of the type of person with whom they are dealing. For instance, upon hearing the chief complaint of dyspnea, they spend a great deal of time properly eliciting all the pertinent material relating to cardiac function, yet completely fail to recognize the fact that the symptom has occurred only in certain anxiety-producing situations to which the patient is extremely sensitive.

Fortunately there are many physicians who see their patients properly as whole individuals attempting to function in a particular environment. Further, they realize that the psychology of the human being is hardly more than an extension of his physiology. The mature, wise surgeon, for instance, recognizes the important effect of his patient's emotional state upon his tolerance of and ability to recover from operative procedures. He recognizes that undergoing a hysterectomy involves emotional as well as physiological adjustments for a woman. He does not hesitate to encourage his patient to verbalize feelings and ideas about this procedure and to help her understand it and therefore allay anxiety. He knows how much effect this will have upon the postoperative course. Similarly, the well-trained and mature pediatrician is as conscious of the psychological development of the children under his care as he is of their physiological development. He keeps a watchful eye not only on physiological nutrition but also on emotional nutrition. Such a physician recognizes his responsibility for the total well-being of his patients. He realizes that the psyche and the soma are so closely interwoven as to make it impossible to treat one and exclude the other.

Essentially there should not be any difference in the physician's approach to a person suffering from a psychiatric condition from that to any other patient. For whatever reason a person seeks medical help, the physician should consider him as a total person and should strive to become as thoroughly acquainted as possible with that total person. To do so requires a certain basic knowledge on his part of some of the fundamental principles of psychodynamics. These enable him to evaluate more readily and efficiently the stresses and strains to which the patient is subjected as well as the psychic and somatic reactions which result. The so-called "art" of medicine applied so well by many physicians, particularly in the past, is an essential part of the armamentarium of every well-trained physician today. The ability to apply it can be greatly enhanced and expanded by a knowledge of some of these basic fundamentals of psychodynamics. The approach may then be put on a firm scientific foundation and no longer remain the property of a few lucky individuals who happen to have considerable intuitive ability. It is to be stressed that the application of these principles is not to be limited to purely psychiatric patients. Those who suffer from organic ills are still human beings and if these psychodynamics are taken into account when dealing with such patients, the physician will find that they are much more able to co-operate and use whatever therapy he outlines.

The patient-physician relationship is one which involves two personalities, and psychiatry has clearly shown that the physician must literally know himself as well as know the patient. Whereas it is possible to use the stethoscope confidently or to palpate an abdomen efficiently regardless of one's own personality, this does not hold true in dealing with the whole patient. In his daily work the physician is subject to an infinite variety of emotional reactions on the part of patients. Some are belligerent, some tearful, some are anxious, and, unfortunately, only a very small number are mature and realistic in their attitudes. Physicians, on the other hand, vary remarkably in their own emotional attitudes toward patients. Some are constantly authoritarian in their attitudes and maintain this behavior regardless of the type of patient with whom they are dealing. Some pride themselves on how blunt and frank they are with patients, again regardless of the type of person with whom they are dealing. It is possible for a specialist, such as a busy orthopedist, to become calloused in his approach to his patients. While he may have seen several hundred fractures recently, it is important for him to remember that the patient has seen only one and that is the one from which he now suffers. Emotional complaint on the part of patients stirs up a negative, resentful attitude on the part of certain physicians. They look upon such patients as "only neurotic" and unwisely prescribe sedatives over a long period of time. It is as if they fear or resent giving the patient any opportunity to discuss his problems, since they do not feel equipped with solutions to them.

Essentially what is required on the part of the physician is a healthy, friendly curiosity about the emotional reactions of his patient and a critical watchfulness toward his own emotional reactions. Unreasonable belligerency, for instance, on the part of the patient should result in the physician's asking himself why this reaction is taking place, rather than producing a childish, hostile response. Unfortunately, graduation from medical school does not automatically confer maturity upon an individual with the same regularity that it confers an M.D. Each physician has his own emotional problems, even though they may be small, and he should be willing to look introspectively at his own emotional responses, always striving to make them more mature.

HISTORY TAKING

It is a common attitude among physicians today that to miss an organic ailment while making a functional diagnosis is an unforgivable sin. On the other hand, it is not considered of great importance should the physician reverse the procedure and miss a functional diagnosis while making an organic one. The general attitude is that the patient may suffer severe consequences from a missed organic diagnosis while this is not true for functional problems. Obviously such an attitude is erroneous. Certainly there is no more convincing evidence than those patients who commit suicide during an involutional melancholia, after having been treated for many months for mild anemia or chronic constipation. It is impossible to measure the amount of family disturbance and monetary loss that results from treating functional ailments as if they were organic. Ordinarily, even the lay person has little difficulty recognizing the appearance of a full-blown psychosis. This does not require medical education. The physician should be able to differentiate accurately and efficiently the less obvious varieties of emotional disturbance from organic ailments and should at the same time be competent to at least carry through the initial evaluation.

The best psychiatric history is obtained, as in any branch of medicine, by allowing the patient first to tell his own story in his own words. Most individuals, whether they suffer from organic or emotional problems, have thought a good deal about their complaints prior to coming to the physician, and if they are allowed to tell the story themselves, the physician gains additional insight into the situation. While the patient is telling his story, the astute physician utilizes all his powers of observation. He notices the patient's general characteristics as well as the presence or absence of tension. He is aware of the particular way in which the patient approaches this new situation. He is able, for instance, to sense rigid compulsiveness in an individual who comes with a too-well-prepared and possibly even documented story. The initial interview is particularly important, since it provides an opportunity to observe the patient meeting a new situation.

The various subdivisions of the ordinary psychiatric history do not differ markedly from the ordinary medical history. These subdivisions concern the various areas of the patient's life which will provide an over-all insight into the patient's life situation and personality functioning. First, as in any history, the physician is interested in the chief complaint and is particularly interested in it as expressed in the patient's own words. The process of elaborating this chief complaint leads to the usual history of the present illness. This includes the onset, the length, severity, and type of complaint for which the patient comes. It also includes an evaluation of the environmental situation under which the symptoms developed. After these facts have been elicited, the physician should probe into the past history. If the patient is psychotic and unable to give a coherent history, much of the material may have to be obtained from close relatives and friends. If, on the other hand, the patient is able to give it, the material is that much more useful since it indicates the patient's own attitude toward his illness and what things he considers to be most important. Generally speaking, rather broad questions are asked and the patient himself is allowed to pick what he considers to be the most important elements.

Under "Past History" several large headings are useful. In the first place, the physician is interested in the patient's family history, which involves, particularly, his parents and siblings. This not only includes such statistical data as births and deaths, but perhaps even more important, the emotional atmosphere within the family and the various interpersonal relationships. Next comes a personal history of the patient, beginning at birth and extending through the formative years of early childhood. Then comes a school history in which the educational achievements of the patient are inquired into. Once again, this not only includes academic performance but also an evaluation of the patient's sexual development and adjustment. Obtaining a sexual history requires considerable tact and judgment on the part of the physician. Some patients are perfectly willing to give a rather full and complete sexual history in the initial interviews, while with others resistance occurs if this material is discussed too rapidly. Therefore, the intuition, experience, and judgment of the therapist must be skillfully utilized. First, one is interested in finding out how the patient's early sexual knowledge was obtained. Also of importance is the patient's adjustment to himself and to the opposite sex during adolescence. Following this there is the matter of courtship and, where applicable, marital adjustment along with its sexual components. In the obviously rigid and inhibited individuals these matters will be elicited only through further interviews. In the more articulate, outspoken person it may be possible to elicit many of them in the initial interviews.

The medical history, including diseases, injuries, and other pertinent medical data, is an integral part of the complete psychiatric history.

The final division of the psychiatric history is an inquiry into the premorbid personality. By this is meant an elicitation of the various signs and symptoms of emotional and mental disorders prior to the onset of the present illness. Much of this material may become evident in other portions of the history. For instance, during the school history it may become very clear that the patient was maladjusted in school, unable to get along with his contemporaries, embroiled with his teachers, and failing in his academic work. Such a lead should be followed at the time that it arises during the history taking and further probed in an attempt to form an adequate and complete picture of the premorbid personality somewhere during the interview.

A physician may be called upon to see a psychiatric patient suffering from a full-blown psychosis and consequently incapable of giving a complete and accurate history. In such a case it is necessary to rely upon relatives and close friends to obtain all the possible information about the patient. It must be stressed that this procedure is not to be undertaken at the expense of spending time with the patient and evaluating his verbal productions, emotional reactions, and behavior patterns. Even in the case of the most disturbed and psychotic individuals a physician who is willing to listen will gain valuable understanding about the personality of his patient. A mother, father, brother, or sister who gives a history to the physician about the patient may be quite sincere in attempting to give a clear picture of the illness, yet, on the other hand, such an informant could not possibly know or understand thoroughly the various factors which have been the most important in the patient's own personality formation and subsequent breakdown.

Outline No. 1 provides a complete psychiatric history which we have found useful in our own work. It must be stressed that rigid adherence to such an outline is inadvisable. Rather it is preferable that the physician familiarize himself with the general areas to be covered and yet maintain sufficient flexibility to delve more deeply into the particular points which are most fertile in providing a complete understanding of the patient. With one patient it may be necessary to expand a particular portion of the outline, while with the next patient some other portion may prove far more useful. Whether the patient himself or a relative is giving the history, it is necessary to allow considerable leeway in how it shall be conducted. Ample opportunity must be given the informant to enlarge upon any particular point in the history which to him seems most important.

Outline No. 1—Outline for Study of the Mental Patient, Temple University Medical School, Department of Psychiatry

INTRODUCTION

It should be kept in mind that almost every mental disorder is a problem in maladjustment of the individual to his environment. Such an adjustment may function adequately during physical health and only break down with the stress of acute or chronic physical disease. Therefore, a prerequisite and essential adjunct to an accurate mental examination is a careful and complete somatic history and examination. These examinations, physical and mental, should be designed and oriented always to initiate the establishment of the primary *therapeutic aim,* namely, *rapport.* To this end, an informal, friendly approach is most efficacious and above all *the patient,* at all times, *must be allowed to talk freely,* unrestrictedly, and at first more or less on his own terms. During this procedure, a constant evaluation of the patient, in terms of his attitudes, volubility, neurotic manifestations (tic, tension, gaze, blushing, etc.), affect, suspiciousness, claim for sympathy, etc., should be made. The purpose then is to adopt a special type of history in order to bring out *dominant personality traits, the focal points of vulnerability in association with the defense techniques used* by the individual, and *the emotional conflicts.* Then we can formulate a diagnosis based on the psychodynamics present and not merely a descriptive classification, and so initiate an effective therapeutic approach.

STATEMENT OF THE PROBLEM

Here a brief, concise statement of the patient's presenting complaint and symptoms should be given.

HISTORY

In order to obtain a satisfactory history of personality development, a supplementary history when possible should be obtained from the nearest and yet most objectively minded relative of the patient. It is often *advantageous* to *have a history from more than one source* in order to develop a more complete picture. However, patients who are themselves able to present the facts of their past life and reactions to them in many cases may readily give material of utmost value in understanding the illness.

I. CHRONOLOGY OF SYMPTOMS' APPEARANCE. When feasible, the primary injunction of allowing the patient to talk spontaneously and without interruption is of paramount importance. *Only when the patient's urge to present his complaint in his own way and at his own pace has been completed, should questions designed to obtain a coherent chronological development of the illness be interjected.* Here, comparison with the ward record, medical and social service histories, will yield important data such as any important additional material, any gaps filled in or any details of medical or personal history omitted (repressed), together with an estimation of their relative importance by virtue of their stress or omission by the patient.

II. PERSONAL HISTORY—BIRTH, INFANCY, AND EARLY CHILDHOOD
   1. Date of birth.
   2. Type of birth, i.e., normal or abnormal (complicated).
   3. Mother's condition during pregnancy. Was child planned for? Desired before, during, after pregnancy; or undesired? Any undue physical, mental, or environmental stress during pregnancy?
   4. Breast- or bottle-fed; age and circumstances of weaning; any unusal reluctance of child to be weaned or symptoms developing after weaning?
   5. At what age was sphincter control begun? Reaction of child and parents? At what age was control established; any relapses? If so, how were these managed by child and parent?

6. At what age did walking and talking begin, respectively?

7. When and how was interest first manifested in sexual difference? Reaction of environment?

8. Adaptation to older and younger siblings? How did patient adapt to other children?

9. Any childhood neurotic manifestations, such as convulsions, tantrums, sleeplessness, nightmares, thumb-sucking, feeding problems, fears of darkness, animals, etc.? How managed by parents?

III. FAMILY HISTORY

1. Father and Mother—age, occupation, birthplace, social status, personality traits, previous illnesses with special emphasis on neuropsychiatric determinants.

2. All other near relatives who have lived in close proximity to the patient or have played any special role in his life.

3. Special emphasis should be placed on the patient's position in the order of birth, empathy or antipathy to either parent or to any of the siblings.

4. Present family and environmental situation.

IV. LATER CHILDHOOD AND ADOLESCENCE.

Examination at this point should be directed toward eliciting a comprehensive picture of the patient's reaction to his childhood situation, including where he lived, financial situation, relationship of the parents to each other, the patient, and other siblings, the patient's relationships with his siblings, and above all *an accurate estimation of the patient's emotional adjustment to his childhood situation.*

A. School History:

1. Age on entering school.

2. Adaptation to teachers and playmates.

3. Intellectual progress and attainments.

4. Any truancy or any type of delinquency.

5. Actual amount of education obtained. Whether under duress, free choice, with or without financial obstacles, etc.

B. Sexual Development:

1. Patient's earliest recollections of any sexual experiences and emotional experiences. Parents' attitude toward masturbation or any of the sexual experiences recollected by the patient. In this connection much important and etiological information should be obtained from collateral sources concerning the environmental and parental attitudes.

2. If the patient is a female, was there any fear, shame, or any other reaction surrounding onset of menstruation? Was the patient prepared in any way by the mother or sister?

3. Note particularly the patient's attitude toward sex and sexual discussion, e.g., reticent, prudish, embarrassed, frank.

C. Work Record:

1. What jobs has the patient held (along with information concerning financial remuneration)? Has there been any improvement or regression in earning capacity, especially in recent years? The patient's relationships with his employers and coworkers should be explored thoroughly. What was parents' and patient's attitude toward financial contributions to the family income? If married, what was the patient's reaction and attitude toward financial responsibilities incurred?

V. MARITAL HISTORY

1. Age at marriage. Length of courtship. Any marked disparity in age between the partners?

2. If marriage was unusually early or late, what was the reason? Previous engagements.

3. Sexual adjustment. Frequency and degree of sexual satisfaction. Premarital relationships? Any type of sexual difficulty in either partner, e.g., impotence, frigidity, ejaculatio praecox, perversions, etc.? Any change in sexual adjustments since marriage? Recent attitude and frequency?

4. Contraceptives? Attitude with reference to religious, aesthetic, or other standpoints?

5. Number of children and respective ages? Health of wife during pregnancy? Were children wanted? If no children, why not?

6. Attitude of parents and family of each partner toward the marriage? Any extraneous pressure for or against the marriage both at its inception and at the present time?

7. Any problem of infidelity, jealousy, divorce, or venereal infections?

8. Present home environment? Who lives at home? Any boarders? Sleeping arrangements? Any older children sleeping together or with parents?

VI. MEDICAL HISTORY

1. Any severe illnesses, operations, injuries? Sequelae of each? Special reference to head injury. Habits regarding use of drugs, alcohol, and tobacco. If in middle-life inquire about climacterium and whether or not any accompanying symptoms.

VII. PREMORBID PERSONALITY. It will be evident that the interview up until now has been designed to build up an over-all, comprehensive view of the total personality and that a fairly accurate picture of the premorbid personality will have been estimated by the foregoing details of the history. However, there are certain features of great aid in understanding the development and dynamics of the patient's illness which should be stressed. Therefore, for purposes of accurate personality review, some estimation of the patient's goals, ambitions, drives, interests, leisure, and work arrangements and actual state of emotional adjustment should be estimated in line with the following, as points of departure.

1. Was there any special attachment or antagonism displayed by the patient to any member of the family both in early life and later?

2. How did the patient react to losses and separation from the family?

3. What was the patient's disposition? Capacity to experience pleasure?

4. How did he react to criticism? Was he a good loser? Fondest daydreams?

5. What special interests or abilities did he display? Actual accomplishments of any goals?

6. Any anxieties, fears, or special concern over his health?

7. What special views were held, religious, philosophical, or other? Was there any unusual demand for system and order?

8. Did the patient display any feelings of inferiority? Was there any indication of any tendency to suspicion or disparagement of others?

9. Onset of illness. Complete details should be obtained concerning dates, changes noted, desire or reluctance to seek treatment, the immediate cause for treatment or hospitalization and the patient's reaction to hospitalization or treatment. *Of primary importance is an evaluation of the current situation in relation to the onset of the illness.*

EXAMINATION

The next important element in the evaluation of a patient is the mental examination or so-called mental status. This psychological examination of the patient should be accomplished and recorded in such a way that it gives maximum information about the patient's mental functioning. Unfortunately there has been a tendency in psychiatry to perpetuate the old and now outdated Kraepelinian system of formalized description. Many mental hospitals still utilize this type of mental status. Whereas it may give a superficially complete picture of the patient's mental functioning at the time he is examined, it unfortunately adds little to the over-all understanding of the patient's dynamics. In addition to this, it is oriented much more toward the hospitalized psychotic patient.

In our own work we have found a need for a different type of psychological examination which is capable of giving a more dynamic understanding of the patient. At the same time such a mental status should be one which is of practical use to the medical student or nonpsychiatric physician. Since the human psyche is complicated, such a mental status could not be exceedingly simple and still fulfill its purpose. The student who spends as much study and practice in the evaluation of the structure and workings of the minds of his patients as he does in the evaluation of physical signs and laboratory studies will be successful in dealing with emotional problems in his practice. Too many students and physicians have said to themselves "I know about people already, so I don't need to study their minds," or they have said, "A knowledge of personality is too difficult for me; let the specialist do it," but like all other branches of medicine, psychiatry is neither too easy nor too difficult and can be mastered with sincere interest and application. We feel, therefore, that the most useful and practical mental status examination which has been suggested to date is the one published by Dr. Karl Menninger in the *American Journal of Psychiatry,* February, 1952.[1] This is reproduced in Outline No. 2.

Outline No. 2—Outline for Organizing and Recording Data

I. GROSS IDENTIFICATION (General Observations)

A. *Circumstances of the Examination.*—State where, why, when, how, and by whom the examination was made. If, for example, the examination was of necessity limited to a 30-minute observation of the patient, or to a single Rorschach testing interview, say so. If it was more complete, indicate how complete. This is the place to indicate the level of confidence ascribable to the report.

B. *Visualization.*—Describe the patient impressionistically in order to

---

[1] Reprinted by courtesy of Dr. Karl A. Menninger and Grune and Stratton, Inc., Publishers.

orient the reader—mentioning such things as appearance, posture, clothing, and voice, including accessibility and general reaction to examination. Try to create a visual picture in everyday terms to which the reader or listener may attach the technical material to follow.

C. *Quotation.*—Give a brief quotation that expresses the patient's problem and/or his attitude toward it in his own words.

II. PART PROCESSES

A. *Perception*

1. Normal features: alertness, accuracy, direction of attention (inward or outward).

2. Deficiencies: sensory (anesthesia, anosmia, amaurosis, etc.); attention (distractibility, dullness, cloudiness); confusion, disorientation (time, place, person).

3. Excesses and distortions: sensory (hyperaesthesia); attention (hyperalertness); false perceptions, illusions, hallucinations, disorders of body image, estrangement, depersonalization.

B. *Intellection* (cognitive functions)

1. Level and range—(a) Normal features: intelligence, memory (remote and immediate), capacity for abstract thinking, information and knowledge. (b) Deficiencies: stupidity, amnesia, hypomnesia, concretism. (c) Excesses: hyperintelligence, hypermnesia, syncretism. (d) Distortions: disorders of judgment ("common sense"). (Do not include delusions here.)

2. Thought processes—(a) Normal features: tempo (rapidity of association and ideas), rhythm (spontaneous, hesitant, halting), organization (constricted, coherent, relevant; relation to goal). (b) Deficiencies: retardation, blocking, incoherence, irrelevance. (c) Excesses: press of associations, excessive intellectualizing, garrulousness, circumstantiality, flight of ideas. (d) Distortions: perseveration, condensation, neologisms, word salad, echolalia and stereotypy, autistic logic.

3. Thought content—(a) Normal features: prominent preoccupations, phantasies, and dreams. (b) Deficiencies: meagerness, impoverishment.

C. *Emotion* (affective processes)

1. Normal features: intensity, depth and modulation of emotional response; quality of prevailing mood (cheerfulness, somberness, irritability, etc.)

2. Deficiencies: inertia, stupor, paralysis, apathy, coldness.

3. Excesses: tendency to prevalent or oscillating elation, rage, depression, panic, worry, fear, apprehensiveness, suspiciousness.

4. Inappropriateness: disharmony between affective response and its provocation, incongruity of feeling and action, dissimulation.

D. *Action* (expressive behavior)

1. Normal features: energy level, vigor, persistence, constructiveness.

2. Deficiencies: inertia, stupor, paralysis, inability to initiate action, inhibition, rigidity.

3. Excesses: restlessness, hyperkinesis, agitation, assaultiveness, impulsiveness, destructiveness.

4. Inappropriateness: compulsions, tics, rituals, mannerisms, peculiar habits (eating, smoking, excretory, sexual, others), stereotypy, catalepsy, posturing.

III. INTEGRATED FUNCTIONING
(Relations to Integrative Opportunities)

A. *Relations to self*

1. Self-concept: What does the patient consider to be his "real" self? Does he feel he is being "himself"? What are the important activities and values that comprise the structure of the self? On what models has the patient based his ego-identity? (*See* Erikson.) How much stability is provided by the ego-identity?

2. Ego-ideal: Goals, level of aspiration, chief identification figures. Ethical standards and how justified. Degree to which ego-ideal has supplanted superego.

3. Superego: Strength, actual and relative. Predominant model (if known; e.g., father, aunt, brother). Characteristic type of placation required (penance or penitence, mourning, physical suffering, gestures, deprivation, bribery).

B. *Relations to others*

1. Quantitative aspects: range, diversity, intensity, constancy, flexibility, etc.

2. Qualitative aspects: selectivity (type of object choice), prevalent modality (parasitic, predatory, possessive, patronizing, domineering, cruel, cooperative, negativistic, exploiting, masochistic, protective, tender, considerate), overt sexual patterns.

3. Love-hate pattern: dominance of which, and in which relationships; ambivalence manifestations (evidence of contrary unconscious attitude).

4. Transference paradigm: In what characteristic way does the patient relate himself to the examiner over and beyond the reality determinants?

C. *Relations to things* (sublimations)

1. Attitude toward possessions—his own and those of others.

2. Work patterns: interest, intensity, variety, consistency, skill, efficiency, satisfaction.

3. Play patterns: interest, intensity, variety, consistency, skill, efficiency, satisfaction, sportsmanship.

4. Philosophic, social, and religious interests and values: form, scope, intensity, satisfaction.

IV. REACTIONS TO DISINTEGRATIVE THREAT
(Degrees of Dysfunction)

A. *Normal reactions to mild threat:* simple tension-relieving devices, other than sublimation, ordinarily used (humor, tears, fantasy, dreams, acting to alter, proud self-control, passive acceptance, activity, overeating, excretory acceleration, plus increased integrative effort)

B. *Emergency reactions*

1. First Order (alarm and mobilization)—Hyperrepression, plus

Hypersuppression (determined effort at "self-control")
Hyperalertness (up to and including "jitteriness," "nervousness," insomnia)
Hyperirritability (touchiness, stubbornness, irascibility, brief rage attacks)
Hyperemotionalism (oscillating depression, fearfulness, anger, euphoria, etc.)
Hyperintellection (purposeful to pointless preoccupation, worry, loquacity)
Hypercompensation (new reaction formations, self-reproach, identification with aggressor, fantasy elaboration, etc.)
Hyperkinesis (inefficient or pointless overactivity, restlessness, etc.)
Hyperwithdrawal (avoidance, denial, contact severance)
Hyperlability of sympathetic system (minor somatic dysfunction such as tremor, flushing, enuresis, etc.)

2. Second Order (partial detachment and attempted compensation)

Dissociation—fainting, isolation, narcolepsy, amnesia, fugues, depersonalization

Displacement (substituted objects)—phobias and counterphobic phenomena, obsessions, strong aversions, projection, provocative transilliency, persistent unmanageableness, simulation (conscious or unconscious)

Substitution (substituted modalities and symbols)—compulsions, rituals, "kleptomania," fire-setting, etc., perverse sexual objects or modalities.

Sacrifice—self-abasement and self-imposed restriction, asceticism; body mutilation (intentional, "accidental," surgical); intoxication or narcotization; somatization in fantasy, sensation, or function (list symptoms); exploitation of somatic affection.

3. Third Order (transitory ego rupture, with prompt restoration; episodic phenomena)

Panic attacks
Catastrophic demoralization
Transitory dereistic excitement
Assaultive violence—homicidal, suicidal, sexual
Convulsions

4. Fourth Order (persistent ego rupture or exhaustion, with marked detachment)

Excitement with erratic, disorganized behavior
Hyperthymia with stupor, agitation, retardation, delusion formation
Autism with flaccid, incoherent, silly, bizarre reactions
Apathy (extreme) with (usually) mutism and/or hallucinations
Delusional preoccupation with one or several themes, usually persecutory, with defensiveness, suspiciousness, grandiosity, etc.
Confusion: bewildered, uncertain, forgetful disorientation.

5. Fifth Order (complete ego failure)

Continuous, uncontrolled violence ending in physical exhaustion and death.
? Some other forms of dying
"Aphanisis" (paralysis of mental functioning) (Jones)

C. *Aspects of the present disequilibration*

1. Sequential chain
2. Anxiety feelings

3. Insight
4. Façade
5. Intact assets for therapeutic exploitation

V. DIAGNOSTIC SUMMARY

A. *Principal features of the examinational findings*
B. *Diagnostic impression (differential)*
C. *Prognostic indications*

DIAGNOSIS

After the history and mental status and physical examination have been completed, the physician should be in a position to record a diagnostic impression. In some instances it will be impossible to make a definite diagnosis, at least immediately following the first interview. It must be stressed that the procedure of making a diagnosis by no means ends the psychiatric approach to the patient. Years ago, patients were catalogued into various diagnostic categories and then promptly forgotten. At the present time, however, much less stress is laid upon the nosological procedures and much more upon an understanding of the underlying dynamic picture presented by the patient. However, there are certain advantages to being able to recognize various syndromes efficiently. In the first place, such recognition gives the physician a more general understanding of the patient's underlying conflicts. Secondly, it allows a clearer and more accurate estimation of prognosis. For instance, if at the end of an initial interview the physician is able to successfully diagnose the patient as suffering from a conversion reaction, then he can foresee certain generalities in future therapy which tend to hold true for the majority of people who have this particular syndrome. He will, for instance, know that the transference is apt to be much more clear and marked than would be true in some of the other neurotic conditions and can be on the lookout for such manifestations. If, on the other hand, the diagnosis is that of an obsessive-compulsive reaction, the physician will recognize at the outset that ambivalence will play a large role in the therapeutic process. Knowledge of such factors early in the therapy will allow the physician to anticipate and handle the various reactions which will in all probability come up during the course of treatment.

The physician should be able early in the contact with the psychiatric patient to make some evaluation of prognosis. The patient, as well as other members of the family, is interested in obtaining some general picture of what therapy will entail and what the ultimate result will probably be. At the time of formulating some idea of the prognosis, the physician should have an over-all plan of treatment in mind. In the case of the ordinary neurotic individual it is often possible to deal solely with the patient and to give him some initial idea of what must be done in order to relieve his problems. In the psychotic patient such information should be given to a responsible family member who may then decide upon the practical aspects of pursuing a recommended treatment.

A formal, complete, and yet efficient classification of a mental disease is difficult to establish. Innumerable factors are capable of influencing the personality, characteristics, and behavior of an individual. A pure syndrome is rarely if ever found, but rather there tends to be an admixture of several syndromes, with one predominating. Many attempts have been made to classify mental and emotional disorders and it is fairly safe to say that all of them have certain deficiencies. However, there are many obvious advantages when a branch of medical science has its own standardized method of classification. The most thorough and widely accepted of these, in psychiatry, is that of the American Psychiatric Association.[2] We reproduce it here in the form in which it was adopted in 1951.

Outline No. 3—Classification of Mental and Emotional Diseases, The American Psychiatric Association

DISORDERS CAUSED BY OR ASSOCIATED WITH IMPAIRMENT OF BRAIN-TISSUE FUNCTION

ACUTE BRAIN DISORDERS

Disorders Due to or Associated with Infection

Acute Brain Syndrome associated with intracranial infection. *Specify infection*

Acute Brain Syndrome associated with systemic infection. *Specify infection*

[2] Diagnostic and Statistical Manual. *Mental Disorders*. Washington, D.C. American Psychiatric Association Mental Hospital Service, 1952.

Disorders Due to or Associated with Intoxication
Acute Brain Syndrome, drug or poison intoxications. *Specify drug or poison*
Acute Brain Syndrome, alcohol intoxication: Acute hallucinosis, Delirium tremens

Disorders Due to or Associated with Trauma
Acute Brain Syndrome associated with trauma. *Specify trauma*

Disorders Due to or Associated with Circulatory Disturbance
Acute Brain Syndrome associated with circulatory disturbance. (*Indicate cardiovascular disease as additional diagnosis*)

Disorders Due to or Associated with Disturbance of Innervation or of Psychic Control
Acute Brain Syndrome associated with convulsive disorder. (*Indicate manifestation by Supplementary Term*)

Disorders Due to or Associated with Disturbance of Metabolism, Growth or Nutrition
Acute Brain Syndrome with metabolic disturbance. *Specify*

Disorder Due to or Associated with New Growth
Acute Brain Syndrome associated with intracranial neoplasm. *Specify*

Disorders Due to Unknown or Uncertain Cause
Acute Brain Syndrome with disease of unknown or uncertain cause. (*Indicate disease as additional diagnosis*)

Disorders Due to Unknown or Uncertain Cause with the Functional Reaction Alone Manifest
Acute Brain Syndrome of unknown cause

CHRONIC BRAIN DISORDERS [3]

Disorders Due to Prenatal (Constitutional) Influence
Chronic Brain Syndrome associated with congenital cranial anomaly. *Specify anomaly*
Chronic Brain Syndrome associated with congenital spastic paraplegia
Chronic Brain Syndrome associated with Mongolism
Chronic Brain Syndrome due to prenatal maternal infectious diseases

---

[3] The qualifying phrase "Mental Deficiency" (mild, moderate, or severe) should be added at the end of the diagnosis in disorders of this group which present mental deficiency as the major symptom of the disorder. Include intelligence quotient (I.Q.) in the diagnosis. [Footnote in original.]

Disorders Due to or Associated with Infection

Chronic Brain Syndrome associated with central nervous system syphilis. *Specify as below:* Meningoencephalitic, Meningovascular, Other central nervous system syphilis

Chronic Brain Syndrome associated with intracranial infection other than syphilis. *Specify infection* [4]

Disorders Associated with Intoxication

Chronic Brain Syndrome associated with intoxication: Chronic Brain Syndrome, drug or poison intoxication. *Specify drug or poison*

Chronic Brain Syndrome, alcohol intoxication. *Specify reaction*

Disorders Associated with Trauma

Chronic Brain Syndrome associated with birth trauma

Chronic Brain Syndrome associated with brain trauma

Chronic Brain Syndrome brain trauma, gross force. *Specify (Other than operative)*

Chronic Brain Syndrome following brain operation

Chronic Brain Syndrome following electrical brain trauma

Chronic Brain Syndrome following irradiational brain trauma

Disorders Associated with Circulatory Disturbances

Chronic Brain Syndrome associated with cerebral arteriosclerosis

Chronic Brain Syndrome associated with circulatory disturbance other than cerebral arteriosclerosis. *Specify*

Disorders Associated with Disturbances of Innervation or of Psychic Control

Chronic Brain Syndrome associated with convulsive disorder

Disorders Associated with Disturbance of Metabolism, Growth or Nutrition

Chronic Brain Syndrome associated with senile brain disease

Chronic Brain Syndrome associated with other disturbance of metabolism, growth or nutrition (Includes presenile, glandular, pellagra, familial amaurosis)

Disorders Associated with New Growth

Chronic Brain Syndrome associated with intracranial neoplasm. *Specify neoplasm*

[4] When infection is more important than the reaction or mental deficiency, specify the infection. If both infection and reaction or mental deficiency are important two diagnoses are required. [Footnote in original.]

Disorders Associated with Unknown or Uncertain Cause
Chronic Brain Syndrome associated with diseases of unknown or uncertain cause (Includes multiple sclerosis, Huntington's chorea, Pick's disease and other diseases of a familial or hereditary nature). *Indicate disease by additional diagnosis*

Disorders Due to Unknown or Uncertain Cause with the Functional Reaction Alone Manifest
Chronic Brain Syndrome of unknown cause

MENTAL DEFICIENCY [5]

Disorders Due to Unknown or Uncertain Cause with the Functional Reaction Alone Manifest; Hereditary and Familial Diseases of this Nature
Mental deficiency (familial or hereditary)—Mild, Moderate, Severe

Disorders Due to Undetermined Cause
Mental deficiency, idiopathic—Mild, Moderate, Severe

DISORDERS OF PSYCHOGENIC ORIGIN OR WITHOUT CLEARLY DEFINED PHYSICAL CAUSE OR STRUCTURAL CHANGE IN THE BRAIN

PSYCHOTIC DISORDERS

Disorders Due to Disturbance of Metabolism, Growth, Nutrition or Endocrine Function
Involutional psychotic reaction

Disorders of Psychogenic Origin or without Clearly Defined Tangible Cause or Structural Change
Affective reactions
Manic depressive reaction, manic type
Manic depressive reaction, depressed type
Manic depressive reaction, other
Psychotic depressive reaction
Schizophrenic reactions
Schizophrenic reaction, simple type
Schizophrenic reaction, hebephrenic type
Schizophrenic reaction, catatonic type
Schizophrenic reaction, paranoid type
Schizophrenic reaction, acute undifferentiated type

[5] Include intelligence quotient (I.Q.) in the diagnosis. [Footnote in original.]

Schizophrenic reaction, chronic undifferentiated type
Schizophrenic reaction, schizo-affective type
Schizophrenic reaction, childhood type
Schizophrenic reaction, residual type
Paranoid reactions
Paranoia
Paranoid state
Psychotic reaction without clearly defined structural change, other than above

PSYCHOPHYSIOLOGIC AUTONOMIC AND VISCERAL DISORDERS

Disorders Due to Disturbance of Innervation or of Psychic Control

Psychophysiologic skin reaction. (*Indicate manifestation by Supplementary Term*)

Psychophysiologic musculoskeletal reaction. (*Indicate manifestation by Supplementary Term*)

Psychophysiologic respiratory reaction. (*Indicate manifestation by Supplementary Term*)

Psychophysiologic cardiovascular reaction. (*Indicate manifestation by Supplementary Term*)

Psychophysiologic hemic and lymphatic reaction. (*Indicate manifestation by Supplementary Term*)

Psychophysiologic gastrointestinal reaction. (*Indicate manifestation by Supplementary Term*)

Psychophysiologic genitourinary reaction. (*Indicate manifestation by Supplementary Term*)

Psychophysiologic endocrine reaction. (*Indicate manifestation by Supplementary Term*)

Psychophysiologic nervous system reaction. (*Indicate manifestation by Supplementary Term*)

Psychophysiologic reaction of organs of special sense. (*Indicate manifestation by Supplementary Term*)

PSYCHONEUROTIC DISORDERS

Disorders of Psychogenic Origin or without Clearly Defined Tangible Cause or Structural Change

Psychoneurotic reactions

Anxiety reaction
Dissociative reaction

Obsessive compulsive reaction
Depressive reaction

Conversion reaction   Psychoneurotic reaction, other
Phobic reaction

PERSONALITY DISORDERS

*Disorders of Psychogenic Origin or without Clearly Defined Tangible
Cause or Structural Change*
Personality pattern disturbance
    Inadequate personality
    Schizoid personality
    Cyclothymic personality
    Paranoid personality
Personality trait disturbance
    Emotionally unstable personality
    Passive-aggressive personality
    Compulsive personality
    Personality trait disturbance, other
Sociopathic personality disturbance
    Antisocial reaction
    Dyssocial reaction
    Sexual deviation. *Specify Supplementary Term*
    Addiction—Alcoholism, Drug addiction
Special symptom reactions
    Learning disturbance
    Speech disturbance
    Enuresis
    Somnambulism
    Other

TRANSIENT SITUATIONAL PERSONALITY DISORDERS

Transient situational personality disturbance
    Gross stress reaction
    Adult situational reaction
    Adjustment reaction of infancy
    Adjustment reaction of childhood—Habit disturbance, Conduct
        disturbance, Neurotic traits
    Adjustment reaction of adolescence
    Adjustment reaction of late life

PART II

Child Psychiatry

PART II

Child Psychiatry

CHAPTER 5

Child Psychiatry

A LARGE PART of the psychopathology which the psychiatrist has to understand and treat in the adult is regression to childish thinking and behaving. If the physician is to understand the thoughts and feelings of the neurotic and psychotic adult, he should know something of the thoughts and feelings of the child. Such understanding, however valuable it is, has been slow in developing, in part because of the tendency to believe that children's problems are temporary and can be outgrown. In fact, the study of emotional disorders in childhood has evolved slowly from the study of psychic disorders in adults. Logically any study of psychiatric disorders ought to put the child and his emotional illnesses first and then proceed to the study of disorders of later life where time, bringing added frustration, failure, disappointment, physical ailments, and deterioration, has further complicated the problem. It has been neurotic and psychotic adults, with their enormous amount of suffering, who have forced the medical profession to make greater effort to understand the child in infancy and at those early ages when trouble is just beginning.

Every mentally sick adult has had his share of childhood emotional illnesses, though they may have been unrecognized. Just as autopsies of a high percentage of adults with pulmonary tuberculosis show the evidence of childhood infection, so in the histories of emotional illness there is the evidence of childhood psychic disturbance. If we screened closely enough the signs and symptoms of pulmonary disease in childhood, we would institute treatment earlier and save much suffering, incapacity, and economic loss. The same holds true for emotional disease; yet the signs and symptoms of emotional distress are everywhere—in homes, in schools, in doctors' offices—unrecognized and untouched because not enough is known about what to do or because somebody does not care to take the time to do it.

The treatment of psychiatric disorders in children is comparatively new in medicine. Until recently the custodial care of mentally defective children comprised the major effort in child psychiatry. However, both Freud and Meyer gave great impetus to the development of child psychiatry by their recognition of the importance of the early years in the formation of the human personality. It was not until a few years after the turn of the century that there was any concerted move toward the study and adequate care and treatment of children suffering from emotional disturbances. As we have come to understand the extreme importance of these earliest years of life in the development of the personality, there has been increasing attention paid to the prevention and treatment of psychiatric disorders in children.

In about 1920 the Commonwealth Fund first helped organize and finance a few pilot child-guidance clinics in the United States; since then many more have been established. Their main orientation has been helping families create an improved emotional atmosphere in which their children may grow, and providing psychotherapeutic techniques designed to meet the problems of already disturbed children. Family agencies have played an important role, especially in the preventive aspects of child psychiatry. Teachers have become better acquainted with the emotional needs of the developing personality, and school systems have added psychological and psychiatric personnel. Pediatricians have also taken a new interest in psychiatry and have incorporated many psychiatric principles into their armamentaria. Books on the principles of modern dynamic psychiatry have been widely read and many parents are becoming increasingly aware of the effects of environment upon the future personalities of their children.

Much of the pioneering in the treatment of emotional disorders in children was originally spurred by the National Committee for Mental Hygiene, now known as the National Association for Mental Health, which was established in 1909. It was also about this time that William Healy [1] began utilizing various principles of dynamic psychiatry in working with delinquent children in Chicago. Psychological tests were formulated which would more accurately determine the level of intellectual endowment, particularly by Binet and Simon in France. Methods were evolved enabling mentally defective children to be taught in a manner making optimum use of their endowments.

Both educators and pediatricians became interested in the then new psychoanalytic technique propounded by Freud, and they gradually worked out methods of applying it to children, particularly through play techniques. Much of the original work which utilized psychoanalytic principles with children was done in Europe. Freud's daughter, Anna, was a pioneer in this field and has made great contributions. Melanie Klein in England and August Aichhorn in Vienna provided this field with rich knowledge. In our own country an increasing number of child-guidance and child-psychiatry clinics began to function. The Judge Baker Foundation in Boston and the Philadelphia Child Guidance Clinic under Frederic H. Allen became centers of research and treatment of the emotional disorders of children. In 1959 the American Board of Psychiatry and Neurolgy, Inc., formally established a subspecialty of Child Psychiatry which requires two years' training in adult work followed by two years in child psychiatry for eligibility for examination.

There is still a marked lag in the field of child psychiatry, both in the training of professional personnel and the development of services. Only a relatively few of our state hospitals have adequate children's units. They are certainly unable to provide care for the almost 14,000 children who are in our public mental institutions. Residential treatment centers for children are being established in growing numbers, particularly in university medical settings, but the number is small. Probably the greatest contribution such centers make is in the area of training.

Any approach to the understanding of the emotional problems of children must be based upon the dynamic concepts of personality growth. The child is an immature human being who is gradually forming what will eventually be an adult personality. The basic

[1] Healy, William. *The Individual Delinquent*. Boston, Little, Brown and Co., 1915.

constitutional ingredients are present at birth; from then on the environment plays a large role. The child is extremely dependent upon his parents and the emotional atmosphere which they create, particularly during the first five or six years. Thereafter he begins to come in contact with an increasingly wide variety of adults who contribute to his final and total personality. It is well to remember that the natural tendency of the child, given proper surroundings, is toward maturity. When deficiencies or excesses hamper this natural growth process, emotional problems begin to develop.

It is, therefore, much easier to grasp the various psychiatric difficulties which are seen in children if we keep in mind the developmental phases through which they pass and the cardinal characteristics of each phase. The infant under a year who is in the oral phase is dependent upon his mother for his every need. This dependency is powerful, since his life literally depends upon his receiving from her what he needs. The mother who does not "give" both physical comfort and emotional security will stir up insecurity within her child. His immature psychic system will be flooded with greater tensions than he can withstand, and an emotional problem will result. Crying will become excessive, sleep will become poor, and eventually his entire physiology will become disorganized with resultant gastrointestinal upsets. Such an infant lies within the province of psychiatry, although not necessarily within that of the psychiatrist. The infant's need in the "emotional problem" cannot be solved by a simple, reassuring statement that he will "settle down in time" or "grow out of it." Since at this time in life he relies on his mother to meet his needs, the wise physician spends sufficient time with her to determine how adequately she is meeting them and to help her to understand her infant and herself well enough to do a good job.

In the anal phase the child is essentially rebellious, ambivalent, and nonconforming. He obviously must be helped to bring some of these reactions under control and to become a more socially acceptable, stable personality. The parents, who are responsible for helping him learn these lessons, recognize, if they are mature, the need to go slowly and to provide a great deal of love, reassurance, and attention in their approach. They are patient, consistent, and calm in their efforts to help the youngster bring himself under control. If they go too rapidly the youngster may either rebel in the form of an exaggerated aggressive reaction, or he may so completely capitulate as to become a passive, fearful child.

As the youngster moves on and becomes involved in his oedipal struggle, he makes some of the basic decisions and foundations for his ultimate relationships both with members of his own and of the opposite sex. The mother of a boy, for instance, recognizes his increased attentions to her and responds to them in a warm, understanding way that is neither seductive nor rejecting. The father recognizes in the boy a certain amount of competition with himself and accepts a reasonable amount of this without excessive punitive action and without bowing to every demand on the part of his son. If mature, each parent presents to the child during the oedipal phase a good example of what it means to be a member of the parent's sex and, therefore, helps the child to be willing to accept both his sex and the other.

In addition, throughout these earliest years, mature parents encourage their children to achieve an increasing independence and ability. They are quick to praise and to understand and yet do not try to push the youngster into a degree of independence beyond his capacity.

METHOD OF APPROACH

The child, being essentially a dependent individual, rarely comes to any physician of his own volition, but is brought when and if his parents decide that it is advisable. The youngster also is unable to give a clear and complete picture of his own problems, and for this reason most information—organic or emotional—about a child is obtained from the parents.

When the parents consult a physician about a child's emotional problems, it is preferable that the child not be present during the interview; if possible, not even be in the waiting room. The physician obviously cannot get all the information that he wants in his presence because of the parents' reluctance to expose the child to a discussion of himself, while if the child is left in the waiting room, he is apt to become bored, anxious, or angry that he is being excluded from an interview that primarily concerns him. Therefore, when a complete evaluation of the emotional development of a child is needed, the interview should be so arranged that the parents come to the physician's office without the child. Such an interview may follow an initial briefer history and physical examination of the child. The interview with parents should elicit the usual medical history, including the chief complaint and present illness of the child. It should cover his development and the important events in his life and include the backgrounds of the parents, since the physician must evaluate their personalities and the atmosphere of the home.

Physical examination of a child can give not only knowledge about his organic development, but also many impressions of his emotional development. The astute physician can carry on a running conversation during the examination which draws out the child's own feeling about the various parts of his body. What does he think about his height? Would he rather be taller, or is he satisfied? What does he think about his weight? Is he too heavy or too thin? What does the young girl think of her hair? Is it the right color or would she prefer another? Over a period of time the physician can develop a relaxed and fruitful technique of conversing with children during physical examinations which will provide him with considerable understanding of their emotional development.

Psychiatric evaluation of the child involves, as it does with the adult, a composite of the many impressions received by the physician during his contacts with the child. Many of these impressions are gained during the physical examination, others by the brief observation of the child with his parents as they wait for the appointment or as they leave after the examination. A more thorough understanding of the emotional status of the child can be attained by seeing him in a situation in which he is comfortable. The child psychiatrist does this by providing a playroom free of medical atmosphere and filled with a variety of sturdy toys. If the youngster is fearful of meeting and staying with a strange physician, as is often the case, he can be reassured that no examinations or injections are to be given and that the doctor is merely interested in having him look over the playroom and toys. He can be allowed a reasonable degree of freedom and encouraged to use whatever toys he chooses, and thus considerable information can be gained by watching his reactions in the play. The inhibited child is apt to be fearful of touching anything. The compulsive child may sit stiffly in his chair as if unable to allow himself the pleasures of childish toys. The aggressive child may quickly reveal his overt hostility and lack of inhibitions by becoming destructive, or in his choice of toys of an aggressive nature, such as guns.

Verbal questioning of a child about his difficulties, especially in a direct manner, is ordinarily not very productive; it is important to try to understand the behavior and type of play in which the child becomes involved. This is not an easy procedure and usually involves more time and patience than is given in a diagnostic interview to the adult patient, who can readily answer whatever questions are put to him. The older the child, the more use can be made of the question-and-answer method.

PSYCHOLOGICAL EXAMINATION

Additional valuable information regarding a child's psychiatric condition can be obtained through psychological examination, ordinarily performed by a formally trained psychologist. Such information may be restricted to the determination of an I.Q. or may be a more complete psychological personality evaluation, giving detailed information on the kinds of fears and conflicts the child has and the mechanisms used for their solution. (See Chapter 20, "Mental Retardation.") The results of psychological testing are, in a sense, comparable to the results of the laboratory examination—that is, they require evaluation on the basis of clinical judgment. They are by no means a substitute for clinical examination, but are an adjunct to it. Obviously, the more competent the psychologist who performs these examinations, the more reliable will be the findings, but such reports must always be viewed in the light of the clinical examination.

DIAGNOSIS

Before diagnosing emotional problems in children, the physician must first be well acquainted with the emotional characteristics of the normal child at various age levels. He should recognize that the compulsive mother who complains that her eleven-month-old child resists her efforts toward toilet training and smears his excreta whenever he has an opportunity is actually describing the normal characteristics of an infant at this age. The same holds true when the mother of a five-year-old boy reports that she notices increasing frequency of masturbation in her son. She is observing, of course, another instance of normal behavior.

The physician must also recognize that psychosexual development in the child does not take place in a smooth progression, but in fits and starts, and that some children have constitutionally stronger tendencies during one developmental phase than another. For example, certain children are more aggressive from a constitutional standpoint and others tend toward more passivity. Therefore, as the physician evaluates his patient, his first concern is whether the child's emotional development seems to be appropriate to his chronological age. In other words, is this child of six still struggling with prominent anal characteristics? Is he at age five still showing evidences of orality far greater than the range of normality? If abnormalities are noted, the physician evaluates why they are present in terms of the family environment and the background of the child. He is especially interested in the important personalities that have surrounded the child—the mother and father, or their surrogates— and how these have reacted upon the child's development. Did the mother provide adequate security during the infant's earliest years and did the parents then take a mature approach to the child's conformity training during his anal phase? What were his relationships to each parent during his oedipal struggle and how did the parents help him with this problem?

Obviously the total diagnosis rests upon the evaluation of many facets, not only of the child, but of the entire family unit. In addition, the physician must consider other environmental factors which have played an important role in the child's past, such as severe physical illnesses, frequent moves, the presence of other individuals within the immediate family unit, the ordinal position of the child in the family group, etc. Last, but perhaps most important, is the evaluation of the parental personalities.[2]

CLASSIFICATION OF DISORDERS

Although numerous attempts have been made to classify emotional disorders in children, unfortunately there has been little agreement as to how this should be done. Children are in a process of rapid psychic change and development and their emotional disturbances are less satisfactorily categorized than those of adults. Certain emotional disorders such as paranoia and true depression rarely appear in children. Other emotional disturbances are seen with great frequency in children, but rarely in adults: enuresis is a typical example.

Emotional problems in children result primarily from pathological environmental situations, especially the emotional atmosphere created by the immediate family, but also the socio-economic culture in which they live. The exact type of emotional problem which the child eventually develops depends essentially upon two things: (1) the type of pathological environmental influences to which he is subjected at various ages, and (2) his specific reactions to these situations.

In the broadest sense, the child may do any one of several things when he meets a difficult problem in his environment: he may rebel against it and demand of it what he feels he should have; he may acquiesce and make every attempt to keep from himself and those around him the true nature of his disappointment and inner frustration; he may apparently acquiesce only to establish an "under cover" passive-aggressive type of resistance; he may somatize the difficulty, developing a psychophysiologic disorder; or finally, if the problem is too great, he may lose contact with reality and develop

---

[2] The student interested in further reading on this topic is referred to The Group for the Advancement of Psychiatry Report #38, *The Diagnostic Process in Child Psychiatry*.

a psychosis. These possibilities are simply the basic choices, and many variations exist. Why one child chooses one path and the next another is not always easily understood.

In our experience it is impossible to classify children's emotional disorders into more than a few broad general groups. We will describe the major types, leaving the reader to consult a textbook on child psychiatry for a more thorough discussion. For the present purpose the following outline serves to clarify some of the most salient problems of childhood.

A. Problems of early years
  1. Feeding difficulties
  2. Toilet-training problems
    a. Enuresis
    b. Encopresis
  3. Masturbation problems
B. Psychoneuroses
  1. Anxiety reaction
  2. Obsessive-compulsive reaction
C. Personality disorders
  1. Chronic aggressive reaction
  2. Juvenile delinquency
  3. Passive-aggressive reaction
  4. Disturbances in sexual development
D. Psychotic disorders
  1. Early infantile autism
  2. Symbiotic psychosis of childhood
E. Psychophysiologic disorders
F. Disorders caused by or associated with impairment of brain-tissue function

It is most important to bear in mind that the child's emotional problems are most often a result of his reaction against his environment. Emotional problems may literally begin in infancy. A simple example is found in the six-month-old child whose mother attempts toilet training at this point. She attempts to force him to control his bowels, first, before he is organically capable of doing so, and second, before he is physically capable of co-operating with such a procedure. The resulting frustration stirs up insecurity as well as anger within the infant. As soon as his neurological apparatus has developed sufficiently to give him control over his bowel elimination, he has generally one of two choices to make in response to his mother's excessive demands: he may give in to her demands, or he may flagrantly disobey her and refuse to conform to her demands at all. These attitudes will form important aspects of the child's growing personality and will usually invade many other areas of his life beyond mere toilet training.

Depending upon the type, severity, and time of onset of pathological environmental conditions, the child who attempts to hold stirred-up emotions within himself will either become neurotic or psychotic, or will suffer from a psychophysiological disorder. If he gives expression, either disguised or free, to his inner feelings, he will most often eventually fall into the classification of personality disorders—those which involve a disturbance in character. It is often difficult to tell before about eight or nine years of age exactly which classification an emotionally disturbed child will eventually come under as an adult.

Bearing in mind the changeability and indefiniteness of emotional disturbances in children, we will discuss some of them under the headings listed above. It is also important to remember that impairment of brain-tissue function can occur in varying degrees of severity and can be associated with any functional disorder.

PROBLEMS OF EARLY YEARS

FEEDING DIFFICULTIES

The infant or child, if in a reasonably healthy emotional atmosphere, will eat in a manner dictated by his own natural appetite. Under such conditions he will eat some of whatever nutritious foods are presented to him, in amounts sufficient to meet his needs. If, on the other hand, the mother is demanding in her attitude about his eating, he soon becomes aware of the fact that his food intake is a matter of great concern to her. While this awareness increases as the infant grows into later childhood, it is present even in the small infant. Whenever the conflict between mother and child builds up and the child needs a means to express his disapproval of her actions or emotional attitude, he simply curtails eating. As the cycle progresses, his food intake is determined far more by the immediate status of the mother-child relationship than by his own nutritional needs. With a continuation of the battle between mother and child, the child's intake of food becomes progressively less, the mother's attitude increasingly demanding, and the entire cycle becomes more vicious. An amazingly large number of infants suffer through repeated formula changes and feeding-schedule variations while the mother and the physician seek some satisfactory means of improving nutritional intake. In many such cases, more profitable results could be obtained by a thorough evaluation of the mother-child relationship and by efforts to improve the emotional atmosphere.

Case History: Feeding Difficulty

A two-and-a-half-year-old girl was brought to the clinic by her mother, who complained that the youngster would accept only liquid or mashed foods and then only if great pressure was exerted by her mother. She often had to spend an hour to an hour-and-a-half per meal coaxing, forcing, and cajoling the child into eating or drinking anything. This problem, according to the mother, had been present ever since the youngster was fed by bottle.

The child was an attractive, alert, intelligent girl who presented no physical defects. She was of slightly smaller stature than average for her age, but well-developed and well-proportioned. The mother gave a history of having been born and raised until adolescence in Poland, where her family had repeatedly suffered from conditions approaching starvation. There had been much attention paid to food as she grew up and, because of its scarcity, the family considered it almost a crime not to eat whatever was available when it was available.

Although the mother had lived in this country for many years and had achieved a relatively secure social and financial status, she nevertheless still kept her old attitude toward food. She demanded that her child finish everything that was placed before her and became extremely anxious if the child did not do so. There then had developed between mother and child a severe conflict in which the child refused to chew or swallow solid food and in which the ingestion of any food was a tedious process for both child and mother.

The therapeutic approach consisted of a few interviews with the mother which helped her to attain a more healthy and reasonable view toward food and also helped her to understand how her past approach to this problem had only intensified the child's emotional problem. A few interviews with the child also helped clear up the problem. During these interviews she had "tea parties" with the therapist, who provided milk and cookies for joint consumption. In the first two or three interviews she obviously tested the therapist as to his reaction to her refusal of food. When the therapist paid little attention to whether she ate and drank or not, she soon joined in the games heartily and consumed at least her share of the food. The mother also was helped to see how this approach diminished the youngster's conflict about the intake of food. The child's eating problem cleared up rapidly under this regimen and did not recur.

TOILET TRAINING PROBLEMS

Enuresis

Enuresis means the involuntary passage of urine. While this term applies also to cases of organic etiology, those discussed here are of functional origin. In a few children both causes coexist. A child with acute cystitis, diabetes, or one of a number of neurological difficulties including epilepsy may urinate involuntarily. Such cases account for a relatively small percentage of the children who wet themselves, and, in them the history and physical findings are ordinarily fairly obvious. The average child who wets himself, however, presents no demonstrable physical abnormalities. Most of such children have been enuretic from birth onward without ever having had a prolonged dry period. A smaller number, however, have achieved adequate toilet training only to relapse subsequently into night wetting, varying in frequency from sporadically to several times each night. Nocturnal enuresis is much more common than diurnal enuresis. The combined occurrence of day and night enuresis ordinarily represents a more severe degree of psychopathology.

The act of micturition itself is a complicated one, involving parasympathetic as well as voluntary neurological pathways. The etiology of enuresis is similarly complicated. There are certain demonstrable neurological centers within the brain which control the act of micturition. In addition, it has been determined that the intracystic pressure within the bladder in the enuretic or untrained infant differs from that of the ordinary nonenuretic individual.

It has been found that from a psychological standpoint, children wet the bed for any one of half a dozen reasons. The important thing to be stressed here is that the physician should direct his efforts toward discovering the particular reason why an individual child is suffering from this symptom and then focus his treatment upon the underlying cause. The most common reasons for bed-wetting are:

1. *Revenge enuresis.* This type of wetting ordinarily results from too rapid and punitive toilet training, as well as other exaggerated discipline. The child is resentful of the punitive measures applied to him and utilizes wetting as a method of revenge against the strict parent. As one little boy said, "You have too many rules around this house and that's why I wet."

2. *Regressive enuresis.* This type of wetting most frequently begins after a child has been successfully trained, and when in some way his security is threatened, he regresses. The most obvious example occurs with the birth of a new sibling. The older child feels insecure in his position, regresses to an earlier age approximating that of his new sibling, may ask for many of the things which he had at that age, and begins to behave as he did previously, including wetting himself. It should be stressed that the proper parental approach to this situation is to gratify the youngster's regressive needs, allowing him to satiate himself for a period of time in order that he may successfully grow out of this phase. Attempts at punishment will only bring further regression.

3. *Enuresis due to lack of training.* In families where enuresis has been common, parents sometimes decide that it is a familial or constitutional characteristic about which little can be done and therefore make no effort toward training the youngster. The latter, patterning himself after his older siblings, continues to wet for a considerable period of time beyond normal. This type of enuresis, in our experience, is relatively rare.

4. *Enuresis due to fancied injury.* This type of wetting occurs when a child has undergone some type of traumatic experience, often physically injurious to him, where he at least unconsciously fantasies that he has suffered some type of injury preventing the

control of his urinary flow. The most common example is that following surgical procedures where the child interprets the surgery as having done him irreparable damage which includes ruining his urinary control.

Interesting studies, including that of Margaret Gerard,[3] have shown that approximately sixty percent of enuretic children identify with the parent of the opposite sex, instead of, as would be normal, with the parent of the same sex. In other words, boys identify with their mothers and girls with their fathers. This has been found to occur in families where the parent of the opposite sex is the more strict, rigid, and feared parent, with whom the child identifies out of fear. In this kind of family, boys tend to be passive, nonaggressive youngsters who retreat from competitive, aggressive activities. Girls, on the other hand, tend to be more aggressive and tomboyish than is usual. Any physician who is caring for an enuretic child should direct his inquiries toward discovering the relationships of the child with his parents, particularly which parent is the more strict and punitive and perhaps feared one.

The treatment of enuresis involves first the elicitation of the cause of the symptom and then efforts toward improving the situation. It is common knowledge that the symptom of enuresis may be suppressed by various measures. It is not unusual that a child ceases wetting after one visit to a physician for this condition, even though only a general physical examination was the total "treatment." Other youngsters stop enuresis following an unrelated surgical procedure such as tonsillectomy or appendectomy. It is wise to remember that such "cures" have not improved the underlying psychopathology, but have only driven the symptom underground. The enuretic child has emotional problems and the proper treatment is directed toward alleviating them and not toward suppression of the symptom.

Case History: Enuresis

Vivian was a six-year-old child referred to the psychiatric clinic from the pediatric clinic, where her mother had brought her with the chief

[3] Gerard, Margaret. "Enuresis, A Study in Etiology." *Am. J. Orthopsychiat.*, IX, 1939.

complaint of bedwetting. Physical studies had been entirely negative. Her mother stated initially that her only complaint about the child was the fact that she had wet the bed ever since infancy. Upon further questioning, it developed that the youngster had various other neurotic traits. However, these had not been particularly bothersome to the mother and, therefore, she had paid little attention to them. The child suffered from frequent nightmares, she bit her nails badly, and she was a fearful and timid child who played poorly with other youngsters. She was reported by the teacher to be somewhat slow in her work, although her intelligence was found to be above average.

Vivian was an only child. Her mother was a dominating, authoritative person who ran the family. The father was a hard-working, sincere, conscientious, but quite passive individual who bowed to all of his wife's demands. He was extremely fond of his daughter, but played little part in her upbringing. All the rules and regulations in the house were made by the mother. As the psychiatric interview progressed, it developed that the mother had begun toilet-training her child at four months. She was proud of the fact that she had accomplished toilet training, with the exception of enuresis, by the time the child was ten months of age. Wetting had continued in spite of all her punitive attempts to suppress it. The mother was particularly disturbed by the messiness involved and by the fact that she herself had to change the sheets as well as wash them. The child adopted a passive attitude about her wetting, as if there was nothing she could do about it. She was an obedient if timid child who obeyed all the commands given to her by her parents and, as far as the mother was concerned, measured up adequately with the one exception of her wetting. The child, according to the mother, had been particularly stubborn in this area.

It was obvious that this child resented her mother's strict approach and, although submitting to it, had allowed herself the one passive outlet of wetting the bed, which she knew was extremely disturbing to her mother, alhough she was not conscious of its rebellious nature.

This child had struggled with a problem common to so many children in her particular situation. She was extremely attached to her mother in a dependent and immature way and yet was resentful of her mother's dominating, authoritative attitude. Her rigid upbringing prevented the release of hostile impulses toward her mother—originally by her mother's prohibition and then by her own developing conscience. The result was that she had to express her unconscious infantile wishes in terms of a passive-regressive type of behavior which, while not overtly aggressive, represented hostile feelings toward the mother. As therapy proceeded, a more flexible atmosphere was provided in which Vivian could live out, without guilt or criticism, her dependent childish wishes, which allowed her to feel sufficiently secure to attain more emotional maturity. The cessation of the enuresis was in a way the by-product of the intrapsychic changes which took place. There was no longer any reason for the girl to express her hostility and her infantilism by means of this regressive symptom. She subsequently became able to express resentment toward her mother in situations where she felt it and yet developed a much healthier positive relationship toward the mother. Her own conscience was made less severe and her mother's restrictions made equally less severe. Eventually when the youngster had worked out a more satisfactory relationship with her mother, the enuresis began to diminish, and finally after approximately a year of treatment during which she was seen once a week, the symptom disappeared.

Such therapeutic endeavors take considerable time, as in this child's case.

Encopresis

Encopresis may be defined as involuntary defecation or soiling which is not due to illness or intrinsic organic pathology. It should not be considered to exist until the child is well beyond the usual toilet-training period. Soiling, while not nearly as common as enuresis, is not only a more bothersome, but a much more serious symptom. The child of grade-school age who continues to soil usually represents a more seriously disturbed child than one who has chosen a less primitive way of showing his problems. The typical encopretic child may or may not have been successfully toilet-trained earlier, but more often than not has shown much resistance to toilet training. He continues to soil himself as often as daily. He may seem at times to show sincere remorse regarding this symptom, yet continues it with a sort of omnipotent attitude. He may hide his soiled underpants in various places around the house, or may behave after soiling as if nothing had happened.

It is generally found that the encopretic child has perpetuated marked anal qualities, usually as a result of parental inconsistency or overdiscipline. For a variety of reasons the child has retained unconsciously the magical concept that defecation has both sexual and aggressive connotations, and may involuntarily soil himself when sexually excited or when angry. He appears to deny the negative reactions toward him which his soiling produces. He often claims that he was busy thinking of something else, or doing something else so that he did not have time to go to the bathroom.

Again it should be stressed that the encopretic child is usually quite disturbed, and may require considerable psychiatric help. When the encopresis has persisted over a number of years there is usually a disturbed physiology of the colon. He may have tended to retain his feces until a "leakage" around an overdistended colon developed, in which case, the bowel distention is obvious by x-ray and Hirschprung's disease must be ruled out. Chronic obstipation leading to fecal incontinence is an extremely difficult problem to handle. When hard-packed feces are retained, defecation becomes painful. Thorough cleansing of the GI (gastrointestinal) tract usually provides only a temporary solution, and a more thorough look into the child's intrapsychic difficulties is essential.

MASTURBATION PROBLEMS

Masturbation is a normal and ubiquitous sexual activity in children, but may reach such proportions as to indicate clearly that the child has an emotional problem, and that he must be helped to find other libidinal gratifications if he is to achieve emotional health. Masturbation is a universal autoerotic activity originating in the child's simple discovery that manipulation of the genital is pleasurable. If the environment does not provide wholesome outlets for his energies, he may fall back upon masturbation with its accompanying daydreams to a greater degree than is consistent with a constructive development of his personality.

The ordinary child in even a relatively permissive family soon senses that masturbation is not accepted as a practice to be indulged in openly and freely. He therefore tends to masturbate only in private, accounting for the fact that many parents do not believe that their children masturbate at all. There are, however, youngsters who masturbate frequently and openly regardless of the circumstance. By the time the parents bring this problem to a physician, they have usually tried various forms of punishment. Some obvious physical conditions may contribute. A child whose clothing is too tight or who has genital irritation will manipulate his genitals in order to end the already generated excitement. Equally simple is the case of the child who is put to bed an hour or more before he is ready to go to sleep and who is prohibited from playing with toys or otherwise amusing himself. He turns to the only source of gratification available, namely his own body.

There are, however, many children who masturbate excessively in whom no such obvious causes are found, and in whom, with some effort, one finds other evidences of emotional problems. Such children often come from families where they received little parental love or other motivation to find pleasure in associations with people. When their relationships with their parents have proved disappointing, they have in a sense retreated to finding pleasure within themselves. There is often added to this a hostile relationship between the child and his parents. When the youngster finds that his masturbation upsets his parents, he may continue it if for no other reason than to produce a reaction in them. Occasionally one finds a child who has been subjected to sexual play by an adult, in which, although he has received some pleasurable excitement, he has not been able to achieve any satisfactory release of tension. His masturbation represents a repeated but unsuccessful attempt to find such satisfaction. There are many more reasons for excessive masturbation which will ordinarily come to light through a more thorough understanding of the family dynamics as well as the dynamics of the child himself.

PSYCHONEUROSES

ANXIETY REACTION

The manner in which anxiety makes itself evident varies considerably. In some children it is bound down in a phobic type of reaction. In others it remains more or less free-floating, pervading much of their activity, making them hyperactive and restless. Sometimes the most prominent evidence is a pronounced learning difficulty, particularly manifested in reading problems, or it may be limited primarily to night-time expression, in the form of frequent nightmares.

In the anxious child whose anxiety is manifest most of his waking hours, we find typically hyperactivity, restlessness, a short attention span, and fearfulness in new situations. The last characteristic may be replaced by its apparent opposite, a pseudo-aggressiveness in situations of potential danger, resulting in relatively poor evaluation of dangerous situations. Most of these children, however, are fearful of possible physical injury and exaggerate the potential harm of any mild infection, disease, or injury. They ordinarily make a rather poor adjustment with their contemporaries because of their hyperactivity and difficulty in joining in the usual games.

The phobic child has managed to collect all of his anxiety, or at least most of it, and attach it to some object, place, or situation so that he can remain relatively free of anxiety in other situations. These youngsters develop extreme panic whenever faced with their phobic object. Actually the phobia has been called "the normal neurosis of childhood" because of its frequent appearance. It is transitory and generally does not interfere with the child's ordinary living pattern. It may be said that the seriousness of the phobia is inversely proportionate to the real potential danger of the phobic situation. In other words, if a child fears butterflies he is probably sicker than if he fears dogs, because there is obviously more real danger from dogs than from butterflies. In spite of his phobic formation, a phobic child is apt to be somewhat restless, fidgety, and tense, much like the child with free-floating anxiety. He also may suffer from sleepwalking, nightmares, or some other conspicuous manifestation of anxiety. The clue to the inner dynamics of such a child is often to be gained from the content of his phobias or nightmares. The little girl who is afraid of witches is in all probability having difficulties in her relationship with her mother. The boy may be afraid of Frankenstein's monster or some other male monster who at least unconsciously represents the male parent, indicating a problem in the boy's relationship with his father.

Frequently the child suffering from anxiety reaction makes a poor adjustment to school and, at least superficially, appears to be a disciplinary problem. He is not, however, an antisocial youngster.

The problem revolves around the fact that his anxiety spills over into his muscular system and produces restlessness—a fidgety type of behavior that makes it impossible for him to sit still or conform to a useful degree. Instead of waiting to raise his hand to give an answer in school, he is apt to shout it out impulsively. As he walks down the aisle of the classroom he may inadvertently knock over another student's book or otherwise disturb the classroom routine. Such acts as these are not perpetrated with any such hostile purpose as that of the aggressive child, but from the teacher's standpoint, the restless child is a behavior problem and is often subject to discipline. This only makes his anxiety worse and increases his restlessness.

Other youngsters may not show such overt restlessness but may be unable to concentrate on one subject for any period of time. These children are said to have a short attention span. Often this interferes markedly with their ability to learn to read, write, or solve arithmetic problems. They often reach second, third, or even fourth grade before the severity of their incapacitation becomes evident to their educators, who then may think of them as mentally deficient. Intelligence testing may prove them to be normal or above, although they may not have mastered even the simplest subject matter. Such youngsters will continue to fail in school work unless some attention is given to the anxiety which has prevented them from learning.

Case History: Anxiety Reaction

An eight-year-old girl was brought to the psychiatrist by her mother because of chronic anxiety, numerous phobias, frequent nightmares, and a general difficulty in adjusting both at home and in school. She was an exceedingly timid child who socialized poorly. She was afraid of many things and some of her fears reached the state of actual phobias. She was unable to go to bed alone at night because of tremendous anxiety, which she had been unable to explain to anyone. She was extremely close to her mother, quite dependent upon her, and worried whenever she was separated from her mother even for a short time.

The mother was a rigid, compulsive, demanding, authoritative, punitive, and unloving sort of person who had had a career of her own prior to marriage which she had given up grudgingly upon the birth of this child. There was one younger brother, age three, of whom the patient was quite jealous. The father was a relatively passive man, who although a professional person had never been able to make much of a success of his work. The relationship between the parents was very strained. The mother had always blamed the father for being a failure at his profession and constantly reminded him that she had had a better job while she worked than he ever had. Clearly it was a matriarchal type of family. The girl's relationship with her father was not particularly close, although it was warm and friendly.

During the first few interviews with the girl it became clear that she had an extremely ambivalent relationship with her mother and, at least unconsciously, resented the mother's demanding, authoritative attitude. However, the girl had developed a severe conscience which did not allow open expression of resentment toward her mother. She also was guilty about her attachment to her father; she would have preferred a much closer relationship to him had this guilt not stood in her way. The constant bickering and quarreling between her parents was a source of great concern to her. On the one hand she would, at least unconsciously, have preferred that they did not get along together so she could have a more complete relationship with her father; and yet, on the other hand, she was so guilty about her negative feelings toward her mother and hopes for parental disagreement that she was unable to express them.

Therapy for this youngster was carried on twice a week for many months and was only partially successful. One of the greatest reasons for the difficulty in treatment was the inability of the parents to work out a satisfactory relationship between themselves. Eventually they separated permanently, after having done so temporarily several times. These parental disagreements and separations kept the child stirred up to such a degree that it was impossible for her to work through her own problems adequately and gain any real security. She did, however, decrease the severity of her superego in some areas, which allowed her to lead a more active and useful life in school and with other children. The problem of her parents' disagreement remained, and since this was her fundamental intrapsychic problem, it could not be worked through as long as the parents presented to her a real division between themselves and thus kept it alive.

OBSESSIVE-COMPULSIVE REACTION

Perhaps the simplest way to describe an incipient obsessive-compulsive reaction in a child is to say that he is "too good." Such a child becomes a "little lady" or "little gentleman" at an age when such behavior and conformity are not to be expected in the emotionally healthy youngster. Such children show none of the relaxed childish characteristics of others of their age. They are meticulous, worrisome, and over-conscientious. They have been forced to build strong and rigid defenses around their natural childishness. They have done so usually for one of two main reasons: either the love given them has been so sparse that they have resorted to this method of gaining what little seems to be available, or punishment has been so unreasonable as to force them into a pattern of excessive conformity. By the time a child reaches six or seven years of age, one begins to see obsessions and compulsions becoming obvious. Transient phenomena of this type are not at all uncommon in normal children during the latency period, but they assume a rigid and conspicuous degree in the obsessive child. These are worrisome children who fret continuously about what is to come. They study more than most children and are greatly perturbed if they do not reach the high scholastic standards they have set for themselves. Parents tend to worry if their child has the lowest academic standing in the class, but unfortunately it is a rare parent who shows concern if his youngster is at the top of his class. While attainment of this position is not per se indicative of psychopathology, it may often be one manifestation of it. The child who achieves almost perfect marks during the latency period may be doing so as a result of an obsessive pattern which allows him little if any outside life, warm relationships and normal childhood activities.

Case History: Obsessive Compulsive Reaction

A six-year-old girl was brought to the psychiatrist by her mother who complained that the youngster was having temper tantrums. As is often true of the parents of compulsive youngsters, the mother initially had no other complaints. As far as she was concerned, the youngster was a "model child and a little lady." Further discussion, however, revealed some doubts in the mother's mind as to the degree which this conformity had reached. The youngster had become concerned with cleanliness to the point where a single spot on her dress would bring her to the house crying and demanding that her dress be changed. The sight of anything at all distasteful to her made her feel faint. She was unable to play with other neighborhood children because she could not enjoy their "childish games." The mother was quite proud that she had been able to take her when she was only a year-and-a-half old to any restaurant and have her behave as if she were an adult. The mother could also take her shopping with her and leave her sitting on a chair for up to an hour or an hour-and-a-half, she said, and would know that the child would be there when she returned. She was proud of the child's vocabulary and polite social attitude with adults.

The mother herself was a rather rigid, compulsive woman who had married relatively late in life and produced this child primarily as a concession to her husband. She made it very clear to the psychiatrist that she had never enjoyed babies because of their messy habits. She had taken pains to toilet-train her child very early, beginning when the child was three months old and feeling that she had succeeded by the time the child was six months old. She was now concerned that the child was constipated from time to time. There were many other evidences that she was both demanding and overprotective. Fortunately, she had sufficient flexibility and understanding to appreciate the psychiatrist's talks with her about the emotional needs of children. She was able to relax her overprotecting and rigid attitude, to encourage the child to relax her own standards and to enjoy messiness and dirtiness, and to tolerate occasional disobedience. At the end of six interviews the mother had achieved sufficient change in her own attitude to produce considerable improvement in the child. At this point she broke off therapy, undoubtedly because she was somewhat threatened by the child's growing tendency toward being childish rather than "a little lady."

This case also illustrates the fact that most children six years of age and under can usually be helped to a greater extent by parental change than by direct therapy with the child. From about age seven, there is usually sufficient solidification of the psychic structure that environmental manipulation alone is less effective.

PERSONALITY DISORDERS

CHRONIC AGGRESSIVE REACTION

The typical child with an antisocial personality pattern is rebellious, unmanageable, and generally does not conform to the social patterns that one would expect in a child of his age. He often steals, fights, lies, and is a disciplinary problem in school. Such a child reveals an inordinate amount of hostility which is readily expressed. He tolerates frustration poorly and reacts to it aggressively. He is selfish, demanding, and lacking in consideration for the rights of others. His social relationships are poor, since he attempts to dominate other children. He learns little by experience, and punishment seems only to make matters worse. The home environment of such children usually reveals a lack of mature parental warmth and affection. Frequently one finds parental bickering and perhaps separation or divorce. Punishment has been excessive and inconsistent. Both the lack of love and excessive punishment stimulate hostility within the child, and as he grows older, he reacts to others outside of the home with this same hostile attitude. Since there is little stimulus within the home to mature and to love, the child continues on the infantile level—loving only himself and incapable of loving others. He functions on the pleasure principle—demanding what he wants when he wants it, regardless of the effect on those about him.

As these children grow older, parents and society react against them with further hostility because of their antisocial behavior. This only reinforces their conclusion that they are unlovable and intensifies their pattern. Rigid, punitive boarding homes and, even worse, the average reform school, only compound the situation.

Treatment of these children is directed toward helping them to establish good relationships. They need to develop a therapeutic relationship with a mature adult with whom they can identify. When punishment is essential, it must be firm, but not brutal, and above all it must be consistent. It is often necessary to place such youngsters in a residential treatment center, since they are able to form the therapeutic relationship only slowly. With outpatient treatment and infrequent interviews, these children usually manage to get themselves into difficulties which result in excessive punishment which compounds the therapeutic problem.

Case History: Chronic Aggressive Reaction

An eight-year-old boy was brought to the psychiatrist by his mother who complained that he was rebellious, unmanageable, disrespectful, and extremely hostile to his little sister. In addition, he was destructive, fought with other youngsters, was often a truant from school, and was a problem to his teacher.

The mother stated that he had been a behavior problem, as far as she was concerned, ever since he was about sixteen months of age, when he began smearing his feces and rebelling against toilet training. She began punishing him at this time, using a variety of disciplinary measures without success. Both his father and his mother beat him severely. The onset of his aggressive rebelliousness coincided with the birth of his younger sister, his displacement from the parental bedroom, and the return of his father from a job in another state. These three simultaneous events had produced both insecurity and resentment within him and he had begun to rebel. His mother reacted to his rebellion with punishment, which increased his acting out. She described herself as an overly clean, overly conscientious perfectionistic person who spent the majority of her time keeping house. She particularly resented the boy's apparent disregard for neatness and order and his flagrant disregard for the regulations which she laid down for behavior within the home. The father was a much more passive, easygoing type of person who alternated his usual pleasant attitude with occasional outbursts of temper during which he punished the boy severely.

The mother also related that the boy was preoccupied with thoughts of violence, death, and accidents, particularly the possibility of these things occurring to members of his own family. He liked to draw pictures depicting scenes of great aggression and violence and would relate fantasies with this theme.

The initial approach to this case entailed considerable time with the mother in an effort to show her ways in which she could improve her relationship with the boy. She was helped to see that he was really an insecure as well as angry youngster because he felt a lack of love and felt she required more of him than he could give. Fortunately, she was able to make the majority of changes required in her own attitude. The boy was seen over a period of months by a woman therapist with whom he developed an excellent relationship. He began gradually to try to please her and his behavior improved in all areas.

Children such as these have failed to develop both superego and ego functions. Expressing their infantile impulses freely, they cannot conform to the usual social expectations, and relate on a level much younger than their actual ages. The treatment requires, in most cases, the formation of a good relationship between the youngster and the therapist in which the youngster identifies with and tries to please the therapist, literally growing through some of the psychosexual development which he has missed. He begins to pattern himself after the therapist, or at least as he expects the therapist would behave, and therefore to introject the therapist in the form of a beginning superego. He learns that the world is not completely filled with hostile, unloving people as he had supposed, but that some, as the therapist, are capable of liking him and helping him.

JUVENILE DELINQUENCY

The foregoing discussion of the chronic aggressive reaction might tempt one to the conclusion that all juvenile delinquents suffer from this syndrome, which, of course, is not true. Juvenile delinquency is not a psychiatric term, but a legal one—a label applied to those youngsters who so seriously or chronically disobey the mores of society as to be legally designated as delinquents. A child with this "diagnosis" may lie, steal, run away, act out sexually, or truant, to consider only a few examples. While the chronic aggressive child may do any one or all of these things, he does not represent all of juvenile delinquency.

Delinquency is a growing problem within our society and one to which every psychiatrist should be willing to devote at least some time and energy. More than half a million children are newly labeled as delinquent each year, and this number is growing. A high proportion of delinquency is contributed by the lower socio-economic group, who are less apt to receive adequate medical and psychiatric help. We do have a large group of youth today who have been referred to by James Conant as "social dynamite," those children who have dropped out of school, whose skills and knowledge are limited, and whose resentment is deep. They have little identification with the mores of our society and form a real problem for social scientists as well as for the government and for all citizens.

The term *juvenile delinquency* covers a variety of acting-out behavior, without a single simple etiology, nor an easy cure. It can be a result of purely medical problems, or in some instances stem from sociological difficulties. The delinquent sometimes is a mildly retarded child who is acting out against the society which has expected more of him than he is capable of giving. Sometimes he is a brain-damaged child whose impulsivity is beyond even potential control. At other times he is a deprived child from a lower socio-economic group who is completely unfamiliar with mature figures of identification. At still other times he is a neurotic delinquent, acting out because of unconscious guilt and arranging his own apprehension and punishment.

Delinquents have been studied by many professions and from many points of view, including the psychiatric view that intra-psychic difficulties lead to delinquency, and the sociological view that social and cultural problems are primary in delinquency. Each has much to be said for it. Certainly a child who is raised in a home in which there is inadequate emotional as well as intellectual stimulation will not progress satisfactorily. If in addition he is ex-posed to an acting-out type of behavior on the part of the adults around him, he himself will be prone to act out against society. However, we also find that delinquents can develop from middle-class families in which the psychopathology may be more sophisti-cated, but nevertheless of equal seriousness.

The answers to juvenile delinquency will undoubtedly prove to be multiple. We already have much knowledge within our possession which could diminish current delinquency. We know that adequate medical and obstetrical care would curtail some of the brain-damage syndromes which we see. We also know that better education for parenthood would enable adults to provide their children with improved opportunities. We know that society's current methods of harsh, punitive rejection of the delinquent would be better re-placed by a more understanding and therapeutic approach. It is essential that all physicians, psychiatrists and otherwise, recognize the need for and be willing to provide their professional help in the problems of delinquency.

PASSIVE-AGGRESSIVE REACTION

The passive-aggressive reaction is one of the most common char-acterological disturbances found in children today. It usually has its roots quite early in childhood and can eventually become an extremely serious impediment to adjustment. The child with this reaction seems to accede to the demands which are made upon him, but in fact passively resists them. While neither aggressive nor openly hostile, the rebellion is real and effective. The passive-aggressive approach may begin early in the child's life in one or another area but usually spreads thereafter to involve almost every aspect of his life. His mother calls him in the morning to get out of bed and he responds affirmatively. She calls him again in fifteen minutes and once more he answers affirmatively. Finally, fifteen minutes later, she has managed to rout him out of bed. A long struggle is involved in getting him to dress, even though he has not rebelled against the idea, but simply procrastinates. When he gets to school, he is pleasant to the teacher but manages not to get done what she has asked. So goes his day. When he is in the bath at night and asked to finish getting ready for bed, he says that he will. Some time later he is found still playing in the tub. A review of his typical day shows that he has managed to irritate most adults with whom he has come in contact, but has never been overtly rebellious against any of them.

The passive-aggressive pattern more often than not is a result of excessive parental demands. The child has been unable, or unwilling, to react with an aggressive pattern. At the same time, he has been unable to bury his own desires and acquiesce to the parental demands. Instead, he has set up a subversive method of behavior through which he can give covert expression to his hostility, at the same time avoiding a direct clash with authority. One of the major difficulties stemming from this type of adjustment is that the child inadvertently penalizes himself by slowing his own education, alienating many people, and generally becoming the recipient of hostility from others. A child of this type usually is shown to have strong oral and anal attitudes perpetuated within himself. He not infrequently vows to improve his behavior, but after a short attempt slides back into the old pattern again.

Case History: Passive-aggressive Reaction

The parents of this ten-year-old boy requested their pediatrician to refer them to a psychiatrist. They felt that their home life had become chronically unhappy and frequently disrupted by the obstinate character-istics of their son. On initial interview they reported that he was a marked under-achiever in school in spite of a superior intelligence. He seemed to avoid every task that was given him both in school and at home. There were short periods where he seemed happy and contented, but most of the time he obviously was not. While he was not considered to be an aggressive behavior problem either by his parents or by his teacher, as his mother put it, "He drives us all to distraction." One of the biggest difficulties in family life occurred with the parents' attempts to help the boy do his homework. These evening sessions stretched to as long as two hours during which the parents became increasingly exasperated while the boy produced little in the way of accomplishment.

The parents were highly intellectual, well-educated people who had devoted a great deal of energy to their child's rapid progression through new accomplishments. They were rather worrisome people who placed excessive demands both upon themselves and their child. During his preschool years they were unaware that he was developing a passive-rebellious syndrome, but after he entered school, the first structured situation in his life, it became increasingly evident that he was unable to accept any authority.

This child's treatment entailed work with both parents and the boy. The parents were encouraged to remove themselves from the homework situation and other similar situations which could be either ignored or delegated to some other authority. They were helped to relax their own goals for him and to be accepting of more ordinary childish behavior from their son. At the same time the boy was helped to understand some of his own needs to resist authority in all forms. He had grown suffi-ciently unhappy with his over-all adjustment that he was a reasonably willing candidate for assistance. Within a period of about six months, during which he was seen weekly, he began to make academic gains with the help of an outside tutor, and his parents began to relax their demands upon him. The number of conflicts within the household diminished, and family life in general was much happier. The child still presented many passive-aggressive features, but these were rapidly diminishing.

DISTURBANCES IN SEXUAL DEVELOPMENT

Sexual identification is a process which begins very early in child-hood and continues into adolescence. The child begins to think of himself as belonging to one particular sex. The degree of sophistication of this knowledge gradually increases as the child grows older and becomes more aware of the differences between the sexes. The parent of course thinks of the child as male or female from the first day of life, and parental attitudes are thus molded from this early date. The meaningfulness to the child of sexual identification is much less in the pre-oedipal period than during and following the oedipal phase.

Problems in healthy sexual identification can stem from a variety of sources, and only a few of the most common ones can be mentioned here. One example is to be found in the mother who has a strong preformed desire to have a girl, only to be delivered of a boy. While she consciously accepts the fact that her child is a male, she may subtly urge and expect many feminine characteristics from him. Another example is the child who is raised in a home with only one parent. A boy raised without a father has difficulty finding adequate figures for masculine identification. Perhaps the most common example, however, is in the home in which the parents assume reversed roles, the mother being aggressive and dominating and the father passive and weak. The children of such a family witness a distorted picture of adult masculine and feminine roles and themselves become confused about their own identifications. Such children are apt to show characteristics similar to those of their parents.

Children may be described as being *polymorphous perverse*. This means that their capacity for sexual enjoyment is not as yet channeled into genital sexuality and therefore they enjoy any generally sexual activity. The term *sexual perversion* as applied to an adult indicates a preference for obtaining sexual gratification by some other means than genital union with a member of the opposite sex. In the child the sexual focus is not that of the mature adult, but consists of a general seeking for pleasurable activity of a sexual type. This may include looking, being looked at, touching, and being touched, and encompasses all of the erotic areas of the body. It is not limited to a heterosexual orientation, and the autoerotic or self-stimulating element is much larger in the normal child than it is in the adult.

Children are capable of being led into various perverted sexual activities. At times, however, one sees a child who has from a fairly early age shown overt evidences of a homosexual orientation. This in a boy may have resulted in a feminine demeanor, choosing girls as playmates, a desire to wear feminine clothes, and obvious identification with the opposite sex. The psychological reasons for this inversion are more thoroughly discussed in Chapter 12, "Personality Disorders."

Case History: Homosexuality

A twelve-year-old boy was brought to the psychiatrist by his parents, who complained of his difficulties in school, poor social adjustment, and occasional facial tics. Leo had few friends and was frequently involved in fights. Further inquiry revealed that he usually plagued other boys to the point where they finally attacked him physically. He rarely defended himself and was usually beaten up by the attacker, even when the latter was smaller than he. He also utilized similar behavior toward his father, often to a degree that even when the father tried to hold his temper, eventually the boy "won out" and the father punished him.

Leo was an only child of rather intellectual, socially active parents. His mother had relegated much of his care to nursemaids during his early years, and several of them had been severe with him. His father was an ambitious, hard-working, successful man who demanded a great deal of himself and of the boy. Prior to the boy's entrance into school, the father's demands had been excessive and were often accompanied by severe physical punishment when they were not met. After the youngster entered school, he continued to be punished periodically by his father. By the time he was six or seven he had developed a few transient tics, as well as his repeated tendency to become involved in fights in which he was beaten up.

The boy was slender and unmasculine-appearing, and not particularly attractive. He had an irritating, needling manner, constantly belittling the office and playroom of the therapist and making derogatory remarks about the therapist's appearance.

This boy unfortunately could be seen only for a few interviews before the departure of his family to another city. However, it developed during these visits that he had a masochistic approach in his relationship with other boys or men. He was particularly feminine in his interest in play activities. He showed no ability in sports and preferred the company of girls. Whenever he was attacked by another boy he became almost completely passive and submitted himself to being beaten. This youngster's illness was quite severe, and he showed a marked homosexual orientation which would eventually lead him either to an overt homosexual pattern or, if this was subsequently repressed, to a paranoid type of pattern.

Sexual curiosity in children, as well as their seeking for pleasure, often leads to sex play between members of the same sex. This cannot be labeled true homosexuality. However, we occasionally do see strong overt elements of the opposite sex in children. The boy may from an early age display feminine physical characteristics and mannerisms, and may even prefer dressing as a girl. This is a condition whose origin and dynamics are similar to those of the overt adult homosexual (Chapter 12). Leo had originally been stirred to a great deal of resentment toward his father by the father's demanding, punitive attitude. All competition and rivalry with the father had been made impossible by the father's brutal treatment of the boy. In a sense the youngster had covered up his inner aggressiveness with passive behavior. He had pleasurized the beatings which he received from his father. Such a pattern as this is an extremely difficult one to treat because the patient tends to continue to act out his problem rather than to benefit by therapeutic assistance.

PSYCHOTIC DISORDERS

Functional psychoses in children differ from those in adults not only to some extent in type, but also in manifest symptomatology. Manic depressive and paranoid psychoses are almost unknown in children, at least prior to puberty. For many years it was felt that juvenile schizophrenia was extremely rare, so rare in fact that such a diagnosis was ample reason for reporting it in the literature. However, since 1943 when Kanner [4] described the syndrome which he called *early infantile autism* there has been increasing attention to psychotic reactions of children, and considerable literature has been devoted to this subject. At the present time there is a general tendency to think of these children as schizophrenic.

The child with early infantile autism is one whose ego growth

[4] Kanner, Leo. "Early Infantile Autism." *Journal of Pediatrics*, XXV, 1944.

has been markedly hampered from the very beginning of his life. In Kanner's original series there was a significant percentage of parents of a highly intellectual type who seemed unable to provide the adequate warmth and affection necessary for ego growth. Subsequent studies have indicated that such parents are not necessarily those with considerable academic background, but may come from any educational level. The present-day concept of this condition presumes the importance both of a constitutional weakness and a lack of adequate parenting. Accurate evaluation of the constitutional factor is difficult, but it would seem that some children are born with a poor integrative capacity for the formation of personality. They cling tenuously to life, make slow progress in the acquisition of new skills, and react to frustrating situations by withdrawing. Presumably the degree of constitutional weakness varies from one child to another as does the degree of the parents' inability to provide adequate warmth and affection.

The autistic child with his lack of ego development has difficulty in learning to differentiate himself from his environment. As the word autism implies, he lives within himself—a world of his own. He has problems in separating animate from inanimate things. Other people, even his mother, are relatively unimportant to him. His development of speech is slow and irregular, and he does not use it to communicate with others. He tends to screen out many incoming stimuli and this has often led to an erroneous diagnosis of deafness. Prior to Kanner's description of this syndrome these children were often labeled as mentally retarded and placed in institutions for the retarded. Their motor skills, however, usually develop normally and they are often graceful and even attractive youngsters. The mothers often describe these children as having been unresponsive from birth. They not only made few demands for attention, but tended to respond "woodenly" to cuddling.

Mahler[5] in 1952 described what she called a *symbiotic psychosis of childhood,* which she considered quite different from early infantile autism. These are children whose first two, three, or four years of life seem superficially to have been uneventful. Ego de-

[5] "On Childhood Psychosis and Schizophrenia," in *The Psychoanalytic Study of the Child,* Vol. VII, New York, International Universities Press, 1952.

velopment appears to proceed on schedule with the development of speech and the ability to relate meaningfully to others. At some point, however, usually following a traumatic incident, such as the birth of a sibling, there is a relatively rapid ego disintegration. The child gives increasing evidences of mounting anxiety and even panic. A powerful regression sets in and many achievements are lost. Speech begins to deteriorate and become filled with neologisms. The process more clearly resembles the onset of a functional psychosis in an older individual. If untreated over a period of time, many of these youngsters develop increasing similarity to the autistic child. The cause of this syndrome lies in the pathology of the early mother-child relationship. The mother has been unable to provide the youngster with sufficient security and ego growth to enable him to separate and individuate himself and he can only function in a symbiotic fashion with the mother. A traumatic event which threatens or ruptures this symbiotic attachment throws the child into a regression and eventually a psychotic pattern.

As our knowledge of functional psychoses in childhood has increased, there has been increasing recognition of the existence of so-called borderline psychotic children. These are children who at times seem to function in contact with reality, and although quite anxious and easily upset, do not always appear psychotic. At other times, because of internal or external stresses, they become overtly psychotic, with disorganized thinking, bizarre speech and other such symptoms. They are basically extremely immature and their weak egos cannot cope with reality demands during conditions of stress. In general, the child with early infantile autism has the poorest prognosis; next comes the child with a symbiotic psychosis; and finally the borderline psychotic child. In actual practice such a separation between these syndromes does not usually occur. We are more apt to see a mixture of autistic and symbiotic features.

The treatment of the child with a functional psychosis is extremely time-consuming and difficult. In many instances it requires institutionalization in a treatment center which provides a round-the-clock therapeutic milieu and which is staffed with adequately trained personnel. During recent years a number of day-care centers have been developed which accept these children for treatment. The prognosis is guarded under the best circumstances, but the earlier the treatment is begun and the more treatable the parents, the better the prognosis. Every effort should be directed toward improving the mother's emotional ability to relate warmly to her child. While some of these patients have been restored to a reasonably adequate adjustment in the community, many others have gone on to state hospitals and eventually, as they grew older, presented the picture of adult schizophrenics.

PSYCHOPHYSIOLOGIC DISORDERS

The intimate connection between psyche and soma is even more evident in children than it is in adults. The immature psychological equipment of a child is incapable of mastering excessive levels of tension and readily allows such tension to spill over into the physiological systems. This is most apparent in the infant, who if allowed to experience increasing hunger tension, begins to cry and becomes increasingly upset. If this condition is allowed to persist, the infant's entire gastrointestinal tract becomes disorganized to the extent that when he is finally fed, he may vomit or show some other GI disturbance. This is in contrast to the adult's ability to withstand a mounting hunger tension until the proper time for eating arrives.

The psychophysiologic disorders in children which have received the most attention are obesity, neurodermatitis, mucus colitis, ulcerative colitis, and asthma. While it cannot be said that we completely understand any of these, our knowledge about them is rapidly increasing. Physical anomalies, in addition to certain chronic emotional disorders, must probably exist in the etiology of any one of these disorders. A number of studies, however, have shown the repetition of certain kinds of family patterns and intrapsychic emotional conflicts in each of these groups of children.

Children with ulcerative colitis tend to be pseudo-mature, perfectionistic and compulsive, with brittle personalities and marked inner immaturity. A smaller percentage of them show gross characterological defects rather than neurotic symptoms. It is important, however, to remember that many children have compulsive traits or characterological difficulties similar to those seen in children with ulcerative colitis and yet do not suffer from this disorder. The presumption is that certain children have a proclivity to reflect the results of chronic emotional tensions in specific physiological systems. The child with asthma may have mild to severe allergic factors predisposing him to this condition. This then can be magnified by the existence of more or less specific emotional problems.

The treatment of children with psychophysiologic disorders is one of the most difficult challenges facing medicine today. We have much yet to learn about both the psychiatric and pediatric factors which contribute to these conditions. Co-operation between physicians of different specialties is important, since each tends to view the child from the standpoint of his own specialized knowledge. In a case of ulcerative colitis, the psychiatrist will see in the child and his family the evidences of psychopathology, while the pediatrician meantime is concerned with the degree of anemia, of weight loss, and the whole distorted physical growth pattern. The surgeon's attention is directed to not only the general physical condition of the patient, but specifically the bowel itself and the possibility of massive hemorrhage or perforation. To arrange an effective working "team" is no easy matter.

The interested student is referred to the Bibliography for further reading on psychosomatic disorders in children. Also, additional material is presented on this subject in Chapter 13.

DISORDERS CAUSED BY OR ASSOCIATED WITH IMPAIRMENT OF BRAIN-TISSUE FUNCTION

The functioning of the central nervous system may be impaired by organic, toxic, or traumatic insults at any time during the life span of the individual. Such difficulties, however, are more common in children and may begin even prior to birth itself. The syndrome resulting may be acute or chronic in nature.

Space does not permit a complete discussion of all the organic, traumatic, and toxic syndromes of childhood. Many are similar to those found in adults. (See Chapters 18, 19 and 20.) There are, however, certain generalities which can be made regarding brain-damaged children.

Despite the advances in knowledge concerning prenatal care, delivery and postnatal care, many children are born without such advantages. Birth injuries can occur when obstetrical care is inadequate. Serious febrile illnesses, especially early in infancy, can result in diffuse central nervous system damage. The eventual effect of any brain damage will depend upon the degree of injury as well as the age and level of personality development at which it occurred.

The child with moderate to serious brain damage usually reveals a number of specific characteristics. He may or may not be mentally retarded, but is usually quite impulsive. His emotional controls are weak, and he is subject to temper outbursts. He is restless, hyperactive, and shows a short attention span. His impulsive acts are often followed by brief periods of remorse, although he is vaguely aware that he is unable to control himself. It is important to bear in mind that the child suffering from chronic anxiety may in many instances be mislabeled brain-damaged.

The therapy of the brain-damaged child is difficult and lengthy. It involves patient, consistent retraining, in some cases in an institution. These youngsters have difficulty dealing with frustration and tension, and wherever possible their lives should be arranged to diminish these problems. It is not at all unusual that the patient with brain damage also suffers from emotional problems, and the careful evaluation of the interrelationship between these two factors is essential in any case. It has been found that certain drugs such as the amphetamines are often of value in the treatment of brain-damaged children. The exact mechanism by which they create a diminution in the hyperactivity and restlessness of these children is not known, nor do all such children respond favorably to these medications.

The acute brain syndromes of childhood are usually associated with some other medical condition such as a febrile disease or an intoxication of one type or another. The basic medical condition usually dictates the type of therapy and when the underlying disorder is removed, the psychiatric symptoms disappear.

PSYCHOTHERAPY FOR CHILDREN

Since the term "child" is used to encompass youngsters from birth to mid-adolescence, it is impossible to outline any single therapeutic regimen. One of the primary differences between the psychiatric treatment of children and that of adults is the necessity in the former of working actively with the parents. In general, the younger the child, the more the parents must be considered in the therapeutic program. Whereas in the child of one or two years of age, the parents are the major focus of the therapeutic approach, in the adolescent of fifteen or sixteen the parents have become less important, but still usually need to be involved in the treatment process. The degree of parental psychopathology is an important determining factor in deciding how the child's difficulties are best to be handled. The more distorted the parents' emotional lives are, the more effort must be spent in the direction of helping them. There are some instances in which a child's psychopathology is essentially unrelated to the parents' emotional adjustments and in which even the very young child is himself the primary recipient of the treatment process, as in the case of the death of a sibling or of some other immediate family member, or a traumatic attack by an adult on the child.

Several factors influence the plan of treatment of a child with emotional problems. First, obviously, is the age of the child and as a corollary to this, his degree of dependency upon and the importance to him of his parents. A major consideration is the extent to which the child has internalized the psychopathological atmosphere of the family. External influences upon his growth and development, including his neighborhood, his family's socio-economic level and his school may also affect the treatment plan.

In the preschool child, the parents are clearly the most important influences in his life, and if their approach to him is pathological, only with a favorable change in their emotional attitudes can the child improve. By the time a child has reached school age, there is usually sufficient internalization that direct therapy for the child is required in addition to work with the parents. The psychiatric treatment of children must be preceded by the following questions:

(1) At what level are the child's primary "fixations" in his psycho-sexual development—in other words, what levels of earlier emotional development are still predominant within his personality? (2) Why has he become "fixated" in these areas? (3) What can be done for him and his environment so that his emotional maturation can resume? The answers to these questions will be determined in part by his age, his family situation, his constitutional endowment, and even his neighborhood, school, and other social considerations.

Occasionally one finds a home situation in which the emotional psychopathology is so great as to require removal of the child from the home. This is a major move which should be undertaken only when all other measures have proven fruitless. The vast majority of parents will, if approached correctly, try to the best of their abilities to participate in the treatment program. Most communities in our society lack good residential treatment centers and adequate foster homes, and it is preferable that a child remain in his own home where this is at all possible.

TREATMENT OF PARENTS

The majority of emotional problems in children are created by emotional problems of their parents. While there are exceptions to this, particularly where the child's formative years have been marred by accidental occurrences, it is the parents' personalities which largely determine the degree of successful maturation of their children. The average parent plans and attempts to do a successful job of raising his children, and is prevented from achieving this goal only by his own emotional problems. Even where these problems do not markedly inhibit success in the adult world, they may reflect themselves in the distorted growth of the child. Parental discord may also add to the child's problems. A child cannot mature successfully in an atmosphere of constant bickering and quarreling or mutual cruelty. Many adults who are capable of reasonably successful careers and even relatively satisfactory marital adjustments still are incapable of providing the necessary security and warmth required for raising emotionally healthy children.

The physician who is consulted about a child with emotional

problems must first direct his attention to the personalities of the parents and to ways and means by which he may improve their relationships, especially to the child. If their emotional problems are deeply ingrained and represent established neuroses or even psychoses, major psychiatric treatment may be required to effect improvement. In some instances, however, their shortcomings as parents may be a result of ignorance or of mild emotional problems which are amenable to short-term psychotherapy easily carried out by a general practitioner or pediatrician. Obvious defects in the parental attitude may sometimes be removed by a few discussions. The over-demanding mother who has ritualized some routines may be sufficiently flexible to accept the physician's advice in the direction of more leniency. The father who spends little time with his children, feeling that his role as a parent is unimportant, may be stimulated to greater activity by a physician's well-chosen comments.

One of the most common pathological family conditions to be seen today is that of the dominating, authoritative, ruling mother figure, with the father the more passive and, at least emotionally, less contributing member. Such a condition has become increasingly prevalent in our culture and, unfortunately, is tolerated by both men and women. Some discussions with parents regarding the unfortunate results of this situation will often suffice to produce considerable improvement.

The physician who perceives adverse parental influence upon a child patient must guard against any impulse to deliver a stern lecture on the necessity of being good parents. It must always be borne in mind that parents, even though they may show no overt signs of severe neurosis, have their own emotional problems. The compulsive mother has a severe conscience and is already guilty about the neurotic child and her failure as a mother. If she is approached aggressively by the physician and told that she has done a poor job, she will either become so angry that she will not want to return, or so guilty that she will not be able to return. The successful physician attempts to obtain as good and solid a relationship with the parents as possible, so that trusting him, they will be willing to act on his advice and suggestions without fear of criticism and hostility from him.

PREVENTION

The absence of treatment or inadequate treatment of the childhood disorders discussed here means that the emotionally disturbed child will someday be another adult suffering from emotional problems, making a poor adjustment, marrying unwisely, and doing a poor job of parenthood. Psychiatry first clarified adult emotional problems, but as our knowledge increases it becomes clearer that the psychopathology of the individual is an interrelated process and that any attempt to classify it too arbitrarily by age is misleading. Even though certain minor emotional problems may well disappear during the process of growing up, many others persist indefinitely to plague the adult in his later adjustments. An unhappy, chronically frustrated child may become an antisocial offender, a paranoid personality, or a psychophysiologically ill person, depending upon the many factors which have structured his personality before the age of ten plus the various things that happen to him during adolescence. It would seem obvious that an increasing amount of time and attention should be paid to the emotional problems of children and toward helping parents to do a better job with their youngsters. Prevention, therefore, in its best sense encompasses: on the parents' part, a knowledge of the child's needs; on the child's part, love for his parents; and on the physician's part, the willingness to teach, aid, and abet any effort that will help bring these things about.

Psychoneurotic Disorders

CHAPTER 6

Anxiety Reaction

ANXIETY reaction is a type of psychoneurosis characterized primarily by the presence of a chronic, diffuse anxiety. This anxiety remains more or less constantly present, waxing and waning to some degree according to the particular situation, but rarely entirely disappearing. It is not confined to certain objects or situations as is the anxiety in the phobic reaction, nor is it bound strongly or even rendered unconscious as in some of the other types of psychoneurosis.

Overt anxiety is an extremely common symptom in our population, suffered in at least a mild degree at various times by almost everyone. We classify an individual as having an anxiety reaction (neurosis) when anxiety becomes more or less chronic and reaches a sufficient intensity to become at least partially incapacitating. The presence of such chronic anxiety interferes with many of the pleasures of ordinary living and markedly impairs the patient's ability to relate to others. It also decreases his working ability and efficiency.

ETIOLOGY AND PSYCHOPATHOLOGY

Anxiety is a basic and fundamental symptom of every type of psychoneurosis. Differentiation of one type of neurosis from another is made primarily according to the methods by which the particular patient attempts to deal with his anxiety. For instance, the obsessive-compulsive patient builds an intricate system of "magical" ritualistic thoughts and actions in an attempt to defend himself against his anxiety. As long as he is able to maintain these thoughts and actions, he remains comparatively free from anxiety. However, if he is pre-

139

vented from going through the rituals, anxiety appears immediately. The phobic patient binds his anxiety to certain objects or situations and then assiduously attempts to avoid the objects. Once again, as long as this can be successfully accomplished and he does not come in contact with his phobic object, the patient remains comparatively free from the unpleasant sensation of anxiety. However, in the typical patient with anxiety reaction, there is no such clear-cut and "successful" defensive mechanism. An almost constant diffuse anxiety is present.

Since anxiety is so fundamental in anxiety reaction, as well as in all other psychoneuroses, a further elucidation of the origin and components of anxiety is advisable. Anxiety has been discussed at some length in Chapter 3, "The Development of Mental and Emotional Disorders." The psychological and somatic components of anxiety are similar to those of fear. However, anxiety differs from fear in that the object of dread is unknown to the person who is experiencing it. Psychologically, there occurs a feeling of impending disaster, which is uncomfortable by nature. Somatically, there are preparations for fight or flight. The pulse becomes more rapid and there is an outpouring of adrenalin. There is increased muscular tension. Pupils dilate, blood sugar rises; these, as well as other similar phenomena, put the body on an "alerted" basis.

The essential purpose of fear is to warn the individual that he faces some sort of realistic external danger which requires a mobilization of his energy so that he may either overcome it or flee it. Anxiety gives the individual a similar sensation or warning that some threat or danger, the nature of which he does not consciously know, is present within himself. Unfortunately, this inner "danger," because it is unconscious, cannot be dealt with or fled as can outer realistic danger. The patient recognizes that he is uncomfortably fearful, yet does not recognize what he fears. His ego is really a victim of forces that it cannot understand.

Anxiety can be better understood from the standpoint of the three mental constituents, the id, the ego, and the superego. The ego receives impressions from the environment through the five special senses. For instance, a threatening sight or sound is immediately transmitted to the ego, where a sensation of fear arises and serves as a warning to the individual that he must take some action either to combat this dangerous situation or to extricate himself from it. The ego also, however, receives impressions from the inner psychic world, that is, the unconscious. Whenever a dangerous or unwelcome impulse threatens to intrude itself into the conscious ego from the unconscious, anxiety results.

The question then arises of what constitutes a "dangerous" impulse and also of what would occur should such an impulse become conscious. The answer lies primarily in the events of the formative years of childhood. It is during these years that the growing child establishes his ego and lays down the pattern of its relationship both to his inner impulses and to his outer environment. In the infant and very young child the ego structure is still comparatively weak, and any rise of body tension threatens to overwhelm the embryonic ego. The child is unable to master such unpleasant tensions and postpone their gratification, just as he is unable to exert sufficient mastery over his voluntary musculature or the environment to succeed in obtaining gratification. Simply put, if the infant becomes hungry, the rise of the unpleasant sensation of hunger threatens the stability of his ego; yet he is incapable of seeking out and obtaining food by himself. Thus, the ego's earliest relationship to inner impulses is one of inability to control or master them and of passive inundation by these impulses. Needs which cannot be gratified become threats in themselves. The wise parent recognizes the infant's helplessness and does not allow unpleasant tensions to repeatedly give rise to powerful anxiety. In summary, then, it may be said that the earliest origins of anxiety are in infancy and consist of a threat to the ego of being overwhelmed. Gradually, as the child grows older and his ego becomes stronger, he is capable of dealing in a more efficient way with instinctual impulses. However, the balance between instinct and ego is again upset at puberty, when there is an upsurge in the strength of the instincts. At this time in life anxiety may develop again as a result of the ego's fear of being overwhelmed by instinct.

Anxiety stemming from the ego's fear of being overwhelmed by instinct is recognized as the earliest type of anxiety, dating back to infancy. There is another source of anxiety which appears somewhat

later, but is equally important. This type is a result of the relationship between the ego and the superego. Whenever an impulse which
is unacceptable to the superego threatens to intrude into consciousness, anxiety results. The ego fears the painful weapon of guilt
which the conscience utilizes if its dictates are transgressed. Many of
the superego's demands are not only unconscious but are unrealistically exaggerated, having been laid down during the early years
of childhood. There may exist then, within the unconscious, both a
perpetuated childish wish or impulse and an exaggerated superego
restriction against the impulse. The wish is strong and hence the
expected punishment is unconsciously imagined to be great. The
impulse and the conscience's reaction against it have existed in a sort
of frozen state in the unconscious since childhood and have never
been exposed to the more mature judgment of the adult conscious
ego. Whenever the impulse threatens to become conscious, anxiety
results, lest the ego be punished with guilt. It is not at all unusual
that fulfillment of the unconscious impulse, if made conscious
through treatment, is no longer really desired by the adult, and
hence need no longer be defended against. For example, the neurotic man may have perpetuated incestuous feelings toward his
mother within his unconscious and have spent many years and
much mental energy defending himself against conscious recognition of this impulse. If, however, during therapy, the defenses are
removed and the impulse becomes conscious, the patient's more mature ego no longer truly desires gratification of this childish impulse
and he is thus freed from continued defense against it. He may then
transfer his positive feelings to a more suitable and mature love
object.

The roots of both types of anxiety lie in childhood. Lack of an
optimum emotional atmosphere in early family life hampers and re-
tards healthy ego development. Generally speaking, the more emotional security which is present during the formative years, the less
anxiety an individual will have. The parents of an anxious person
have been unable to show him a constant, mature type of affection
and protection against stressful stimuli, so that he has suffered repeated unnecessary exposure to unpleasant tension. Such parents
have not been able to provide their child with a comfortable and

stable emotional atmosphere in which he could learn to face some of the dangers and responsibilities of ordinary living. Such an unhealthy atmosphere impedes ego development and perpetuates immaturity. When, as so frequently happens in this kind of upbringing, an unhealthy and rigid conscience is formed, further anxiety is engendered through the relationship of the conscience to the continuing childishness. The ego, already hampered in its development, is further beset with problems in its attempt to maintain some semblance of peace between the severe conscience, demanding renunciations, and the inner childish needs, constantly striving for expression.

A simple example of such a situation is to be found in the person who suffers from "stage fright." He is, at least unconsciously, an egocentric individual who hopes for and requires the admiration and attention of his entire audience. He wants to be looked at and he wants to dominate his audience. Yet his severe conscience prevents conscious awareness of these desires and makes him feel even less capable, worthy, and lovable than he actually is. Therefore, whenever he appears before a group of people, there is a progressive rise in the level of anxiety, and this may result in his attempting to avoid such situations altogether.

SYMPTOMATOLOGY

The primary symptom of anxiety reaction is, of course, the anxiety itself, with its psychic and somatic components. Anxiety may best be described as an extremely uncomfortable sensation of dread. Most people who have known both severe anxiety and organic pain would much prefer the latter because they have found it less disturbing and uncomfortable. A contributory fact is that organic ailments have a "known" and "understood" quality, while the source and cure of anxiety seem mysterious. Patients with anxiety reaction suffer from what has been referred to as *free-floating anxiety*. This term indicates that the anxious condition is chronically present and not limited to certain times or situations, although it may be enhanced by some environmental conditions. The anxious person worries about many things. If he is to meet someone, he fears he may be late. If he is to be with a group of people, he fears he will not make the proper impression. If he is alone, he is fearful because there is no one with him. Whatever task engages him at the moment produces anxiety lest he not perform it properly, and he is constantly insecure and unhappy about the impression his work will make on others. Consequently, there is a tendency for him to go rapidly from one task to another. This person figuratively keeps running, but he does not know from what he runs. He is never entirely satisfied with his performance, no matter what he is doing. His anxiety is to be distinguished from the "morbid" variety which is bound to certain situations, places, or things. This latter is the type of anxiety seen in the phobic reactions. The phobic patient has, in a way, found a partial solution to the constant discomfort of anxiety, even though he has actually added to his illness in so doing.

Anxiety is not limited to the daytime hours. Many patients suffering from this symptom have difficulty in falling asleep, and after sleep comes, it is frequently restless or disturbed by nightmares—symptoms which are merely another evidence of the constant presence of anxiety. The threatened, unmastered danger of childhood recurs in the nightmare. The fear of the jealous parent of the opposite sex is present in the normal person in the oedipal period and also at puberty, but in anxious patients it reappears chronically. Nightmares are often precipated by some events during the preceding day which bear a slight resemblance to the original oedipal situation and thus can be used as vehicles to express unconscious fear. During later childhood it is not uncommon for youngsters to see a frightening television or movie program and subsequently have nightmares containing some essentials of the plot. Parents usually consider this to be part of the normal process of growing up, and yet such nightmares usually represent some of the deeper unconscious fears which the child has long had.

An acute anxiety attack is of sudden onset and may begin without any apparent precipitating event. The patient is suddenly extremely apprehensive. He is aware of palpitations. Perspiration becomes profuse and breathing is difficult. There is a feeling of impending nausea or perhaps diarrhea. The patient often fears that a medical calamity is taking place within his body. Particularly during the first such attack, the patient is apt to feel that he will faint, or die, or lose control of himself or of his mind. In the severe anxiety attack, the patient literally reaches a panic state where he feels overwhelmed and completely helpless. He is aware of a tremendously strong impulse to run away. However, he does not know what he is running from, or where safety lies. Even following the attack, the patient remains chronically apprehensive lest he suffer another such unpleasant attack. This, of course, creates a certain amount of additional anxiety which tends to precipitate further attacks.

The patient who has suffered from a chronic anxiety reaction for a long period of time often begins to show an increasing concern about his bodily functions. Diarrhea, indigestion, headaches, and palpitations may all have their roots in the anxiety condition, but are viewed by the patient as indicative of developing organic diseases. Such a belief only intensifies the anxiety and also the symptoms. Most of such patients have an unnecessary and exaggerated apprehension about their health. They are apt to become preoccupied with the possibility of getting cancer if there is a cancer fund drive going on. They are concerned about the possibility of poliomyelitis during the season when this disease is most prevalent. Minor cuts and bruises are a source of anxiety to them. They observe many health rituals and maintain numerous medications which they feel have been helpful at one time or another. They often fear visits to physicians and dentists and yet are frequent visitors, particularly to the former, because of numerous somatic preoccupations. Such preoccupations may serve as attempts to rationalize and thereby "bind" the anxiety.

The anxious woman is apprehensive about whether she will be accepted by others and about her ability as a mother and a wife. She worries unduly about the health of her children. She, of course, cannot help but perpetuate the same type of insecurity and apprehensiveness in her children, since it permeates the entire emotional atmosphere of the family.

TREATMENT

The physician responsible for the treatment of a patient with anxiety reaction must first assure both himself and the patient of the absence of organic disease. Should any such disease be discovered, its careful evaluation and prompt, adequate treatment are of great importance. The manner in which the physician communicates to a patient of this type the results of his physical examination often has far-reaching effects on the future course of the condition. The examination must obviously be of sufficient thoroughness to convince both physician and patient of its adequacy. If no organic findings are present, this fact should be presented to the patient in a direct and unequivocal manner. If minor organic problems are discovered, the patient should be told of their nature and treatment in such a way as not to enhance the already present apprehensiveness. It is of extreme importance that the physician be clear, concise, and simple in his discussion with the patient concerning his physical condition, so that the patient cannot possibly misunderstand and misinterpret, thus becoming alarmed. It must be remembered that such patients are chronically worrying, pessimistic, apprehensive people who find dangers in everything and will exaggerate the slightest hint that they suffer from any organic ailment. It is extremely difficult, if not impossible, to successfully treat a patient suffering from emotionally rooted palpitations by psychotherapy if he has been convinced in the past by some other physician that he suffers from cardiac disease.

The patient with anxiety reaction usually believes that his condition is comparatively hopeless as well as serious. Once the emotional nature of the syndrome has been determined by the physician, considerable benefit can be produced in the patient by simple reassurance. The patient may be told that his condition is not a result of organic pathology, but rather of emotional problems. He may be reassured that his condition will in no way shorten his life span and that although from time to time it may be quite uncomfortable, it will, nevertheless, do him no permanent or serious damage. Finally he can be assured that the condition is not particularly uncommon, and has a reasonably good prognosis if adequately treated. Such initial reassurance does not effect a cure, but is an important preliminary to further treatment.

PSYCHOTHERAPY

As soon as the physician has convinced himself of the emotional origin of the patient's condition, he should orient both himself and the patient toward a psychotherapeutic approach. The patient must initially be helped to understand how his difficulty stems from emotional problems and to see that the alleviation of the condition will depend upon bringing to light, understanding, and working them through. It is necessary for the patient to understand that neither the administration of medication nor simple manipulation of the environment is the answer to his difficulties. To put it simply, the patient must become much better acquainted with himself, and this can only be accomplished through discussions with the physician about all the aspects of his adjustment, both past and present. It is wise to explain to a patient early in treatment how close the relationship is between body and mind, and how disturbances in the emotional sphere are quite capable of producing physiological discomfort. Simple examples can be presented to the patient and should be of a type that the patient himself has experienced. Everyone is acquainted with the somatic reactions in fear and the reactions make an excellent example by which the patient can be shown how his own emotions affect his heartbeat, respiration rate, and other physiological phenomena. The patient can be helped to understand how his own condition is similar to that of fear, producing the same body reactions, and yet stems from a somewhat different psychological mechanism. Charts showing physiological mechanisms may be used to clarify the patient's understanding of some of his symptoms. One of the greatest concerns in the average patient with anxiety reaction is that he has a new and not understood or perhaps even incurable malady. It is of considerable reassurance to him to recognize that the physician has not only seen similar conditions previously, but has a rational explanation for the ailment. The fearful mystery is thus removed from the condition and the patient is given something constructive to think about in regard to improving himself.

As soon as the patient has been convinced of the emotional origin of his illness, he is encouraged to express himself freely and completely concerning all the areas of his life. These include everything from his childhood and early family life to his present marriage, occupation, and friends. As this material begins to unfold, it usually becomes evident that the patient has made a poor adjustment from childhood onward. Histories of difficulties in school, inability to adjust socially, and poor relationships with parents and siblings are examples of past emotional problems. Present-day relationships are usually found to be equally distorted. The patient is leading a remarkably inhibited life, due to his anxiety and his preoccupation with himself. His ability to relate to and love other people is distorted and disturbed. His circle of friends is small and his interest in hobbies and other pleasurable activities lacking. He is investing most of his mental energy in himself, to the exclusion of friends and other interests.

Ordinarily, as the patient talks about his feelings and his experiences, it becomes increasingly clear both to him and to the physician where many of his difficulties lie. He begins, for example, to see that he suffers from a great deal of insecurity about his job and his relationships with his boss. Perhaps he finds that there are many similarities between his mother and his wife and that he has always unsuccessfully sought excessive care and attention from both and been angry that he has never received it. Many patients, during the therapeutic process, spontaneously remark that they feel like "a little child" and are somewhat at a loss as to how to function as an adult in the adult world. At times patients bring forth exaggerated and previously unrecognized severe conscience restrictions which they have placed upon themselves. Verbalization of all of these factors helps bring them into the more mature part of the adult ego. Then the illogical and unrealistic aspects can be discussed by patient and physician and more mature solutions can be found. Such patients may be helped to understand how they are perpetuating or attempting to relive their own childhood circumstances as if the same factors and even the same people were still present in the current situation.

Treatment of the patient with anxiety reaction involves not only therapeutic interpretations and encouragement toward verbalization but also positive support and encouragement toward leading a more full and rounded life. Many patients have voluntarily limited themselves in their activities for fear they might suffer anxiety attacks in various situations. As the patient's trust in the physician's understanding of his condition grows, he becomes more willing to accept encouragement to broaden his activities. He becomes desirous of pleasing the physician and thus more willing to attempt new ventures from which he has previously excluded himself. He gradually comes to see that the conditions of his childhood no longer prevail. He finds that security can be gained in his present-day living situation if he proceeds in a reasonably mature manner. He is gradually helped to understand that, on the one hand, he has been making unconscious excessive demands upon the environment and, on the other, that his conscience has been extremely intolerant of his inner childish demands. He is helped to find a more satisfactory, middle-of-the-road adjustment wherein he can more successfully meet his needs and at the same time make an honest and sincere effort to relate more maturely to others. There is much therapeutic benefit as the patient begins to invest in other people more of his mental energy, since this, at the same time, means he spends less of it upon himself in a worrying, apprehensive way.

It is frequently comparatively easy to convey psychiatric concepts to a patient from an intellectual standpoint. However, the important advances in the therapeutic process come through true emotional understanding on the part of the patient and a real inner conviction and awareness of the truth and meaning of the concepts which he and the therapist discuss. As with the treatment of any other emotional disorder, much of the patient's emotional conviction comes through the transference, which, briefly, is the tendency to relate emotions and attitudes originally developed toward people in childhood to persons in the immediate, present-day environment even though they do not fit the present situation.

It is well to remember that the patient suffering from chronic anxiety does not relate fully and maturely to others. This means that all of his relationships, including the one to the therapist, will be colored and distorted by the various immaturities and difficulties from which he suffers. He may react by feeling misunderstood when the therapist is making the most sincere efforts to help him. In many of these individuals there is a heightened sensitivity which is the result of frequent rejections and defeats suffered from childhood onward. Such patients are extremely hesitant to relate closely and warmly to anyone, lest they be hurt in the process. There is ordinarily considerable unconscious resentment against people who they feel have not gratified their wishes and who have treated them unfairly. There is a tendency toward excessive dependency which, if allowed to express itself, results in a clinging, parasitic type of relationship that demands a great deal and gives comparatively little. The physician must be constantly on the alert for evidences of these characteristics in the patient, both in the therapeutic relationship and elsewhere. Optimum emotional conviction on the part of the patient is most apt to occur when one of these distorted emotional attitudes can be shown to him as it relates to the transference situation. He can be helped to see how, in spite of the understanding, friendly, and encouraging approach of the physician, he has reacted to him in an unrealistic and childish manner, as he does in many other situations.

The physician must understandingly and slowly help the patient to see how these various immature traits are undermining and destroying the very love and acceptance which the patient is seeking. Children do not relate on a purely give-and-take basis, but instead require more than they give. The same is true of the patient with anxiety reaction. He may or may not be consciously aware of it and may or may not express it openly, but it is nevertheless true, and he must slowly be helped to become aware of the fact that adult mature relationships exist on a give-and-take basis. He must be helped to see that there is more gratification to be obtained from such a relationship than there is from the archaic, childish methods which he has perpetuated within himself and tried unsuccessfully to use. As one patient early in treatment said, "I don't know how anybody could be interested in me. I am never interested in them."

It can be seen that the psychotherapy of a patient with anxiety reaction requires considerable patience, time, and effort on the part of both the patient and the physician if the outcome is to be successful. A cornerstone of treatment is, as mentioned, the relationship between physician and patient. As the latter learns slowly, within the framework of this relationship, where his own immaturities and difficulties lie, he learns to handle such problems better not only in the treatment relationship but with others in his environment. Such a patient will obviously require the constant support, attention, and understanding of the physician, particularly during his early attempts toward maturity and independence. In many instances the patient's life outside the treatment situation improves considerably, while he remains excessively dependent upon the physician. He often requests extra appointments or calls the physician at home frequently. If a situation of this type is to be handled correctly, the physician himself must be mature and stable. If he becomes irritable, demanding, or sarcastic, the entire therapeutic effort will fall by the wayside and the patient will be even more convinced of the dangers of growing up. If, however, the physician can maintain his friendly, understanding attitude and yet slowly help the patient to see his immaturities as well as correct them, the therapeutic result will be worth while.

It is not unusual for medical students' or physicians' reactions to patients suffering from severe or mild anxiety to take any one of several unfortunate directions. A common attitude is that the symptom is "nothing but neurotic" and therefore not within the physician's province to treat. They may also feel that since the symptom is not threatening to the longevity of the patient, the doctor need not be concerned about it. Other physicians decide that immediate suppression of the symptom is indicated and they resort to the use of some type of medication for this purpose. The wide and questionable use of tranquilizers is an example of this attitude. The patient who has chronic anxiety may be put on an ataractic drug, with resultant diminished anxiety. Such medication, however, leaves the basic problem unsolved. It may be compared to giving codeine to a patient who has a cough without bothering to find out whether he suffers from tuberculosis or some temporary, innocuous condition. It is true that there are occasions when sedative or tranquilizing drugs are indicated in neurotic individuals, but such medication should be utilized only as a temporary crutch and never to avoid the necessity of looking further into the underlying causes of the condition.

Another not uncommon approach among physicians to patients with anxiety is to give them a "lecture" pointing out the unreality of the anxiety. They will carefully tell the anxious patient how little there is, really, in his life to become apprehensive about. When immediate cessation of the anxiety does not occur, such physicians are

apt to become irritated with the patient, feeling that he is not sufficiently grateful or is resistant or is just generally unwilling to listen
to medical advice. Such approaches as these are unfortunately far
too common in medicine today. The physician who would treat
the patient suffering from any type of anxiety must first of all recognize that the individual is ill. It must be kept in mind that severe
anxiety is often a more painful and intolerable condition than the
most severe physical incapacitation. It also should be remembered
that the patient is not consciously or willfully causing his own condition. If he avoids certain situations or if he seems timid and frightened, he is not doing so because he wants to, but because he can't
help himself. It is unfortunately frequent, particularly with the anxious patient, that the physician's own emotional reaction, called
countertransference, causes him to react in a thoroughly unscientific way. This particular phase of treatment is discussed more
thoroughly in Chapter 21, "Principles of Psychotherapy."

Essentially the proper orientation of the therapist toward a patient suffering from anxiety is that of helping to clarify the problems from which the patient suffers and helping him to work these
problems through, both in the therapeutic relationship and in the
outside environment. This can only be accomplished over a period
of time during which the patient has ample opportunity to discuss
his own feelings and his background and to try, in his daily living, to utilize what he is learning in the treatment. Whenever the
physician is willing to sit and listen and understand he will soon,
with the aid of some knowledge of psychodynamics, begin to see
more clearly where the roots of the patient's difficulty lie. With considerable frequency, patients with anxiety reaction present in their
initial interview a history which seems fairly normal, with the exception of the outstanding complaint of anxiety. They often describe what seems to be a fairly happy family life with good relationships with other people and a satisfactory working adjustment.
However, within a very few interviews, it becomes evident that the
marriage which has originally been painted as so satisfactory has
many elements of unhappiness in it. It also may become clear that
the occupational history is not as placid and contented as originally
described, but that there is a background of a great deal of resent-

ment toward superiors. The "popular" social relationships are clarified so that they are found to be based more upon an ingratiating attitude than upon mature emotional relationships. Such difficulties as these cannot always be elicited during the initial few minutes of the first interview. If the physician is in a hurry and his time is limited, he may quickly resort to a prescription for a sedative or tranquilizers rather than going on to attempt to understand why the patient suffers from his particular symptom.

The physician by virtue of his knowledge of psychodynamics is able to deduce certain unconscious attitudes and drives of the patient before the patient himself becomes aware of them. It is important, however, that the therapist not impart too much of his own intellectual understanding of the illness to the patient until the latter is willing and able to accept this knowledge. To tell the patient during the first or second interview, "You have difficulty with your boss because you had the same sort of difficulty with your father," does not help the therapeutic process and may only postpone eventual working through of the problem. Such a statement, if accepted by the patient, gives him only what is known as "intellectual insight" and such insight lacks the real conviction of emotional understanding. It is not productive of the gains that accrue to the latter.

In general, the rules for interpretation to the patient with anxiety reaction are similar to those for any other psychological condition. Initially, the relationship between therapist and patient must be fairly good, so that the patient is willing to accept and think about what the physician says. Secondly, the interpretation should be based, as much as possible, upon material which the patient himself has produced during the interviews. Thirdly, the interpretation should not involve deeply unconscious material, but should reflect a depth which the patient, at his particular point in treatment, can understand. Interpretations may become progressively deeper as far as unconscious significance is concerned only as the patient gradually works through some of his defenses against recognizing his own unconscious tendencies. In the example first given, the patient should have an opportunity to recognize the difficulties which he has experienced with various men in authority and then gradually, with some therapeutic help, begin to see the similarities between these present-day difficulties and those he experienced with his own father.

PROGNOSIS

The prognosis of anxiety reaction can, in a way, be compared to the prognosis of the patient with pneumonia. Some patients, whose affliction is not severe and whose symptoms are not a result of overwhelming pathology and who are treated rapidly and efficiently, respond well. Others, who have long suffered from severe pathology of a refractory type, respond slowly. The patient with anxiety reaction has been unsuccessful in erecting even pathological defense mechanisms to a sufficient extent to prevent the chronic appearance of anxiety.

The prognosis is dependent upon several factors. One is the matter of the strength of the ego. Another is the severity and chronicity of the anxiety. There are, for instance, patients who develop an anxiety reaction only under prolonged and marked stress from which they have not been able to escape. If a way out of the environmental situation is found, they lose most of their anxiety. Other patients have anxiety reaction most of the time even though they are leading reasonably quiescent and predictable lives. Certainly the prognosis is far better in the first than in the second group. Ego strength is not always easy to evaluate, but past accomplishments are often a reasonable criterion. The patient who, even though suffering from anxiety and struggling with realistic problems, has attained worthwhile goals has a better prognosis than one who has bowed to this painful affect and accomplished little or nothing. It is often necessary to begin a sort of "trial" treatment period with the patient suffering from anxiety reaction. This allows the therapist to become sufficiently acquainted with the entire personality structure of the patient before an accurate prognosis is attempted.

Case History: Anxiety Reaction

A twenty-two-year-old married woman was referred to the psychiatrist by a friend of hers. She was an attractive, intelligent young woman who, although very anxious, was quite sincere in her efforts to find a solution to her problems. She had for some time recognized that her difficulties were on an emotional basis. She said that she feared insanity and that she had become increasingly nervous and disturbed about a multitude of things for the previous six months. Her final decision to seek psychiatric consultation had been precipitated by an anxiety attack which had lasted for about five days. She had been forced to quit her work because of this anxiety and had become increasingly fearful about everything which she had to do. She was apprehensive about such simple things as leaving her home, meeting people, going to bed, greeting her husband, or even answering the doorbell.

She was accompanied to her initial interview by her husband, a merchant. Because of her anxiety, she had been unable to come to this interview alone. Her repeated anxiety attacks during the previous week had frequently necessitated her calling her husband from his work. She had been able to achieve some measure of comfort only when he was sitting near her. She had often awakened him during the night when she had been unable to sleep and on numerous occasions had called the family physician at all hours of the day and night.

This patient's history, which she herself gave, revealed that she had been married for about six months and felt that her marriage was a successful and proper one. Her husband was the head of a thriving business and was obviously quite attached to her and interested in her well-being. She had been a laboratory technician prior to marriage and had graduated some two years previously. She said that she had always performed her work adequately and had left her job only because of the gradual increase in her apprehensiveness. Her family history revealed that she had one sister, three years her senior, who apparently had no emotional problems of consequence. Her parents were living and, as she stated in the initial interview, were happy and well-adjusted people.

The patient spontaneously went on to say that she had always been a moody person who had either been "way up or way down." She said that she had also been inhibited and made friends rather slowly, but got along with them quite well after she established good relationships. She had always been timid in her initial contacts with people for fear of possible resentment or rejection. She was unable to say why they might resent or reject her, but she always refrained from thoroughly accepting others until she had convinced herself that they were truly friendly toward her and that there was no chance that she might be snubbed or ignored.

As the patient described her childhood and adolescence, it soon became evident that in addition to being the youngest child she had also been the favorite, particularly of her father. He had showered many gifts upon her and had never hesitated to show his preference for her. Her mother had been more of the disciplinarian in the family, and in spite of the patient's occasional attempts to be friendly with the mother, the relationship had always been distant and cool. Further elucidation of this area showed that the mother had never been excessively demanding, but had certainly been less permissive than the father. The patient had been able, in the majority of situations, to obtain whatever she wanted and had rarely denied herself anything. If she was unable to obtain whatever she wanted from her mother, it was usually possible for her to get it from her father. As a result, whenever she had run into frustration, she had always turned to her father. He had constantly praised her and had frequently been her ally against her mother.

This patient said that the majority of her complaints had begun soon after her marriage. As she talked, it became evident that she felt that her husband was not as understanding as she had hoped that he would be. She had discovered, soon after marriage, that their financial status, though adequate, was certainly not unlimited. At times it became necessary for her to deny herself things and such a deprivation had rarely occurred to her prior to marriage. She had also begun to discover that there were many responsibilities which fell to her after marriage that were of a type she had never experienced or expected. Actually these responsibilities stemmed from her husband's normal tendency to expect her to share their marital responsibilities. There had been numerous occasions when the patient had become extremely angry at her husband, stamped her feet, and screamed at him, as she had previously done at her own parents. However, she soon found that her husband did not respond to this in the same "understanding" way her parents had.

As succeeding interviews passed, it became increasingly evident that she was an extremely narcissistic, selfish, and immature woman, who had never been given the opportunity to learn to carry responsibilities herself. From childhood, she had always been able to turn to her father in times of difficulty and he, in turn, had always provided her with an easy solution, often removing the difficulties of the situation in which she was involved. She had expected the same sort of treatment from her husband, and when it was not forthcoming, had found him wanting in good qualities. She had become increasingly angry at him and, at the same time, entertained some doubts as to the wisdom of choosing him as her marital partner. She had always assumed, unrealistically, that marriage would be a utopian type of existence, and she had fantasied that there would be few responsibilities. Actually, without realizing it, she had expected to get the same kind of treatment from her husband as she had from her father. When reality was presented to her in the form of her husband's reasonable demands, she had become extremely hostile. Much of this hostility remained within her, with only portions of it being expressed in occasional temper outbursts and the remainder of it remaining within her on an unconscious level. It gradually came into conflict with her conscience's demands, and thus she began to feel guilty. The result was that instead of feeling the resentment itself, she began to suffer acute anxiety attacks which, without psychotherapy, might have merged into a true chronic anxiety reaction.

After approximately a dozen interviews, the patient began to recognize her immature strivings and to improve her adjustment in marriage. She could accept her husband's demands more and was willing to attempt to fulfill at least some of them. As her understanding of her own immaturities and unrealistic expectations increased, her anxiety symptoms diminished. She ceased hating and began to use her aggression constructively and to receive the strengthening benefits of love and approval which a healthy environment always gives to maturely behaving people.

In summary, then, this patient had reached adult life and marriage with an immature and unrealistic outlook. Because of her childishness she made excessive demands upon her environment. These had always been sufficiently satisfied in the past, particularly by her father, so that there had been no great reason for the weaknesses of her personality to reveal themselves in the form of anxiety. However, when she married and had to face additional responsibilities, she became chronically dissatisfied and frustrated. This stirred up a great deal of inner resentment, some of which appeared in explosive outbursts, but much of which remained within her, stirring up considerable guilt. Her anxiety appeared as a warning signal to keep the true extent of her inner resentment from becoming evident to her. As is true of many neurotic conflicts her anxiety gradually spread to involve new areas of her life until she became almost totally immobilized. However, and this is also typical in many such cases, as her understanding of her own personality and her relationships increased, her anxiety diminished. Her symptoms disappeared and her own desire to mature became more prominent as well as more gratifying.

CHAPTER 7

Conversion Reaction

CONVERSION reaction is a type of psychoneurosis characterized by the individual's tendency to represent his inner psychological conflict by means of symbolic, somatic disturbances. There develops within the individual, because of his immature personality, a gradually rising level of tension which, at a propitious time, is "converted" into expression through a somatic symptom. Often this occurs in a dramatic and sudden manner. In previous nomenclature this syndrome was referred to as "conversion hysteria." The physiological channels through which the conversion phenomena are expressed are most frequently the voluntary systems, but may be the involuntary. The sudden occurrence of a paralysis of an extremity, or a stockinglike type of anesthesia, or perhaps total incapacitation of one of the special senses such as seeing or hearing is typical of conversion reaction. It is not uncommon, however, to find involvement of the involuntary systems as in certain types of vomiting. It might even be said that the latter involvement is more common today than it was fifty years ago and involvement of the voluntary systems less common.

The cornerstone of conversion reaction is the ability of the individual to express in some portion of his body the unconscious conflict from which he is suffering. The symptom then, as is true of any neurotic symptom, represents the patient's attempt to find a solution, though a distorted and pathological one, of his unconscious conflict. While the obsessive-compulsive patient tends generally to confine his neurosis to psychological spheres, the conversion-reaction patient utilizes his physiological mechanism to represent his conflict. It is typical to find a sudden onset of symptoms in conversion reaction, and these most often occur in a setting of marked emotional crisis. The picture is thus a dramatic one, with an abrupt occurrence of an obvious symptom in a particularly emotional and meaningful environmental setting.

The frequency of conversion phenomena is difficult to ascertain. In past years the occurrence of what was then called conversion hysteria was quite prominent. The sudden loss of sensation of an extremity, or paralysis, blindness, or deafness was not uncommon. However, such histrionic symptoms are not as common as they were and there is more chance at the present time of finding patients developing a more subtle and insidious involvement, such as an autonomic phenomenon. In Victorian society these conversions were apt to occur in naïve individuals whose upbringing had been extremely strict, particularly from a sexual standpoint. The present-day trend in our more sophisticated society is toward less dramatic and less obvious acting out by the body, and to include even involuntary-system involvement. It has become increasingly frequent to find such symptoms developing in situations involving workmen's compensation and in medicolegal situations. There has been so much written and portrayed in cartoons about the emotional factors involved in paralyses and other such symptoms that these become less "available" to most potential psychiatric patients today.

The term *conversion hysteria* has become sufficiently ingrained in the vocabulary of psychiatry that a word of explanation concerning its origin is advisable. The word *hysteria* is derived from the Greek word *hystera,* meaning womb. The medical term arose when, in the early days of medicine, physicians thought the condition due to a wandering of the uterus through various parts of the body, producing symptoms wherever it came to rest. Only by this rather peculiar method could early physicians explain the dramatic and sudden onset of such remarkable symptoms. While the emotional origin of hysteria had been suggested by many, it was Freud who originally, just prior to the turn of the century, began to develop our modern dynamic understanding of this syndrome in his early researches in psychoanalysis. Hysteria was the first psychoneurosis to be studied using this technique and fortunately proved to be the easiest and simplest for the new science to utilize in building some of its basic concepts.

As our knowledge of psychodynamics has improved it has been deemed advisable to eliminate the old word *hysteria* from the official classification. Patients suffering from phobias and amnesias, as well as from conversion phenomena, were originally grouped under "hysteria." It would seem more efficient, as exemplified by the present classification, to group patients with psychoneurotic disorders primarily according to the particular methods of defense which they utilize in dealing with their anxiety. Thus the term *conversion* is now used to indicate those patients who express their psychic conflict symbolically through the sensory and motor body activities, and occasionally through an organ system. The basic differences between conversion phenomena and psychophysiologic disorders will be discussed in Chapter 13.

PSYCHOPATHOLOGY AND ETIOLOGY

The patient with conversion reaction, like any other psychoneurotic, suffers essentially from an impeded and incomplete psychosexual development. This implies that he has within his personality areas of immaturity with which he still struggles. As with any other psychoneurosis, we are interested in two factors: first, where in the level of psychosexual development the individual primarily is "fixated," and second, how the patient attempts to defend himself against this immaturity so that certain characteristic symptoms occur as a result of these defenses.

The conversion-reaction patient has fared reasonably well in his psychosexual development compared to other psychoneurotics. Theoretically, at least, his oral and anal levels have been surmounted without obvious "fixation." In other words, he has passed through both periods, reasonably satisfied his desires, and moved onward into the genital period. It is here, in his attempts to solve the oedipal conflict, that his difficulties arise. A word should be said against oversimplification. Actually the conversion patient usually still presents both oral and anal characteristics, particularly the former. However, it is in the struggle with the oedipal conflict that he has come to insoluble difficulty. Rather than resort to regression to an earlier oral or anal level, this patient tends to remain "fixated" in the oedipal level of development and continues to struggle unsuccessfully with the problems which are attached to it.

At this point let us pause to consider the most essential elements of the child's personality development in terms of his psychosexual phases. The oral child during the first year is an extremely primitive individual whose needs can be characterized as being primarily dependent and whose relationship with others is built upon this strong dependency. The individual who retains such oral characteristics into later life will have certain problems involving this type of dependent relationship. The youngster who is in the anal phase relates in an entirely different way to those about him. He is capable of being extremely positive in his relationships and yet the next instant extremely negative. We refer to such relationships as *ambivalent,* indicating that they contain at the same time both strongly positive and negative feelings. So it is that the person who remains "fixated" at this level of development will, in later life, show a difficulty in loving because of the coexistence of hating and loving in all of his relationships. The oedipal situation offers the child still another type of relationship. At this time there is the beginning of a sexual tinge to the situation, even though this is an immature manifestation rather far removed from adult sexuality. The child during this phase has reached a stage of personality development closer to maturity than those which have gone before. However, there is still a noticeable childishness about all of his relationships. He needs to be helped to feel that love of the mother is acceptable and that the father does not have to be feared.

The oedipal phase may be clarified by considering a hypothetical example. Let us assume that we are considering a five-year-old boy. This youngster has felt an attachment to his mother since birth, but this attachment has recently taken on a somewhat different tinge. The child is now much more aware of the fact that his mother is of one sex and he of another. His desires toward her, while still those of complete possession and total love, have become tinged with this newly acquired awareness of masculine-feminine relationships. This obviously means that the youngster comes into some conflict about his mother's relationship with his father, and he feels that the latter hinders his own relationship and total possession of his mother. In order to further clarify the situation, let us assume that this boy's mother loves him in a somewhat immature way so that she is seductive toward him and invites and encourages a much closer relationship with him than is consistent with psychological health. To complete the picture we may also assume that the boy's father is a rather distant and punitive person who frightens the youngster and discourages any competition between himself and the youngster. The boy then faces the decision of either giving up his mother as an object of his secret childish longings or of hiding them from himself. In the neurotic child the latter decision is apt to be made. The chances that it will be made are increased particularly if the oral and anal phases have not been quite successfully surmounted. This means, of course, that the youngster has entered the oedipal phase with a somewhat insecure background, leaving him to face the new dangers with an inadequately constructed personality. He does not retreat to the previous levels, but nevertheless is unable to successfully surmount the oedipal strivings. The result is the relegation of the incestuous feelings (which are natural and appropriate for his age) to the unconscious, where they remain in a frozen state to further disturb his future relationships, particularly with the opposite sex, but obviously of course with the same sex. When such a youngster reaches adult life any relationship with a woman will be tinged with this same forbidding, frightening, incestuous aura which characterized his difficulty with his mother. Such an adult has literally never given up his mother and still seeks her, at least unconsciously, as a love object. He is therefore unable to accept any other woman on a basis which includes mature love. Even in our enlightened society today there are all too few children who are helped through this phase of development in their love relationship to the point of feeling free to love a person of the opposite sex and able to establish and easily maintain a friendly relationship with one of the same sex.

The relationship of oedipal conflict to conversion symptoms needs some elucidation. Because of the persistence of unconscious oedipal, and therefore sexual, conflict much of the patient's existence is a conflict between expression of and defense against oedipal sexual feelings. In terms of mental energy there is a large proportion directed toward expressing the immature sexuality and an equally large proportion against expressing it. Many comparatively innocuous activities and situations are, at least unconsciously, viewed by the conversion patient as potentially sexual and hence conflictual: to see, to be seen, to touch, to be touched are examples often only remotely related to sexuality. The body then becomes the means by which the patient reveals his conflict: to do or to prohibit—to allow or to deny.

SYMPTOMATOLOGY

The symptoms of conversion reaction are remarkably protean in type. They can mimic almost any condition, although usually in a crude way. As we have mentioned, the onset of these symptoms is often dramatic, occurring during a period of emotional stress. Therefore, it is not uncommon to find a widespread outbreak of conversion symptoms during such catastrophic environmental situations as earthquakes, fires, and wars. Not infrequently, however, in the neurotically disposed individual the conversion symptoms gradually become evident as an outgrowth and superimposition upon a physical injury or disease which has, in the meantime, been cured. This is an example of *somatic compliance* where the body, through injury or illness, "complies" with the needs of the neurosis by providing an expression of the neurotic conflict.

Conversion symptoms are divisible into several categories, depending upon the particular body system involved. They will be discussed under headings of motor, sensory, and autonomic symptoms.

MOTOR SYMPTOMS

These disturbances involve the voluntary muscles of the body. Most characteristically they involve an entire extremity, as, for example, a paralysis of one or both legs or arms. The causative stress is apt to be a situation particularly difficult for the patient, who feels that he wants to take a certain course of action and yet feels a prohibition against the action. An example is the soldier at the front lines who, on being ordered to attack, finds himself unable to move his legs. On the one hand he is deeply fearful of injury if he goes with the attacking forces, and yet his conscience unrealistically forbids him conscious realization of his fear. His particular solution to the conflict is the paralysis which comes on as an unconscious "answer." It is literally impossible for him to move, even if his life is threatened. It is interesting, however, that the person suffering from what obviously seems to be a severe and incapacitating paralysis of this type does not seem to show the deep, fearful concern that is ordinarily found in an organically paralyzed person with similar incapacitation. It is as if the conversion reaction patient realizes that his paralysis is not necessarily a lifelong nor life-endangering condition. This emotional detachment was noted years ago by French observers and called *la belle indifférence*.

Neurological examination shows that the conversion paralysis does not result in an absence of the deep reflexes. At times one may find some exaggeration of these reflexes, but not to the point of clonus, nor are there Babinski signs. The paralysis is usually of a flaccid type, but lacks the complete flaccidity found in organic paralysis. For instance, if the "paralyzed" leg is raised from the prone position and suddenly dropped, the individual with conversion reaction is apt to reveal an involuntary and unconscious response, so that there is a contraction of the voluntary muscle with the result that the leg does not flop downward as it would in true organic paralysis. Another important differential is to be found in the reactions to faradic and galvanic currents. In conversion reaction there is a retention of normal electrical responses, while these are gradually lost in the flaccid organic type of paralysis. There is, incidentally, no fibrillation to be found in conversion reaction. Wasting may eventually result after years of complete conversion-type paralysis, but this is primarily an atrophy of disuse. Skin temperature and circulation remain normal in conversion phenomena.

It is not unusual to find conversion paralysis occurring at or near the site of some traumatic injury. A typical example is the complete paralysis of one leg following a mild, glancing bruise of the external surface of the leg. As the traumatic event is subsequently reconstructed, it becomes obvious from the neurological standpoint that such a total paralysis could not possibly have resulted from the injury. Such knowledge combined with the presence of a conversion-type personality should guide one in diagnosis.

Sensory disturbances involve either various areas of the surface of the body or one of the special senses. The sudden development of a stockinglike type of anesthesia or hypesthesia is typical. Here again the dramatic, rapid onset occurring under particular emotional circumstances is characteristic. Also of importance is the nonphysiological distribution of the anesthesia. Organic damage to the larger roots of the peripheral nerves will not result in a stocking-type anesthesia. While it is true that certain organic ailments, such as peripheral neuritis, are capable of producing this stocking-type anesthesia, they usually have a history that is easily recognized and they do not produce the sharp line of demarcation that is commonly seen in conversion reaction.

It is important to stress here that the symptom is produced through the unconscious of the patient, and therefore he is not aware of its true meaning. The symptom is "successful" in that painful sensation produced in the involved area is literally not transmitted to the consciousness of the patient and thus it is possible to prick such an area in a manner that would ordinarily be quite painful without producing any visible signs of discomfort in the patient. There is an unfortunately common attitude on the part of physicians that since the symptom is not truly organic the patient may be only "pretending" not to feel the stimulation.

The obvious reason for the occurrence of stocking-type anesthesia lies in the patient's lack of knowledge concerning the sensory distribution of peripheral nerves. If, for instance, one were to assume the existence of a conversion reaction syndrome in a trained neurologist, it might be expected that the anesthesia would occur in a proper neurological arrangement which closely simulated true organic disease. It is not unusual in the typical conversion patient to find a hemianesthesia which literally includes one entire half of the body in a sharply demarcated line. However, again because of a lack of knowledge in the patient, there does not exist the typical organic overlap into the involved side which is seen in true organic disease, but is a straight line of anesthesia extending down the middle of the body and including all of the face and the head. Such a syndrome, of course, would be impossible as a result of organic damage. The physician well grounded in neurology ordinarily has little difficulty in differentiating between a conversion and an organic anesthesia or hypesthesia.

Various other special senses may be involved in conversion disorders. The individual may develop anything from complete blindness to hemianopsia. However, again, at least in the latter, the physician whose knowledge of ophthalmology is adequate will have little difficulty in differentiating true hemianopsia from the conversion type. Generally speaking, it is well to remember that the peripheral sensory apparatus in the conversion-reaction patient is working perfectly well. Impulses are transmitted to the central nervous system, but there they are denied access to consciousness. The senses of hearing, smell, or taste may be either partially diminished or completely absent as a result of conversion.

Repeated examinations of the conversion patient will usually reveal a difference existing from one examination to another. This difference is of a type which is not ordinarily found in organic disorders. Strong suggestion employed by the physician during the examination may produce such changes or exaggerate them to a degree that will clarify the diagnosis.

AUTONOMIC DISTURBANCES

Conversion symptoms, although ordinarily lending themselves more easily to voluntary systems and special senses, may occasionally be expressed through the vegetative nervous system. The conversion symptom itself represents, as we have mentioned, an expression of a forbidden impulse and at the same time the prohibition of this impulse. The symbolic representation of this conflict can be more dramatically and meaningfully portrayed, as a rule, through the voluntary musculature or sensations, or through the special senses. For instance, hysterical blindness is an obvious possibility in the patient who "will not see" a given unpleasant situation. The autonomic nervous system is less obvious in its manifestations and less dramatic, and therefore, its choice as a symptom site in conversion reaction is perhaps not as "expressive." Of course, hysterical vomiting is a frequent symptom in one who is "sick of" a certain person or situation. However, other factors enter into this picture. In the first place, such almost theatrical and totally incapacitating symptoms as general paralysis are more widely recognized by both the medical profession and the laity today as frequently being manifestations of emotional problems. The general practitioner who visits a home in which the eager, developing adolescent has a sudden paralysis in a healthy body almost automatically begins to wonder what frustration phenomena are going on. Relief from dreaded or hated responsibilities may reveal itself as the source of a fishbone "accidentally" swallowed or a minor food poisoning. Another factor which may focus a conversion reaction in the autonomic system is the existence of an injury or a minor organic ailment. An example is the individual who receives a blow on the head of minor severity, but in a situation of great emotional stress. If the patient has a conversion-type personality, it is not unusual for him to develop a chronic cephalalgia of a functional nature as a result of the initial blow.

The primipara who has great difficulty with her pregnancy, in particular suffering constantly from nausea and vomiting, is often a conversion reaction type of person. Her conflict lies in the difficulty which she has in accepting her pregnancy. She literally "cannot stomach it." Her gastric disturbance is a symbolic expression of her unconscious conflict concerning her own sexuality and all of its manifestations, including her pregnancy. This condition differs considerably from a gastric ulcer, the psychophysiologic condition of which is based on an emotional conflict which eventually leads to organic pathology. The ulcer patient is typically concerned with the conflict of dependency versus independence. He has within himself a great deal of unaccepted, and to him, intolerable dependency which he attempts to overcompensate by presenting to himself and to the world a pseudo-independent attitude. However, his inner infantile needs chronically stimulate hyperactivity in his upper gastrointestinal tract and this leads eventually to ulcer formation. The ulcer itself does not really express anything symbolically, at least with the same degree of clarity as does the nausea and vomiting of a pregnant woman with a conversion reaction. The ulcer patient's upper-gastrointestinal hypermotility and hyperacidity represent a normal physiological response to an inner type of "hunger."

It is possible to demonstrate the effect of the unconscious upon the autonomic as well as the voluntary systems in a dramatic manner through hypnosis. The hypnotically engendered unconscious conflict is similar to one which may occur in conversion reaction. In a hypnotic state a suggestible subject may be touched by the hypnotist with a cold object. If the subject is told that this object is red-hot, a visible and typical blister may be produced which would ordinarily result only from the application of heat. It is also possible, in a suggestible individual, to produce different pulse volumes in right and left extremities through hypnotic suggestion. The person who is in a hypnotic trance may be told that his right leg is extremely cold and the result will be a blanching of this leg due to a constriction of all the arterial vessels in the leg. Such artificially produced physiologic changes are not as dramatic as production of blindness or paralysis, but are certainly convincing evidence of the importance of the unconscious in autonomic function.

It is important here to say a word about differential diagnosis between malingering and conversion reaction symptoms. Malingering is a *conscious* attempt to simulate some condition which is not actually present, while conversion reaction involves the *unconscious* production of a symptom so that the patient is unaware of its emotional origin. Malingering is most often seen in military service, or in civilian compensation cases. It is resorted to by an individual with a severe personality disorder for the purpose of evading some distasteful situation or of gaining some preferred situation. For instance, the distinction must be drawn between the soldier who consciously feigns paralysis of some type, realizing that he is doing it in order to evade duty, and the conversion-reaction person who develops a paralysis without conscious awareness of the reason for his paralysis. The first individual is punishable under military law, while the second is considered to be emotionally disturbed and therefore a medical problem. Actually, the individual who malingers is a sick person from the standpoint of psychiatry, but the fact that he adopts his symptoms on a purely conscious basis makes him punishable in both military and civilian law. It is ordinarily not difficult to distinguish between these two reactions. While conversion paralyses and sensory disturbances, as well as other similar symptoms, may be of an odd and bizarre type and not fit any organic pattern, they tend to remain constant and the patient cannot be "tricked" into losing them. An example is to be found in the person who claims deafness without demonstrable organic cause. The physician may be initially uncertain as to whether this is a malingering or conversion phenomenon. It may be possible to get a reaction from the patient by the production of an unexpected and loud noise if he is malingering, but not in the case of true conversion reaction. It is worth stressing here that malingering is not nearly as common as is ordinarily believed. Even in military service the number of proven cases of malingering was quite small compared to the number of conversion reaction patients. The average malingerer is often careless in his attempts to maintain his symptoms, and particularly during military service it is often easy to spot the "paralytic" malingerer walking about the ward when he feels he is not being watched. This obviously would not occur in a conversion patient. Again, however, it must be stressed that it also requires an emotionally disturbed personality to produce malingering, but in malingering the difficulty is primarily due to a defect in conscience formation, while in conversion the end result is due to conflicts among the different parts of the personality.

PROGNOSIS

Since conversion reaction is the closest to normality of all the psychoneurotic reaction types, one would expect it to lend itself to therapeutic measures more readily than some of the other types. While this is frequently true, it is by no means a constant finding, since many patients with conversion reaction also present elements of earlier fixations which complicate and prolong treatment. In theory, at least, the typical conversion-reaction patient has advanced with reasonable success through oral and anal levels of psychosexual development only to become enmeshed in the oedipal situation. In practice, however, this situation is often marred by the persistence of unresolved oral and anal tendencies. The oedipal conflict of the typical patient with a conversion reaction persists in the unconscious and interferes with all of his present-day relationships. The chief mechanism of ego defense of these patients is repression. The entire unsolved oedipal conflict is repressed. The major goal of the therapeutic effort is release of the repressed material, which can then be assimilated by the conscious ego and utilized in a more mature way. The typical conversion patient appears immature, histrionic, and narcissistic. Conversion-type individuals are ordinarily quite sociable, but their interpersonal relationships are superficial and lack a satisfactory depth and stability. Women who suffer from this syndrome are frequently attractive and make the most of whatever pulchritude they may possess. They seem warm and friendly, but are soon found to have the typical qualities of immaturity and superficiality in all of their relationships.

The prognosis in the average uncomplicated case of conversion reaction is usually fairly good, especially if adequate treatment is given. Many of these patients, however, reveal a sizable degree of *oral fixation* (dependence) and are more difficult to treat successfully. The prognosis also is affected by the amount of secondary gain which enters the situation. A patient whose symptoms bring him much attention or other reward and remove him from an intolerable situation will not respond to therapy as well as if these factors were less. The conversion phenomenon may be a part of an over-all personality difficulty of greater seriousness, and if so, the prognosis is correspondingly poorer. For instance, a schizoid person may under stress develop a conversion symptom, and while symptomatic treatment may be successful, more complete therapy is difficult. In other words conversion symptoms may occur in a large variety of personality disturbances and it is up to the physician to weigh many factors such as:

(1) history of childhood development
(2) childhood experiences
(3) environmental stress which produced symptom
(4) modifiability of environmental situation
(5) goals and gratifications which future may hold for patient

(6) skill of psychotherapist in integrating these factors with
(7) amount of psychotherapy patient and family will accept
(8) imagination and courage of patient to work through his difficulties to satisfaction and success.

TREATMENT

A wide variety of methods have been used to eradicate the various symptoms of conversion reaction. Some of them have been thoroughly scientific and others have depended totally upon the patient's increased suggestibility. It is often a relatively simple procedure to rid a conversion patient of his particular symptom. The problem, however, of his basically neurotic personality remains, and the patient is more than apt to develop either the same symptom again or some new type, particularly if another environmental situation arises which will enhance his conflict. An authoritative or persuasive approach either commanding or suggesting to the patient that his symptom will disappear will suffice to eradicate the symptoms, at least temporarily.

If, however, the physician desires to accomplish more basic changes in the personality of the conversion patient, rather than merely to provide symptomatic relief, further therapeutic measures are essential. There are three general types of therapy which have been widely utilized in this condition: hypnosis, narcosynthesis, and psychoanalytic psychotherapy. We will discuss these briefly here, although they are covered in greater detail in Chapter 21, "Principles of Psychotherapy."

HYPNOSIS

Hypnosis lends itself very well to the treatment of the conversion-reaction patient, since he is a particularly suggestible person, and hence usually an excellent hypnotic subject. Symptomatic relief can often be obtained by suggesting to the patient who is hypnotized that upon awakening his symptom will have disappeared. A single hypnotic session will frequently suffice to remove a symptom, but if it does not, repeated sessions will in the majority of cases accomplish this. Obviously, however, mere symptom removal has not changed the patient's basic personality structure and he still has the same psychopathology which will predispose him to the development of further symptomatology. Where hypnosis is used, the therapeutic goal is not only symptomatic relief, but also the bringing to light of unconscious material which has led to the original symptom formation. Such unconscious material is accessible to the hypnotist while the patient is in the hypnotic state. The strength of the mechanism of repression is diminished during hypnosis, which allows unconscious material to emerge. However, the hypnotist has taken over some of the functions of the patient's ego, so that the patient does not really assimilate the unconscious material as it emerges as efficiently as he would in the waking state. Unless he is told to do so while under hypnosis, the patient will probably not remember what he has said, since the repression will be re-established when he wakens. If it is suggested to him that he will remember everything that he has said during the trance, the patient may subsequently become quite upset because of the sudden consciousness of much conflictual material which had previously been unconscious and unacceptable to him. This difficulty is usually obviated by telling the patient while he is under hypnosis that he will remember only certain portions of what he has said. The physician uses the additional knowledge which he has gained about the patient to hasten further psychotherapeutic efforts, but without attempting to impart all his knowledge immediately to the patient. Hypnosis has been expanded into hypnoanalysis, which consists of more frequent and thoroughgoing hypnotic sessions oriented toward a more complete exploration of the unconscious. One of the greatest therapeutic deficiencies of hypnosis and hypnoanalysis is in the area of the mechanisms of ego defense. These are not worked through and understood by the patient as happens when treatment is carried on in the waking state. There is, in addition, as already mentioned, the possibility of producing excessive anxiety in an individual by exposing him too suddenly to unconscious material which he is not ready to assimilate. However, hypnosis may be found to be of some use, particularly in alleviating symptoms of the conversion patient and, in certain other chosen cases, for a more extensive exploration of the unconscious. It should be pointed out also that in spite of its potential efficacy in the hands of a highly skilled physician, hypnotism as the sole treatment is not commonly used, and has never gained a wide, everyday application.

NARCOSYNTHESIS

Narcosynthesis, which gained its greatest use in World War II, involves the intravenous injection of a barbiturate solution which produces a state akin to hypnosis. This method is most frequently utilized where either the physician is not adept with hypnotic technique, or where the subject cannot be successfully or easily hypnotized. As a rule, the conversion patient, with his extreme suggestibility, need not be subjected to narcosynthesis if the physician is capable of utilizing hypnosis. Anywhere from five to fifteen grains of sodium amytal, or an equivalent amount of sodium pentothal, are injected slowly intravenously. The patient gradually becomes drowsy, but is still responsive and capable of answering questions. The amount of barbiturate can often be diminished if hypnotic technique is utilized at the same time. Essentially the goal is to reach a hypnotic state, either by the use of strong hypnotic suggestion or barbiturates or a combination of the two. The material which is brought out by narcosynthesis is essentially similar to that brought out during hypnosis. Many of the symptoms seen in combat-reaction cases during the last war were of a conversion type and the underlying dynamics of the particular symptom were brought to light either through hypnosis or narcosynthesis. Symptoms of recent origin—a few days or weeks—are much more amenable to this type of treatment than those of longer duration.

PSYCHOANALYTIC PSYCHOTHERAPY

Any adequate and permanently successful treatment of conversion reaction should be aimed at understanding and eradicating the pathological mechanisms of defense with subsequent expression and working through of the unconscious conflicts. To accomplish this end requires a psychoanalytically oriented type of treatment. While orthodox psychoanalysis is probably the treatment of choice, in many of these cases practical considerations dictate a briefer type of treatment based on similar principles.

Patients with this type of neurosis develop rapid and strong transference feelings. It is important for the therapist to realize that these patients ordinarily romanticize the majority of their relationships and will do the same thing in the treatment situation. A typical example is to be found in the young female patient who becomes enamored of her male therapist. Romantic fantasies and dreams begin to appear in which the patient links herself to the therapist. The wise therapist is quick to recognize the unrealistic, neurotic origin of these feelings and help the patient eventually develop a better ability to form object relationships. The unwise or untrained therapist is apt to react to such positive transference as if it were a realistic attitude on the part of the patient. If this occurs it means that the patient never has an opportunity to work through and understand his or her persisting emotional complexes formed from childhood.

Case History (1): Conversion Reaction

This twenty-seven-year-old single woman was referred to the psychiatric department by the department of otorhinolaryngology. The chief complaint was aphonia. Thorough examination, including laryngoscopy, by the ear, nose, and throat department failed to demonstrate any organic pathology.

Her history revealed that this patient had been brought up in an extremely inhibited family. She was an only child whose parents led a remarkably restricted life. Her parents were reasonably warm and kind but, although they focused a great deal of attention upon the patient, they allowed her little in the way of independence. There was a constant implication by her parents that such things as parties, dancing, and dating, while not actually sinful, held potential dangers and were to be avoided. The patient remained extremely close to both her parents throughout her childhood and adolescence. Her entire living standard revolved around her small, constricted home situation, and she never had an opportunity to see how her contemporaries lived. Her heightened devotion to her parents caused her to acquiesce early to their dictates, even though she occasionally allowed herself conscious desires toward some of the activities in which she felt other boys and girls were engaged. She looked enviously at some of these other youngsters whom she met at school, but never allowed herself to join with them in their parties or dances.

This patient graduated from high school with excellent grades, having made a good impression upon all of her teachers and almost no impression upon any of her contemporaries. She took a secretarial course and, upon graduation, in order to please her parents, obtained a job in a religious organization. Her employer was a man who had many characteristics and views similar to those of her parents. A few months after she began work, she became interested in a man in the organization, but her employer voiced his criticism and disapproval of the budding relationship. The patient became dimly aware of her desire to "speak out" and protest against this disapproval, which was so similar to that which she had always received from her parents. Her conscience, or superego, however, having many of the qualities of the parents, forbade this desire to "speak." Her aphonia developed as a symbolic expression of this conflict about speaking out.

This patient was hypnotized at the time of her initial visit, and it was found that under hypnosis she could speak quite clearly. She was told while in the trance that upon awakening her voice would be perfectly all right, and this suggestion was successful in removing the symptom. She was seen for a total of thirteen more interviews, during which time she was helped to understand the meaning of her symptom and how it related to the rest of her personality adjustment. With the help of a friendly, understanding, and permissive physician she came to see more clearly her exaggerated dependency upon her parents and the unrealistic inhibitions which she had placed upon herself. Her entire attitude became more independent and mature. It is this kind of psychotherapeutic work following symptom removal that strengthens the personality and acts as insurance against return of the same or other symptoms.

Case History (2): Conversion Reaction

A twenty-year-old single, attractive young woman was referred to the psychiatrist by an internist. She had consulted him for recurrent nausea and vomiting spells. He had been unable to discover any organic pathology and felt after studying her that her difficulties were on an emotional basis. She had been quite willing to accept the idea of an emotional illness and, as a matter of fact, had herself entertained this thought prior to consulting the internist. Her nausea and vomiting spells had begun at the age of fourteen when she was kissed by a boy for the first time. She had been very concerned at the time as to whether it was proper to allow this boy to kiss her—feeling on the one hand that it was wrong, and yet wanting him to do so. Subsequently, whenever she had a date she developed nausea and often had to excuse herself in order to vomit.

Her symptoms became most obvious whenever she found herself in a romantic situation with a boy and particularly when the boy tried to make any advances to her. She remarked that it seemed to be most prominent with the boys for whom she cared the most.

This patient came from a family consisting of herself, mother, father, and one older brother. In her initial interview, she described the family life as fairly satisfactory and one in which there were congenial relationships between all the members. She gave the impression that her parents had always gotten along well. They had not been particularly strict and had provided quite well for her and for her brother.

She was a very intelligent young woman and had always done well in school. During adolescence she had been quite popular, but her symptoms had caused her to limit her dates much more than she would have otherwise. She dressed attractively, and on initial impression seemed to be a friendly, warm, pleasant, intelligent young woman.

Of immediate importance to the patient was the fact that at the time she was going with a young man of whom she was very fond and whom she hoped to marry. She was always extremely fearful that she would be unable to conceal her nausea and vomiting spells and feared that they would eventually be the cause of her having to break off the relationship.

As far back as she could remember she had been quite close to her father, with whom she spent a good deal of time. Her mother, although a relatively warm and understanding person, had never shared any of the father's interests and apparently had not had the active desire for social life and achievement which the father had. The patient had always been a rather talented girl with abilities in many areas, which had cemented her close relationship with her father. Her older brother was much more like her mother in that they were both rather quiet and retiring people. There were no serious disagreements or disturbances within the family and when together there was a strong sense of loyalty and friendship between all of them. As far as she was concerned, the patient was equally drawn to both her mother and her father, although she freely admitted that she had much more in common with her father.

As treatment proceeded it soon became clear that the father represented to the patient the ideal but unattainable man. He represented everything that she desired in a man, and she was never able to find another boy in her own age group who measured up to her father's qualities. She always liked the company of boys, but as soon as they became more than casually interested in her, and particularly if they made any advances to her, her symptoms of nausea and vomiting ensued.

Very soon after the beginning of therapy the patient revealed the same desire to please the therapist that she had always evinced toward her father. She became, as far as she was concerned, the therapist's "favorite little girl" and attributed to him all the characteristics which she admired in her father. Gradually during the treatment process, her overidealization of the therapist and also of her father was brought to her attention. She was helped to give up her father and the therapist as sole recipients of her attention toward the male sex. As she gradually released her strong attachment to the therapist and to her father, she became free to seek male companionship of her own age without strong guilt and with a much more realistic attitude. Interestingly enough, as is often true in conversion reactions, her symptoms disappeared quite early in the process because of her rapid development of transference feelings toward the therapist.

Case History (3): Conversion Reaction

This patient was a twenty-year-old private in the Army during World War II who suffered from a particular conversion symptom called "camptocormia." This soldier was assisted by two of his buddies to the dispensary. At the time he was seen he was standing but was bent at a forty-five degree angle forward from the hips. He seemed not to be in great distress, but claimed that he was unable to straighten up. Any attempts to do so caused severe pain and were unsuccessful. Examination revealed no demonstrable pathology. He was taken to the station hospital where further examination still did not reveal any organic difficulty. X-rays of the entire spinal column were negative. The soldier gave a history of having been working on a cleanup detail in his company area prior to final inspection before embarkation for overseas. He had spent considerable time bending over picking up various rubbish in his area when he felt a severe pain in his back and subsequently had been unable to straighten up.

The patient was admitted to the neuropsychiatric service where a more detailed history was taken. He had been the youngest of four children, raised in a rural area. His father was a strict, domineering, authoritative farmer who had run his family "with an iron hand." The mother was a more passive but very warm and maternal person who had always tried to protect the patient from the father's outbursts of temper. Her efforts in his behalf had apparently been much more obvious than any she had made for the older siblings. He had remained quite dependent and attached to her and his first separation from her had occurred six months previously when he had come into the Army. He had been quite homesick upon entering the service and had found the rapidly moving life confusing and disturbing to him. He had never quite learned to hold his own with the more educated and sophisticated urban soldiers with whom he came into contact. The Army had been for him a frightening experience.

The patient was a very sincere, if immature, boy who felt a strong need to fulfill his obligations to his country, but who remained inwardly quite frightened at the new life that he was leading. He had been teased and even mildly ridiculed by many of the men in his company because of his lack of sophistication. He had tried hard to be accepted by them and to hide from them as well as from himself whatever fears he had. It became obvious in the second interview that he had many vague fears about going overseas. Some of these stemmed from exaggerated stories about war which his tentmates had told him. However, he had not admitted fear to himself and had made every effort to hide it from everyone else.

As is often true in conversion reaction, his symptom came on in a period of stress, both physical and mental. He had spent considerable time during the morning bending over to pick up rubbish, in addition to which there was growing the gnawing fear of his approaching embarkation. His conscience refused to allow him to admit his fear, yet underneath he was very frightened and worried about going overseas. His symptom solved the entire situation immediately and spared him the guilt that he would otherwise have had. He was hospitalized and therefore "legally" unable to go to war.

The initial steps in the treatment of this case were two interviews during which the psychiatrist gained knowledge about the patient. The next step was the administration intravenously of seven-and-a-half grains of sodium amytal. While the patient was under the influence of the drug, his symptom disappeared and he talked openly about his homesickness, his fear about not measuring up to the rest of the men in his company, and his great concern about facing what he considered to be unknown dangers overseas. Following his recovery from the amytal, the patient's symptom remained absent. He was seen subsequently in approximately five interviews. During this time he was helped to discuss his various fears and homesickness in a permissive atmosphere. He was shown how many soldiers who came into the Army suffered these same symptoms, that the symptoms were nothing to be ashamed of, and that even the bravest men were often afraid. He was allowed to revisit his unit, whose departure had been delayed for a few days, and his spirit of belonging to the unit was stimulated in every possible way. By the time his final interview came around, the patient was not only willing but quite anxious to rejoin his unit and accompany it overseas.

This particular symptom followed the pattern often shown by conversion reaction in that it chose an area of the body which already had a physical symptom. Undoubtedly the patient developed a certain amount of backache in his strenuous work and this was sufficient to allow his psychic conflict to be expressed in an exaggerated form as a disability of his back.

CHAPTER 8

Dissociative Reaction

DISSOCIATIVE reaction is a type of psychoneurosis characterized by the individual's attempts to deal with his anxiety through various disturbances of consciousness or through walling off certain areas of the mind from consciousness. Examples of symptoms to be found in this category are amnesia, fugue states, somnambulism, and multiple personality. The dissociative type of psychoneurosis, while not as common as some of the others, is probably the most dramatic in its symptomatology. As a result, patients with this difficulty often make newspaper headlines because of predicaments occurring during the course of their disturbed conscious state. Dissociative symptoms appeal to writers as subjects for portrayal because of their dramatic presentation of the human personality in action.

ETIOLOGY AND PSYCHOPATHOLOGY

The various symptoms occurring in dissociative reaction must be viewed as the patient's attempts to deal with his anxiety. The personality of the patient with dissociative reaction is similar in its underlying dynamics to that of an individual with conversion reaction. In past nomenclatures both of these conditions were grouped under the term *conversion hysteria*. From the standpoint of psychosexual development, patients with conversion and dissociative reaction have both fared comparatively well. They have, even with some difficulties, managed to surmount the majority of problems of the oral and anal periods but have eventually become enmeshed in an unsuccessful attempt to love and be responsible to those who have reared them

—or their surrogates. It is wise to restate here that all patients with psychoneurotic difficulties reveal residual immaturities from all levels of psychosexual development. Patients with dissociative reaction have reached their primary stumbling block in the oedipal level of development. Their unsuccessful solution of this oedipal situation is, however, based upon an insecure and unstable working through of oral and anal levels of development. This means that when they reach the oedipal situation they are inadequately prepared to meet it. They have not found it necessary to regress to much earlier levels, as is true, for instance, in the compulsive neuroses, and yet, on the other hand, they have not been sufficiently secure and well-adjusted to surmount the hurdle of oedipal strivings.

Many of these individuals are at times confused with schizoid or schizophrenic patients, particularly when their symptomatology takes on a somewhat bizarre formation. They are badly handicapped by virtue of their symptoms in their relationship to other people. It is not, however, unusual to find the diagnostic error proven to be in the opposite direction. For instance, there are amnesic patients who originally appear to belong to the dissociative-reaction type, and yet ultimately, after more thorough personality evaluation, prove to be schizophrenic.

The patient with a dissociative reaction has a conflict, as do all psychoneurotics. This internal, unconscious conflict is enhanced by any environmental situation which stimulates the conflict. What the patient is attempting to do is escape an uncomfortable, anxiety-producing situation, and this is why he develops his symptoms. Because of his immaturity, such a patient is unable to face some of the usual responsibilities and tasks of ordinary living; when the situation reaches his level of intolerance, dissociative reaction results. The patient may then close off a portion of what had previously been conscious memory and feeling and become totally unaware of a period of his life, or he may disturb his conscious awareness of what is going on about him and enter a dreamlike state in which he reacts without his ordinary reality-testing mechanisms.

Here again, as in conversion reaction, the characteristic mechanism is repression, the method by which small or large segments of the patient's experiences are relegated to the unconscious.

SYMPTOMATOLOGY

The essential feature of the symptoms of dissociative reaction is a disturbance in the quality or quantity of the conscious stream of thought. The symptoms vary not only in the degree to which they interfere with consciousness, but also in the manner in which they interfere with it. Undoubtedly the best-known syndrome in this category is *amnesia*. Amnesia involves a blocking-out from consciousness of a certain portion of an individual's life—a loss of memory of a particular period of time. The patient, by use of the mechanism of repression, is able to blot out incidents or periods of time if they threaten to expose unwelcome material to consciousness. The amnesia may be of various types. It may be "circumscribed," in which case a certain period of time is repressed and all that came before and all that followed is remembered. It is as if the particular traumatic situation did not occur, for the patient has no memory of it. When the amnesia extends backward to cover all events prior to the traumatic situation, it is called "retrograde." When it extends from the traumatic situation forward, it is called "anterograde." An amnesic may live for years in his dissociative state until, finally, some highly charged emotional situation restores his memory, or adequate psychotherapeutic measures release the repression.

Examples of far simpler, and certainly more common, evidences of a minor sort of dissociative reaction fall within the personal experience of almost everyone. These ubiquitous, but pathological, evidences of repression are derived from the same type of mental mechanism that is found in the patient with dissociative reaction. Freud has referred to them as "the psychopathology of everyday life." Examples are the forgetting of an individual's name when one knows the person well or the forgetting of places and dates, only to recall the correct name, place, or time later. Such information has been temporarily repressed because of its association with some unconscious conflictual material. Perhaps a name is linked in some way with an individual whom one does not like, but about whom there is guilt about the dislike. Possibly a place has an unconscious association with a place whose recall would be unwelcome in consciousness.

Amnesia is not invariably due to dissociative reaction; differential diagnosis is important. A head injury may produce a period of amnesia, which can last for varying periods of time although frequently it is not prolonged. Diagnosis of amnesia is ordinarily a secondary matter in these cases, since the history and the physical injury point toward the proper diagnosis. Another type of amnesia is seen in epileptics where the events during seizures are forgotten. There is also an amnesia for the fugue states seen in epileptics. Again the associated history of a convulsive state indicates the proper diagnosis.

Occasionally amnesia is feigned by a patient for one reason or another. It is a result of conscious and deliberate "symptom" formation by which the patient hopes to extricate himself from an uncomfortable situation. The attitude of the patient lacks real sincerity and is either wanting in completeness or reveals an exaggerated histrionic quality not seen in true dissociative reaction. Such a symptom is very difficult to maintain for any great period of time.

Amnesia is seen occasionally as a symptom of schizophrenic reaction. The latter diagnosis may be very difficult to make especially if additional history sources are not available when the patient is first seen. Usually, however, as the patient becomes more talkative and as routine treatment procedures are tried, the seriousness of the personality difficulty becomes evident. Schizophrenic patients do not respond to the measures which are successful with dissociative reaction, even though the amnesia frequently abates.

Somnambulism, or sleepwalking, is another symptom of the dissociative reaction. It is most often found in childhood but may appear in any period in life. In the typical somnambulistic state the person arises from his bed during sleep and, contrary to popular notion, has his eyes open and is apparently aware of much that is occurring in his environment. He seems, however, not to be assimilating and integrating this environment as well as he would if he were awake. He may or may not respond to questions and then may or may not return voluntarily to bed where he resumes his sleep. In such a state, however, he may become involved in a precarious situation, which is even, at times, life-endangering, because of his inadequate ability to evaluate what is going on about him. For instance, he may climb out on window ledges or other high places without apparent realization of the danger involved. If one were to awaken such a patient at this time he might well lose his balance and be severely injured. In general, it is not any more difficult to awaken him while he is somnambulistic than when he is in a normal sleep. Usually, however, there is no good reason for wakening him and the proper solution is to lead him back to bed where he can resume his slumber. The next morning such a patient may or may not remember "vaguely" some of the events of the previous night. At other times he remembers a "dream" which has some similarities to the events which transpired.

Multiple personality is a relatively rare type of dissociative reaction. It involves the alternating of currents of two or more partially or completely separate "personalities" each of which takes turns in gaining access to the current stream of consciousness and thus controls behavior. Probably the most famous and best-described example of this type of personality disorder is to be found in Morton Prince's book, *The Dissociation of a Personality*.[1] The case involved was a young woman who had at various times five separate and distinct personalities which alternated in their appearance, and which varied widely in their characteristics and behavior. A more modern example is *The Three Faces of Eve* by Doctors Thigpen and Cleckley.[2] Essentially, in an individual with such a dissociative reaction one finds the alternate appearance of different facets of his underlying psychic structure. The result is that on one occasion the individual may appear to be shy and inhibited and on another occasion quite aggressive and forward. There is often some awareness in the individual of the different personalities, and they may alternate in the same day, or from day to day, or may persist for periods of months at a time.

Another possible symptom of dissociative reaction is the *fugue state*. This is slightly more common than multiple personality, but still not particularly frequent. The individual so affected wanders

---

[1] Prince, Morton. *The Dissociation of a Personality*. London, Longmans, Green and Co., 1925.

[2] Thigpen, C., and H. Cleckley. *The Three Faces of Eve*. New York, McGraw-Hill Book Co., 1957.

away from his usual environment, takes up residence elsewhere, and may remain for months or years as a personality completely apart from, and usually different from, his former self. He may acquire property, marry, have a family, and become an accepted member of the community, only to suddenly some day "come to" with a more or less complete memory of his original personality situation. More frequently fugue states are of much shorter duration, occupying only a few minutes to a few hours. The similarity here to amnesia is obvious.

Another symptom found in dissociative reaction is that of *stupor*. In this condition the patient withdraws from his environment and does not respond to what is going on about him. This stupor has many similarities to the stupor state seen in psychosis, or occasionally in toxic conditions. If the patient speaks, his words are often jumbled and lack coherent meaning. The completeness of the withdrawal varies: some patients respond to external stimuli more than others. At times the differential diagnosis between a dissociative type of stupor and a more serious psychotic, or even toxic, stupor is initially difficult. However, an adequate history and thorough physical and neurological examination will usually give clear clues as to the proper diagnosis. Many dissociative patients will respond to some degree, although they evince anxiety and discomfort about their responses. It is as if relating to others and talking literally pains them, although not in an organic manner. The history frequently reveals a psychologically traumatic event immediately preceding the onset of the stupor. It is as if the patient does not wish to remember nor to verbalize and communicate to anyone the events of this traumatic situation. The state into which he has plunged himself is a temporary, even though inadequate, "solution" to his problems.

All of the dissociative reaction symptoms are at times confused with organic brain conditions, toxic syndromes, or even functional psychoses. There is, however, as mentioned, an absence of focal neurological signs and a history lacking the indications of organic, toxic, or psychotic personality. There are individuals suffering from epilepsy who have occasional "fugue" states in which extreme aggression, destructiveness, and even homicidal impulses are prominent for a period of minutes, hours, or even longer. Such patients are completely amnesic concerning the destruction they have wrought and may, at times, present a differential diagnosis problem. Here again, the history of epileptic seizures, physical and neurological findings, and the presence of extreme rage reaction are useful points in the establishment of the diagnosis. A careful encephalographic study will help to establish and clarify the thinking of the physician.

Schizophrenic patients at times develop a temporary stuporlike condition, or even reveal periods of amnesia. Here again, differential diagnosis may for a time remain in doubt. Therapeutic measures applied to such patients often reveal the presence of more severe psychopathology in the schizophrenic patient than is found in the dissociative patient.

TREATMENT

The treatment of dissociative reaction may be oriented primarily toward immediate removal of the symptoms, or, preferably, toward gradual improvement of the basic personality structure. The popular concept of treatment of this disorder has been influenced by dramatic portrayals in literature and moving pictures. The general impression of most people seems to be that in an amnesic patient immediate measures should be taken to restore memory. It is as if this restoration of memory will promptly solve all of the patient's problems. Unfortunately, this is no more true of the dissociative reaction than of any other psychopathological symptom. Suppression or selective removal of a particular symptom may temporarily appear to improve the patient's condition markedly. However, in the long run it leaves the patient's basic personality conflict unchanged and he is prone to form a similar symptom under some similar stressful situation. Amnesic or even stuporous symptoms may often be removed through such dramatic procedures as hypnosis or administration of sodium amytal. These measures will ordinarily restore a patient rapidly to contact with his environment and will return to him all of his painful memories. The question remains as to whether or not such a procedure has accomplished much over-all permanent gain for the patient. Similarly, it is not unusual to find such a symptom "cured" when the patient is presented with a close relative or friend whom he has not seen during the period of his illness. Again, this procedure, although often useful, is by no means an answer to the whole problem.

The wise therapist keeps in mind when he is treating a patient with dissociative reaction that he is dealing with a basically immature personality structure, rather than merely with one particular symptom. However, the therapist recognizes the symptoms as a childlike attempt to escape the realities of living. He recognizes that the patient would not have found it necessary to "dissociate" himself from his environment had he been able to find a more mature level of adjustment. The therapist is aware that the patient's basic immaturity stems from an insecure childhood. He realizes that the individual is still, in a sense, attached to his parents' value system in a manner reminiscent of childhood, and is unable to form an adequate and adult type of relationship with other individuals. In the patient's attempts to use an immature, inefficient type of personality in an adult world there has gradually developed an increasing amount of tension with final development of symptoms. The therapist, therefore, not only orients himself toward amelioration of the immediate symptoms but includes longer-range goals. He attempts to help the patient become more mature and more capable of coping with his life situation. The essence of his therapeutic inquiry should be, "Why do you need to do this?"

As has been mentioned, once the immediate symptoms of dissociative reaction have been removed, the underlying personality structure of dissociative patients bears a similarity to that of conversion patients. The immature, dramatic, and somewhat selfish characteristics of the patient become increasingly obvious. There is an extensive repression which must be loosened through therapy, thus helping the patient become aware of and work through some of the immaturities which persist in his unconscious. Once they become conscious these immaturities can be dealt with on a more reasonable basis by the adult ego.

PROGNOSIS

The prognosis in uncomplicated dissociative reaction is comparatively good. Symptoms can usually be alleviated in a relatively brief time. The underlying personality structure can be favorably changed through further therapy, thus minimizing the possibilities of another attack. The most important factors are impressing the patient with the need of further treatment and increasing his motivation to carry it through. The dramatic improvement which follows symptom removal is often so gratifying both to the patient and his family that further treatment is neglected. The prognosis also depends upon the number of symptoms, their chronicity, and the circumstances under which they arose. Generally, the more stressful the precipitating situation, the less serious the neurosis. An amnesia occurring under prolonged battle conditions is less pathological than one which is precipitated by an unhappy job situation.

Case History: Dissociative Reaction

This twenty-two-year-old woman was picked up by the police in a railroad station after she had told them that she did not know who she was nor where she lived. She was unable to give the police any information about friends or relatives. At the time of admission the patient appeared physically healthy and was an attractive young woman, well dressed, pleasant, apparently co-operative, but unable to give any information in regard to her identity or past. She expressed some rather vague concern about her inability to remember anything and yet not in the degree which might be expected of one who neither knew who she was nor from where she had come. It almost appeared as if she was content to remain in the hospital and leave the solution of her problem to others. The patient remained essentially vague in her memory for two days. During this time she was given warm, understanding attention and encouragement by the staff and every attempt was made to help her recognize the kindly interest of those about her. She was helped to understand that the staff were interested in assisting her in her problems and would continue to try to help her with whatever difficulties presented themselves.

At the time of admission of this patient there had been some concern on the part of the staff as to the possibility of a severe degree of underlying psychopathology. Consequently a decision was made against the immediate use of intravenous sodium amytal to restore the patient's memory. The stuporous, mute, or presumably amnesic schizophrenic will sometimes react violently to relatively small doses of sodium amytal and therefore caution is used in administering this drug where the diagnosis has not been established.

This particular patient, by the end of about two days, began to remember a few isolated details about herself and by the end of the third day had been able to fill in most of the details of her past life. As she reconstructed the events leading up to her amnesia, she described herself as having had many guilty and self-depreciatory feelings. She had reached the point where, to her, things had become unbearable and so she had "blacked out."

A more complete history, as supplied by the patient over the next few days, revealed that she had been deprived of her mother's love at an early age through the latter's death. She had been placed in a foster home for two years where her treatment had been cold and unloving. Subsequently she had acquired an austere, uninterested stepmother who had never learned to love her and had always clearly shown animosity toward her. The stepmother rarely paid much attention to the patient, and whenever she did it was of a critical and negative type.

The patient grew up in an atmosphere presided over by the dominating stepmother, who forbade her the pleasures of the company of most other youngsters of her own age. She consequently remained alone and friendless throughout her developmental years. She was rejected and sharply criticized on many occasions by her father and, at an early age, found that it was impossible to please him no matter what she did. She received no support from him in her difficulties with her stepmother. During her middle adolescence the patient vowed that she would leave the parental home as soon as possible. At the age of sixteen she married in order to accomplish this. She had known her husband only a very short time and soon after the marriage he revealed himself to be an antisocial character with a criminal record. It was only a few months until he was again in difficulty with the law. The patient divorced him at this point and began looking frantically for another husband out of fear that she would not be able to make her way alone and would have to return to her parents.

She found another man, established a relationship with him, and subsequently agreed to live with him in the hope that he would eventually marry her. Soon, however, they quarreled and she attempted suicide by jumping in a river. She was rescued, but the man with whom she was living reproached her sadistically with the whole episode. It was at this point that she wandered out of the house and remembered nothing until her memory returned five weeks later in the hospital.

This patient remained in the hospital for two weeks following her memory return. During this time she had daily psychotherapeutic interviews and accomplished some solution of her difficulties. The patient began to develop a beginning understanding of her childish dependency on those about her. She also was encouraged in the direction of more mature solutions of her difficulties with her father and stepmother. She was encouraged to visit them a few times and to understand how, without her previous excessive dependency, she need not be as fearful of a relationship with these two people. The patient was also encouraged to begin building her own life and her own circle of friends. She was reassured that the interest and understanding of the physician, on whom she had become somewhat dependent, would continue after her discharge from the hospital in order to further effect a better adjustment on the outside.

While, at the time of discharge, this patient was by no means cured of her underlying immaturities and dependency, she nevertheless had achieved a much more efficient and stable adjustment. Her continued outpatient psychotherapy eventually resulted in still more improvement as well as final emancipation from the therapeutic situation and the development of sufficient ability to relate to other individuals and establish her own living pattern. The patient remained free of symptoms and satisfactorily adjusted.

CHAPTER 9

Phobic Reaction

PHOBIC reaction is a type of psychoneurosis characterized by the presence of one or more unexplained, severe, and unrealistic fears. Such an individual suffers extreme anxiety to the point of panic whenever he is confronted with the phobic situation. Phobias are much more common in the general population than is ordinarily suspected. Exaggerated fears of high places, animals, closed spaces, dirt, public speaking, and other phenomena are some of the most common examples. Many of them never come to the attention of a physician because the patient literally learns "to live with his fear." He avoids the phobic situation and thus remains comparatively free from anxiety. Medical attention is sought usually when a phobia develops which seriously incapacitates ability to carry on ordinary daily activities. However, a remarkable number of people so arrange their lives for years on end that they need never venture out on the street alone or ride in a public conveyance or attend a crowded function. These self-imposed limitations in order to avoid phobic situations become an integral part of the individual's life. He accepts them, plans his life around them, and in a great number of instances never seriously considers seeking medical help.

ETIOLOGY AND PSYCHOPATHOLOGY

The phobic mechanism is simply another neurotic method by which the individual attempts to deal with his underlying anxiety. The patient with anxiety reaction has more or less constant "free-floating" anxiety. The patient with a phobic reaction has, in a sense, "improved" his situation by focusing his anxiety on certain situations, animals, or things and by then avoiding them. The result is that such patients are often able to remain comparatively comfortable and free from anxiety as long as they avoid their phobic situations.

Phobias have been called the "normal neuroses of childhood" because of their almost ubiquitous appearance during this period of life. Most youngsters suffer at least a transitory phobia or two, with the greatest frequency during the fourth, fifth, and sixth years. It is at this time that the child is involved in his oedipal struggles and a phobia is an attempt to handle the generated anxiety. The youngster is disturbed by unconscious stirrings of feelings of rivalry toward the parent of the same sex. There is, on the other hand, within him a preponderance of love and affection toward this same parent. The little boy who is envious and jealous of his father's relationship with his mother nevertheless loves, admires, and is affectionate toward his father. In order to "solve" this uncomfortable situation of mixed feelings the anxiety engendered by the feelings toward the father becomes detached from the father and displaced onto some external object or situation, which can then be avoided. In this way the father can be more comfortably accepted by the youngster. The little boy may suddenly develop an exaggerated fear of dogs and refuse to go anywhere near one, even a friendly and harmless puppy. Phobias, particularly in children, may also concern things which exist only in fantasy. For instance, it is not uncommon to find a little girl, struggling with her negative oedipal feelings toward her mother, developing a fear that witches will visit her during the night.

The widespread occurrence of transient phobias during childhood is a phenomenon which owes its occurrence to the immaturity of the growing personality. The ego of the child, as yet incapable of mastering all instinctual impulses, is hard pressed to control oedipal strivings. It therefore follows that even the comparatively normal child, during the process of development, may resort to the pathological mechanism of phobia formation, without such a symptom necessarily indicating the degree of pathology which it would in an adult, whose ego is expected to have attained greater maturity. There are other youngsters, however, who develop more incapacitating, chronic phobias which may last for two or three years or even into adult life. Such children and adults are lacking in security. It is true that they have displaced some of their original fears of childhood onto objects and situations, but it is also true that their earliest years have lacked sufficient security to enable them to thoroughly and efficiently overcome and work through their early fears.

The history of a phobic patient will generally show what might be called emotional neglect during earliest childhood, as well as a lack of intuitive understanding on the part of the parents as to the basic needs for love, security, and stability of the infant. It is not unusual to find a history of overprotection which really represents an attempt on the part of the parents to compensate for a basic lack of concern for the child, as well as a difficulty in comfortably loving the child. Having been neglected from an emotional standpoint, such a child grows into a self-centered adult who cannot love others in a satisfactory manner. He is absorbed in self-love not because he deliberately sets out to become so, but because he has been forced to compensate for the lack of affection and interest from his parents in his earlier environment. Having had to look out for himself during his early years, he has grown up with defects in his ability to love and with exaggerated fears of the rebuffs which he assumes will be forthcoming if he loves. He has great needs for love but at the same time expects disappointment, and is, therefore, inwardly bitter and resentful. He resents his fellow men, who he feels do not sufficiently appreciate and love him, but cannot permit this resentment direct expression by the superego. Such a patient has mixed feelings of love and hate toward everyone. In his attempts to handle such difficult relationships the phobic mechanism is put into effect.

From a psychosexual standpoint such a patient often reveals anal characteristics, including obstinacy and ambivalence. On the other hand, he may resemble more closely the conversion-reaction type of personality. It is not unusual to find many oral characteristics in such a patient, evidenced by extreme dependency on those about him as well as by a general feeling that the world owes him a great deal. In summary, then, it may be said that the phobic patient ordinarily reveals residual oral, anal, and oedipal difficulties in his personality. His superego frequently prevents open expression of the resulting impulses and, in his attempt to handle his anxiety, he projects his difficulty onto an outward object, situation, or place. He then attempts to avoid this object, situation, or place, but if he is confronted with it his anxiety is stirred to a paniclike state.

SYMPTOMATOLOGY

The phobia, as mentioned, is an exaggerated and unrealistic fear. A typical example is the young woman who has a phobia of riding in elevators. She is unable to give any clear explanation of what she fears. She is only aware that whenever she enters an elevator and the doors are closed she becomes panicky. She ordinarily avoids every situation which might require entering an elevator. She would rather climb many flights of stairs than ride in an elevator. Should circumstances dictate the necessity of her riding in one, she becomes extremely apprehensive and fearful. She feels closed in, unable to catch her breath, certain that the elevator will plunge to the bottom of the building, or certain that it will become stuck between floors, trapping her.

There are innumerable possible phobias and only some of the more common ones need be mentioned here. *Claustrophobia,* a fear of enclosed spaces, is one of the most common. A person suffering from this symptom is unable to remain in a closed room or confining space unless, perhaps, he is sitting or standing near an open door and realizes that he may make his exit at any time. However, if he finds himself in a situation where all the exits are closed or where he would create a noticeable disturbance if he should attempt to leave, he then begins to suffer marked anxiety. Such a person can attend a theater as long as he sits near the back of the theater and in a seat next to the aisle, where it is possible for him to leave at any time. The mere recognition that he may leave often is sufficient to forestall the development of anxiety. The essential underlying difficulty is that there is an inner awareness on the part of the patient that he must control his own impulses, while he is sufficiently insecure about his ability to do so to cause him considerable anxiety. If one were to ask such a patient what impulses he fears in a theater, he would not be able to give a clear answer, but would only state that he knows he feels safe if he is certain that there is an opportunity to leave whenever he wishes.

Agoraphobia, a fear of open spaces, is also extremely common. An agoraphobic patient is unable to venture out on the street alone. He also is unable to give any clear reasons for his fear. His childish insecurity is allayed and he feels comfortable only if he has someone accompanying him. He often fears that he will faint or that some unpleasant thing will occur to him which he will not be able to manage unless accompanied by someone. He may, for instance, fear the possibility of heart attack and feel that he will probably die on the street unless accompanied by a friend. Such a patient, like the claustrophobe, fears his own inner, childish impulses. The agoraphobe fears his exhibitionistic and other sexual impulses, as well as the expected hostility of the people in the world. It is as if he feels that he cannot control himself if alone, nor can he save himself from the expected punishment. He feels, inwardly, that the added presence of a more mature ego than his own will save him from giving way to his inner impulses and therefore also from punishment from the hostile world.

While it is possible for an individual to be phobic about almost anything, the basic underlying mechanism is very similar in all phobias. They represent the patient's inner insecurity and conflict. His anxiety is bound to the phobic situation, and if that situation can be avoided, he may make a superficially satisfactory adjustment. There is often a similarity in characteristics between the phobic patient and the conversion patient. They both often appear outwardly to be friendly, warm, attractive people. However, continued association with them usually brings to light their childishness, immaturity, selfishness, and general insecurity. This superficial attractiveness and geniality is a sort of outer layer which these individuals do not ordinarily maintain with close relatives and friends. At home they are prone to be moody, inarticulate, and aloof, and they know little of the simpler joys of living and little of the potential security that lies in close friendships with and trust in others.

As the phobic defense reaction spreads and becomes more severe, it begins to include more situations and things. The patient loses himself in preoccupation with himself and his own problems and his own state of mind. Eventually many of these patients literally limit themselves to their own homes, avoiding people, avoiding the outside world, and avoiding work. They become increasingly dependent upon those about them and yet more difficult to please. All of this makes a vicious circle because, although the patient is seeking security, his own tendency to be wrapped up within himself prevents others from providing even a minimum of his sought-for security.

A word should be mentioned here about the hostile element of a phobic reaction. The patient, by virtue of his incapacitation, often immobilizes those closest to him and warps their lives as well as his own. A housewife who is unable to shop, unable to answer the door, fearful of the telephone, or phobic about entertaining guests may constantly harass her husband with innumerable and unreasonable requests. She may require that he come home from the office to quiet her anxiety. She may find herself developing a panic if she attempts to go out, and "solve" this by requiring her husband to be her chauffeur constantly. Such patients are ordinarily completely unaware of the underlying hostile element in their phobic living pattern.

TREATMENT

The formation of a phobia itself is, in a sense, the patient's own attempt at self-treatment. He has, by virtue of his use of the phobic mechanism, been able to tether his free-floating, and bothersome anxiety and literally fix it upon certain objects, situations, places, or animals. Then, as long as he can avoid these, he remains relatively free from anxiety. He has traded chronic anxiety for the necessity of avoiding certain things in order to escape even more severe anxiety. Should the patient be able to avoid these situations, he will probably not seek psychiatric or medical help.

As with many other neurotic conditions, the whole pathological structure in phobia is comparatively inefficient and must be constantly reinforced and expanded lest it collapse completely. Phobic patients, as their responsibilities and duties increase, often meet these difficulties with new phobias. The adolescent who is still attending school, dependent upon his parents, and comparatively free from responsibility may be without symptoms although he is basically a phobic individual. As the years pass and he gets a job, marries, begins to raise a family, and develops many other responsibilities, his inefficient personality structure begins to break down. He becomes phobic first about one thing and subsequently about others. When and if the new phobias interfere with the patient's ability to continue a reasonable adjustment, he usually seeks psychiatric help.

The physician who wishes to help a phobic patient must first evaluate the total life situation and personality of the patient. Often the content of the phobias themselves will give clues as to the inner difficulties of the patient. A little girl, for instance, who is phobic about witches is probably having great difficulty with ambivalent, mixed feelings toward her mother. The young woman in her twenties who is fearful of being on the street alone is probably struggling with her own inner confusion about exhibitionistic and sexual tendencies, as well as prohibitions in these directions and lacks a confident conscience.

The phobic patient, like any other neurotic, is still struggling in his adult life with conflictual feelings set up during his childhood. The woman who is phobic about leaving her home without her husband has mixed feelings toward him which, in a sense, have been carried through the years from their origin in mixed feelings perhaps toward her father. It is obviously necessary for the physician to get a fairly clear picture of the patient's present-day life and feelings, as well as those which were prevalent earlier in the patient's life.

Another important element which must always play a role in the treatment of a phobic patient is that of *secondary gain*. This is the additional satisfaction which the patient receives as a result of the symptom. The phobic woman, for instance, who is unable to venture out without her husband requires his frequent presence and attention and therefore, in a sense, gains from her symptom. Wherever the family attitudes allow the secondary gain to reach large proportions therapy of the phobia is difficult. The physician must take care never to require that the rest of the family adopt a negative or punitive attitude toward the patient because of a neurotic symptom. On the other hand, the patient should not be allowed to completely warp the lives of the remaining family members merely because of an illness. As long as the patient can force others or require others to conform to his phobic structure, he will never suffer anxiety and therefore has little motivation to seek help. Remaining family members should be encouraged to lead reasonably independent and individual lives even though this may mean occasional anxiety in the patient. The latter must begin to recognize the reality of the situation and therefore acquire more reason to seek help in ameliorating it.

The physician who has accomplished an improved family attitude also, of course, orients himself to helping the patient understand the origins and meaning of his phobia. Discussions delving into the patient's background, into relationships with others both past and present, are an integral part of the treatment. The patient is helped to understand that his particular phobia, perhaps fear of an open street, is not literally about the street itself, but about his own insecurity and difficulty in managing his childish impulses. Through friendly, kind, and patient understanding, most patients will begin to hazard a contact with their phobic situation. This is continually urged and advised by the physician, although not demanded. The patient is helped to see that although his phobia is an example of psychopathology it is not limited to one particular area but is a result of an over-all living and relating problem that encompasses all of his life.

PROGNOSIS

The prognosis in phobic reaction varies according to several factors. The more numerous the phobias, in general, the poorer the ultimate prognosis. Such patients tend, except with extensive treatment, to form new phobias as existing ones are eradicated. The factor which might be called the "reality element" is also of importance prognostically. The patient with a phobia of large black dogs is probably not as ill as the one who has a phobia of dinosaurs. One fear has more reality to it than the other. Similarly, if two patients have phobias of horses, the healthier patient is the one who was kicked or bitten by a horse while the sicker one has had no contact with horses at all. Prognosis is also influenced by degree of incapacitation and the patient's attitude toward it. Some patients passively accept marked limitations in their lives due to phobias and make little effort to seek help. Some have suffered with phobias since childhood and seem to consider this abnormality a necessary and integral part of their existence. Also prognostically important is secondary gain. The more the persistent secondary gain the worse the prognosis. In general, phobic reaction, unless quite severe because of excessive immaturity and lack of imagination, responds fairly well to adequate treatment.

Case History (1): Phobic Reaction

This thirty-one-year-old married woman, mother of three children, was referred to a psychiatrist by her family physician. She had come to him complaining of an inability to travel alone or even be alone. At such times she developed a feeling of faintness and paniclike anxiety. In addition, she said that she was quite depressed, often with a feeling of the worthlessness of her own life. She had been examined thoroughly and nothing organically wrong was discovered in this examination; therefore she was referred for psychiatric treatment.

The patient, as she presented herself in the initial interview, was a potentially attractive young woman. However, she had given comparatively little attention to her appearance and, as a result, presented a picture of general sloppiness and untidiness. She seemed quite unhappy but extremely anxious to launch forth into her story of numerous complaints and difficulties. She felt, it seemed, that her entire life had been difficult and that many other people had been responsible for her unhappiness. Her history revealed that her mother had died when she was two years of age, and she had been subsequently raised by an aunt. This aunt, a sister of her mother, had overindulged her to a remarkable degree and had never made any effort to have the patient face even the average amount of reality in living. The patient's father had similarly overindulged her and yet, at the same time, had attempted to exercise strict control over her behavior. The result had been a sheltered and yet dominated existence to which the patient reacted with considerable rebellion. She had managed to make a marginal adjustment throughout school, even though she was obviously endowed with much greater ability than she showed. She had never worked at any single task for any great length of time, nor had she particularly enjoyed any type of duty which involved the expenditure of labor on her part.

The patient had married at the age of twenty-four and, following this, had continued to be quite sloppy about her home and her own personal appearance. She was capable of dressing up and enhancing her attractiveness on special occasions, but never felt it necessary to do so within the confines of her own home. She took little pleasure in her house and was a nagging, unhappy, and resentful mother. She had always been, and continued to be, a very shallow person. Even during college she had read only what was required and had shown little interest in this. Her primary enthusiasm was in the scandals of her immediate friends and neighborhood and in the doings of prominent people in the entertainment world. She had undue respect for those who were exceedingly wealthy or had been overwhelmingly successful in some other field. She had little if any concern for ordinary people whom she might meet in her everyday living.

Essentially this patient was an empty person, relating poorly to other people, interested primarily in herself. She could be described as egocentric and narcissistic. It took several sessions in psychotherapy before she began to see that she was extremely self-centered. She had previously assumed that she was sick and that the illness had subsequently given her a personality disturbance. Actually, of course, it soon became clear to her that her original personality disorder had resulted in her symptoms. She was gradually helped to see that the effect of her early life environment upon her ways of thinking and acting had resulted in her present-day difficulties. She was helped to take a more altruistic interest in her home, her children, her neighbors, and the community about her. She became conscious of a great deal of hostility against her early environment, particularly her parents. She began to see how their basic uninterest and overprotection had warped her view of relating to other people. At several points during psychotherapy she expressed difficulty in understanding how the physician could show any interest in her, since she herself had little interest in him. She frequently complained that she was unable to understand how other people were friendly with each other when basically, to her, it seemed as if there were no value in this. Eventually she began to understand that the physician's interest in her, as well as that of many others, was of a basically friendly nature, and that she herself could gain some pleasure from responding to it with equal friendliness. A long period of treatment, aimed at modifying this shallow, self-centered personality, resulted in ameliorating many of her fears concerning traveling and being alone. She gradually began to learn some of the fundamental rewards which accrue to an altruistic type of living. She began to enjoy her children and take an interest in their growth and development. She began to see her husband as an individual who had needs and wants of his own. It became evident to her slowly that her early childhood insecurity, produced through the loss of her mother, had enhanced her later desire to control her father. This had resulted in a remarkable degree of need to control. This need she had taken out on her husband and children with a great show of domination. However, as her insight increased, her ability to relate to other people in a friendly manner improved and she eventually learned to like other people sincerely. She began to take a more useful part in her own home and in community activities. As she did so, she received a certain amount of pleasure in the improved relationships that she achieved. She began to look upon her therapist as an example of more mature behavior and began to seek his advice and counsel in matters regarding her own life.

Essentially, it had been necessary initially to help this patient understand that her own adjustment was lacking in many respects. Then, of course, she needed to understand what maturity means and to begin to desire to move in this direction. Having seen the defects in her personality, she was gradually able to remedy them with resulting confidence and an improved sense of well-being. As her relationships with others improved, the need for her own symptoms subsided and then disappeared.

Case History (2): Phobic Reaction

This thirty-six-year-old married accountant recognized the presence within himself of emotional difficulties and asked for psychiatric treatment. He presented himself to the psychiatrist complaining that he was an extremely nervous person most of the time and that he had found himself recently becoming increasingly irritable. Also of great concern to him was his fear of heights. This fear had reached the point where he was unable to go into a tall building even though he assiduously avoided looking out windows, and therefore had no visual concept of his distance from the ground. The windows themselves held special fears for him even though he might see them only at a distance. He said, "When you have a nightmare you dream of falling from a window. When I'm in a high building, I feel as if I'm doing that even though I'm awake. I look at the window and even if I'm not close to it I'm afraid that I'll fall out." He went on to describe how he remained in a state of chronic anxiety most of the time and had great difficulty even falling asleep. He said that his fear of heights had become particularly marked during the past six months.

Further history elicited during the initial interview revealed that the patient had been an only child of parents who had separated when he was ten years of age. He had continued to live with his mother following the separation until he had finally married at the age of twenty-six. He had been in his present occupation for about six years and had become progressively dissatisfied with it. His job required a great deal more education than he had had. As a result, there was a constant pressure on him to do more and better work of a type for which he was ill prepared. He had tried in every way to meet the standards that were outlined for him but had always fallen short of them.

His marriage had been fairly satisfactory for only a short time and had then become an increasing source of irritation to him, particularly because his wife made more demands upon him than he was able to fulfill. She had criticized the fact that he had not advanced with sufficient rapidity, nor had he made enough money to satisfy her. He had finally reached the state where he felt reasonably comfortable only during the time that it took him to get from work to home or from home to work.

The patient went on to describe how he had always had a tendency to be irritated with minor matters and to show a temper at inconsequential things during his early life. He felt that he had been spoiled as a child, particularly by his mother. His parents had never gotten along well; he had always sided with his mother and had been quite close to her. However, his mother had always been critical of him and had demanded more from him than he was able to produce. He said, "I think my main trouble is that I don't know what I want in life. I try so hard to do something to prove to my family that I can. I was always told that I wasn't good enough at home. Mother even told me that I was too dumb to marry. All these years I've worked to prove that she was wrong. I have worked hard and now I finally get to the point that I have a good job, but I'm still bragging and trying to be something that I'm not. I try to do the right thing, but I always hit a stone wall. Everybody likes me, but I still can't have any fun. I can't relax. I'm very sensitive. I feel other people's feelings. I'm sensitive of hurting other people and yet I still fly off the handle once in a while. When I blow up I'm exhausted and I'm tired and I feel badly afterward."

This patient was seen for approximately thirty-five therapeutic interviews at weekly intervals. Some of the pertinent material which emerged showed clearly that he was unable to relate in a satisfactory, comfortable manner to his superiors. It seemed that they all liked him but he nevertheless harbored considerable resentment against them. However, as he said, "I don't show it." He went on to say, "Lots of times I'd like to tell them off but I don't. I always talk nicely to them. I treat others as I want them to treat me, but they still push me around."

It was during the fourth interview that the patient mentioned the difficulties that he was having with his wife in the sexual sphere. He had begun, during the past few months, to be impotent. This was a culmination of a long accumulation of resentment toward his wife, who had forced him to practice coitus interruptus. He had not thoroughly discussed with his wife the possibility of the use of contraceptives but, because of her desire to avoid pregnancy, she had insisted on his practicing withdrawal. He seemed to feel that his wife nagged him a great deal and demanded more of him than was reasonable or than he was capable of producing.

By the sixth interview the patient elaborated more material in regard to his mother. He said, "I love her whatever I say. I could never live with her—she is too domineering. She bossed me all my life until I broke away and got married. No one could live with her. You can't even talk in her presence." The patient's mother and wife thoroughly disliked each other and he was unable to mediate the conflict successfully. He remained more or less in the middle and refused to take sides. On the one hand he felt guilty about having left his mother, and yet was worried that she might live with him and his wife. On the other hand, he felt himself unable to side with his wife and back her in her more reasonable demands against his dominating mother.

It was about this time in therapy that the patient elaborated some of his relationships at work. He had been transferred to another department under a new supervisor about the time that his symptoms became more acute. His new boss was a more authoritarian individual than his previous boss had been. The patient described the new supervisor as a "dirty, rotten, sneaking person, who would cut his own mother's throat if he thought it would do him any good." The patient went on to say, "I think he's trying to get me out of that department by beating me down, but I'm outfoxing him." In his relationships with his new boss the patient had adopted a quite passive attitude and had rarely shown any aggression or rebelliousness. As he said, "I bend over backwards in politeness to him."

The therapeutic process involved the patient's repeated discussions of his relationships with his wife, his mother, and his coworkers, particularly his superiors. He was gradually helped to see that he, first of all, had harbored considerable resentment toward his mother for her dominating, authoritative attitude. He had been forced to relegate the majority of this resentment to his unconscious and had forbidden himself expression of it. His guilt about having this resentment within himself gradually diminished as he brought it forth during treatment. In addition, he was helped to see how in many ways he had recreated the same situation with his wife. He had assumed a more or less passive role with her and then had accused her of being the same dominating, authoritative person that his mother had been. Actually his wife did have some tendencies in this direction but they were markedly enhanced by his own need to literally force upon her all the aggressive actions of the marriage. At work a somewhat similar situation occurred, particularly in relation to his superiors. He adopted an ingratiating attitude and continued to build up an increasing reservoir of unconscious resentment against his bosses.

This, of course, was intensified when he transferred to a boss who was truly a dominating person. The patient was helped to see how this neurotic pattern worked in his relationships to the therapist. He adopted a similar sort of ingratiating attitude toward the therapist and treated him as if he were a demanding, authoritative person. Numerous situations arose during treatment which revealed to the physician, and subsequently to the patient, the latter's degree of unconscious hostility. Such matters as the forgetting of appointments, coming late, and "forgetting" to pay fees were examples used to gradually help the patient understand his resentment toward the therapist.

As the patient became more aware of his resentment, and at the same time, less guilty about it, he was subsequently able to express it in more reasonable ways. His condition concurrently improved and his phobias diminished. His original phobias could be thought of as his actual fear of his own inner pent-up resentments. As these found release through the therapeutic process, the need for the symptoms gradually diminished.

CHAPTER 10

Obsessive-Compulsive Reaction

THE OBSESSIVE-COMPULSIVE reaction is a type of psychoneurosis in which the patient suffers from unwelcome repetitive ideas or impulses to perform ritualistic acts. Such a patient, for instance, may be tormented by recurrent blasphemous or obscene thoughts or by the need to perform apparently useless acts such as touching certain objects in a ritualistic way, dressing in a particular order, counting doors or steps, or some other such similar gesture. The repetitious thoughts are called *obsessions;* the actions are called *compulsions.* While the patient may realize these thoughts or actions are irrational, he must continue them in order to relieve emotional tension.

The frequency of mild obsessive or compulsive rituals in the general population is much higher than is ordinarily believed. Even superstition falls within this general category. Such things as knocking on wood, throwing salt over one's shoulder, or avoiding walking under a ladder are examples of minor and usually nonincapacitating obsessive-compulsive reactions. Particularly during childhood, in the age group of seven to perhaps eleven, these things are seen with a remarkable frequency. As long as such simple acts or thoughts do not seriously disturb the individual's efficiency, productivity, or love life, they are relatively innocuous. However, if they are magnified and involve much of his daily experience, they can become tremendously incapacitating and interfere seriously with everything he tries to do.

ETIOLOGY AND PSYCHOPATHOLOGY

The obsessive-compulsive reaction stems primarily from difficulties encountered in childhood, particularly during the anal phase. It can best be understood by reviewing the various characteristics of the anal phase and the way the child behaves during this period. The youngster from perhaps one to four years of age is first and foremost ambivalent. By that is meant that he loves when he hates and hates when he loves. He has not yet reached the level of psychosexual development where he can truly be said to love someone. To clarify this, one need only watch a three-year-old with his mother for a short period of time. He accepts, enjoys, and at times even seems to return some of the warmth which she shows him, only in a few moments to be furious with her because she has frustrated a desire of his or made a demand upon him. One senses very clearly that in his relationship with his mother he is the important person and he places his gratification far above hers. The three-year-old girl who is very maternal with her little brother will, a few moments later, show great hostility to him because of something he has done to one of her toys. Such unstable relationships as these, which alternate from obviously positive feelings to severely negative ones, are characteristic and normal at this age. Only gradually during the next few years do relationships begin to reach a more stable and mature level.

The child during this phase is also greedy. Proof of this can easily be obtained by giving two three-year-olds one toy between them. Each will claim it for his own with little regard for the rights of the other. Obstinacy, sadism, messiness, and rebelliousness are other characteristics prevalent in youngsters of this age. In addition, these children show a particular interest in their functions of excretion and gain pleasure from both withholding and evacuating. Such characteristics as these are accepted as being normal during the anal phase. At the same time, however, parents begin to require some conformity from a child to the rules and regulations of society. If parental methods of teaching the child are properly mixed with a sufficient amount of love, the youngster slowly begins to bring under control his impulses to wet and soil and to be generally untidy, and he goes through a slow metamorphosis to the next phase, where he is capable of more stable relationships and more useful and acceptable pursuits. He reaches this next phase much more easily if he is loved and praised than if he is coerced and scolded. If the parental method of teaching is too rapid or punitive or if it is mixed with insufficient love, all of these anal characteristics are perpetuated within the core of the personality of the growing child. A youngster then literally does not get a chance to be loving or cooperatively friendly but feels imposed upon and does things from a cold sense of duty.

If we were magically to transpose this youngster into an adult, leaving these same characteristics, we would find a truly obnoxious person. The obsessive, as an adult, has these characteristics within him and much of his neurosis is built around his defensive efforts to keep them under control. He has set up a multitude of rigid defenses against their ever being expressed. In other words, he develops symptoms in order to keep his undomesticated, punitive, hostile, and unacceptable impulses concealed even from himself. At the same time the symptoms often secretly express some gratification of those drives.

This leads to a discussion of the various mechanisms of defense which the ego of the obsessive patient uses to prevent expression of unacceptable urges. The first is that of *isolation,* which, as mentioned elsewhere, is a separation of the idea from its associated affect, with a subsequent repression of the affect or its expression at some later time. The ultimate result is that ideas appear consciously without their true emotional counterparts and make the individual seem "cold" and lacking the ordinary warmth and emotional flexibility that is associated with most people.

One of the results is that such patients can often remember far back into childhood but their memories are essentially without the appropriate degree of emotion. This is in marked contrast to the typical conversion-reaction patient who utilizes repression and in whom both the idea and the affect are relegated to the unconscious. For instance, one young man with a severe obsessional reaction was able to remember quite clearly all of the details of an incident which occurred when he was five years of age, at which time an adolescent girl had engaged in some sex play with him. From his description it was obvious that the incident had been quite an emotional one and he himself admitted that it was strange that as he thought about it he had no emotion at all. Only gradually, over a long period of time during treatment, did all of the original feelings become reattached to this incident. Had this young man been of a conversion or dissociative reaction type, he might well have converted the conflict into a physical symptom or not have remembered either the emotion or the incident.

Closely allied to the mechanism of isolation is another called *intellectualization*. This refers to the patient's tendency to try to reduce everything to intellectual processes devoid of all emotion. Everything which occurs to him, or to which he gives consideration, is subject to the cold logical scrutiny of the intellect and, as much as possible, divorced from all emotional components. The typical obsessive patient during psychotherapy prides himself upon his extensive knowledge of psychiatric principles and is often able to quote at length from various books he has read or statements he has heard concerning these matters. Generally speaking, however, although the material that he quotes is quite accurate, it means little to him because it is only intellectual knowledge and he is devoid of real feeling about it.

Another important mechanism of ego defense characteristic of the obsessive patient is that of *reaction formation*. This type of defense involves the covering of original unacceptable infantile urges with a more superficial characterological attitude which is usually just the opposite of the original one and is oriented toward preventing expression of it. Instead of showing sadism, for instance, such a patient is apt to show an ingratiating type of behavior. Instead of snarling and berating others, the obsessive will be obsequious and polite. However, in the end his cruelty and hostility make themselves felt. Such patients literally show an *overcompensation* in the opposite direction from their underlying unacceptable urges. Instead of being excessively dirty, they become excessively neat and clean. They do not reveal a preference for disorder and disarray, but a tendency to perfectionism and meticulousness.

Finally, another mechanism of ego defense characteristic of the obsessive patient is that of *undoing*. The use of this particular mechanism rests upon the individual's belief in the omnipotence of his thoughts. He is like the little child who has a belief that his own thoughts have some magical power which will bring forth by themselves certain results in the outside world. A similar magical quality is also attributed to certain ritualistic acts by the adult obsessive patient. Therefore, whenever an unacceptable urge arising within the id reaches the level of conscious thought or symbolic action, the compulsive patient feels the need to perform a ritualistic action or to think in such a way as to magically negate or neutralize the first impulse and hence the entire situation. For instance, in the patient who consciously recognizes, even though without emotion, a hostile impulse toward a presumably loved parent, there arises a tendency to neutralize this with a positive loving thought and thus "undo" the original thought.

Of major importance in an understanding of the obsessive-compulsive reaction is a consideration of the superego. The superego of the compulsive patient may be characterized as rigid, punitive, and tyrannical. His ego is constantly threatened with guilt by the superego lest it transgress the rules and regulations laid down by the conscience. One most often finds that the obsessive person grew up in a house in which rigidity was prevalent. Rules and regulations had to be followed. The parents were generally unloving and overly demanding. Too much was asked too soon from the child, and he was forced to bring under control his early childish urges in order to conform to his parents' rigid standards and gain whatever little acceptance he could find. He was generally denied any overt expressions of childish desires and was early made to feel, in a punitive way, that such desires were unacceptable and unexpressible. The obsessive's superego is an internalization of his concept of his parents. No matter how hard he tried, he could not please his parents, nor can he ever completely please his conscience. Both parents and conscience have always been ready with criticism and lacking in acceptance and warmth.

Therefore, in summary, we see that the obsessive patient is inwardly urged toward messiness, rebelliousness, stinginess, and all of the other anal characteristics, yet his rigid puritanical superego forbids expression of even the slightest tendency in these directions. His ego, therefore, is hard put to maintain intrapsychic peace and resorts to the various mechanisms of defense which have been described. The result is a cold individual leading a rigid, constricted, unemotional life, often filled with numerous ritualistic thoughts and actions. While most of his overt behavior is evidence of the rigid defenses, occasionally one finds certain small areas where the underlying unconscious urge is breaking through. This is possible when the resulting behavior is not of a kind which will incur the wrath of the conscience to produce guilt. For instance, an original interest in excretions may eventually reveal itself in the adult tendency to prolong time at stool. The childhood stingy, greedy attitude may be perpetuated in the adult in a similar tendency to hold on to his money. It may also include the same attitude toward giving and sharing of material things. An adult who is meticulous and perfectionistic about his mode of dress may have perhaps one item of clothing which he wears until it is filthy. Likewise, the ingratiating, superficially pleasant obsessive patient occasionally shows an outburst of temper which approaches a ragelike reaction typical of the very small child and shows large elements of the original sadistic urge.

SYMPTOMATOLOGY

The classical symptoms of this type of psychoneurosis are obsessions and compulsions. The former are repetitively recurring thoughts which the individual feels in some way compelled to have and over which he has little voluntary control. Obsessional ideas vary greatly in their content. They may represent either the unconscious unacceptable urge from which all emotion has been removed or an opposite type of thought used magically to counteract the unacceptable one. In either case the patient is aware only that his ritualistic thinking must be adhered to lest he suffer some terrible but unknown danger. Numerous examples of obsessive thinking are to be found in the patient's unwelcome thoughts about his parents, for instance. He may be tormented by recurring thoughts concerning harm coming to one of his "beloved" parents, for whom, at least unconsciously, he harbors considerable hostility. If, on the other hand, his defences are more successful, such a thought may be prevented or neutralized by a similarly obsessive thought concerning his great love for this "beloved" parent.

Compulsions are similar to obsessions but involve, instead of thought, the performance of a ritualistic act, to which the patient attributes some magical quality. He feels as if the performance of the act will in some strange way prevent an unknown catastrophe of which he is fearful. Compulsions vary like obsessions in their content but stem similarly either from the unconscious unacceptable urge or the more or less magical attempts to defend against it. Often compulsive rituals may contain both of these elements. For instance, the patient who must turn the gas jets on and off several times before he can finally convince himself that they are safely shut off is thereby, on the one hand, giving partial expression to his sadistic, destructive impulses, and at the same time denying them. Other compulsive rituals such as repetitive handwashing are primarily symbolic, magical attempts to "wash away sin" as a result of a severe conscience. It is a sort of a washing away of the dirtiness inside or a decontamination of the aggressive impulse to soil or contaminate.

Generally speaking, the unacceptable impulses with which the compulsive struggles belong to two categories. One is the aggressive, sadistic, destructive type and the other the sexual type; since both are present in the unconscious, we ordinarily find a mixture of the two being warded off by the obsessive patient. The subjects in the outer world with which the obsessions and compulsions deal are ordinarily those which have the strongest mores and codes of ethics surrounding them. For instance, parents are supposed to be loved. Sexuality is to be reserved for certain special and restricted situations and religion is to be accepted unconditionally. The compulsive often finds himself with obsessions concerning negative thoughts about his parents, thoughts about sexual excesses or perversions, and blasphemous thoughts about his religion.

The obsessive patient may be looked upon as having an inwardly childish, sadistic, rebellious nature. Outwardly he has surrounded this with a rigid set of defenses which present to the world the opposite picture, namely that of perfectionism, meticulousness, and ingratiation. From time to time elements of the inner childishness break through, usually devoid of their emotions. The compulsive then tries to deal with them as if by magic, utilizing his mechanism of undoing. Such a patient is ordinarily a worrisome individual, and pessimistic in his outlook. He has been described as ruminative because of his tendency to be excessively doubtful and continuously to think over and over various issues. Such doubtfulness can reach extreme proportions where the patient is unable to make up his mind even about minor matters. Each decision is subjected to long, involved, and usually pointless intellectual processes. As a patient reveals a more severe degree of this type of psychoneurosis, his daily activity becomes increasingly encumbered with obsessions and compulsions, to the point where he is able to accomplish very little. In the milder forms of the neurosis the person is ambitious, striving, and hard working. He drives himself in his work in order to achieve a perfectionistic level, being certain that even the most minute details that he performs are correct. Obviously, such diligence and hard work often result in attainment of a higher position. This then usually requires the individual's delegation of some authority. It is at this point that he runs into difficulty. He is unable to delegate responsibility to those beneath him lest they not accomplish their tasks in his perfectionistic way. He drives himself harder and harder in order to accomplish the tasks himself and eventually, when this becomes impossible, he is overwhelmed by anxiety.

Perhaps the most obvious examples of this process were seen in the last war when certain obsessive individuals, because of their attention to detail and need to do everything perfectly, were promoted rapidly. As a noncommissioned officer, such a soldier could often oversee all the details of each man under him. However, as he rose through the ranks and achieved a higher rating, it soon became impossible for him to take care of all the details himself. Such individuals, in an attempt to achieve the impossible, became extremely anxious. Such things, for instance, as spot checks became impossible because they did not meet the standards of the compulsive. Finally the only possible outcome was a complete breakdown of the rigid compulsive mechanism with a marked increase in anxiety and subsequent hospitalization.

The obsessive patient's personality, stemming as it does primarily from the anal phase of psychosexual development, is marked not only by ambivalence but also by what may be termed *bisexuality*. At the time of life during which the anal phase is ordinarily predominant, namely two, three, or four years of age, a youngster is really not thoroughly masculine or feminine but has, in a sense, elements of both sexes. He is, so to speak, bisexual.

The obsessive adult patient, having encountered difficulties during the anal phase, still retains these elements of bisexuality. He has never been able to reach the level of psychosexual development where he can be said to love someone truly. For love, in the broad sense, requires tenderness, permissiveness, and a capacity to identify with the feelings or emotional needs of others. The obsessive patient has had to invest so much effort in keeping the impulses of the anal period in check, in concealment, that is, that he has not been able to develop mature heterosexual interests. Therefore, though convention may draw him toward marriage, he lacks the ability to love one of the opposite sex fully and he remains bisexual rather than becoming predominately heterosexual.

This does not mean necessarily that he indulges in homosexual as well as heterosexual relationships. It means merely that the burden of conscience put upon him in relation to his oral, and particularly anal, impulses has forced certain love-making fantasies to appear around portions of the body beyond the genital area and has reduced his capacity for normal heterosexual pleasure. To put it another way, he has been led to feel that the psychological trends associated with toilet training, such as duty, punctuality, cleanliness, and order, are more important than love.

TREATMENT

The treatment of the obsessive patient is, as with any other psychoneurotic, oriented toward giving him an understanding of his inner problems in order to help him achieve a more mature level of adjustment. As mentioned previously, these particular patients have, in a sense, a problem stemming from two directions within their psychic structures. Unconsciously, from the id, come infantile anal, sadistic urges striving for expression. Cruelty, messiness, stinginess, and other such qualities are constantly pushing toward the consciousness. On the other hand, harsh prohibitions toward such expressions stem constantly from the tyrannical, punitive, dominating, authoritative conscience which these patients possess. The ego is obviously caught between these opposing forces. The therapist aligns himself with the ego of such patients, constantly attempting to enlarge and strengthen the ego structure itself by making the ego better acquainted with the nature of the id and softening the severity of the superego.

The greatest difficulty in the treatment of obsessive patients lies in the particular mechanisms which they utilize. Isolation involves the separation of an idea from its affect and the relegation of the affect to the unconscious. This, of course, means that there will be a lack of true human warmth in the interpersonal relationship of the obsessive and that he will attempt to deal with everything and everyone on an intellectual basis, which also, unfortunately, holds true in the therapeutic process. The obsessive patient who has read extensively from psychiatric literature and who quotes from such writings wishes without clearly recognizing it, to make psychotherapy another intellectual exercise. Such patients tend to keep the relationship between themselves and the therapist devoid of any emotional display and will, wherever possible, become involved in long, complicated intellectual discussions of their problems. Such tendencies must repeatedly be brought to their attention, especially from the standpoint of the lack of normal affect.

This can most easily be accomplished in situations where one would expect the ordinary individual to have a good deal of emotion and where the patient has little if any. For instance, if a patient has been unavoidably kept waiting for a period of time and then appears for the interview showing no signs of resentment, and seeming to accept the entire situation without emotion, it can be called to his attention that this does not seem to be what might be expected. Ordinarily a person would be rather irritated in this situation and it can be shown to the patient how his own irritation does not reveal itself, perhaps even to himself. At times the patient may tell, during therapy, of occurrences of a type that would have resulted in a great deal of emotion in the ordinary person, but cause the patient little or none. It frequently takes a great deal of laborious work to break down gradually the patient's tendency to use the mechanism of isolation and make him more aware of what is really going on in the way of feelings within him.

Similar handling is often required in regard to the defensive mechanism of reaction formation. Here again, it can repeatedly be called to the patient's attention how his attitude seems to remain essentially the same regardless of external circumstance. He is superficially pleasant, ingratiating, and seemingly altruistic in every situation, even those that would ordinarily lead to resentment or some other reaction. In due time, as these things are repeatedly brought to his attention, he slowly begins to absorb their true meaning and to allow some beginning expression of his own feelings.

Obsessions and compulsions are dealt with by slowly leading the patient into discussions of the various important people in his life, both past and present. As such discussions proceed, the more unconscious feelings that a patient has toward these particular figures usually become more evident, at least to the therapist. Also, the patient's severe superego prohibitions against such feelings become increasingly obvious and can be slowly and understandingly pointed out to the patient. If, as is so often true, the obsessions or compulsions deal directly or indirectly with some of these important figures, the therapist and the patient can gain a clearer understanding of the dynamics involved and can make the changes necessary in the direction of personality help.

For example, one fourteen-year-old girl who had a severe obsessional reaction became preoccupied with obsessive thoughts that she hated her mother. These thoughts she subsequently had to counteract by an undoing process of thoughts of great love for her mother. In discussions with her about her mother it soon became evident that the latter was a very overprotective, dominating, authoritative woman who allowed the patient little if any freedom. As the discussions progressed the patient became more and more aware of how differently her mother treated her from the way her friends' mothers treated them. At the same time she saw how she had always been unable to show any overt irritation toward her mother, and yet on the other hand, her friends had always been able to show some toward their mothers, at least on occasions. As she became less guilty about her hostility and sensed that the therapist would not be critical of it, she began to express a little bit of resentment toward her own mother. As this occurred and the therapist did not disapprove, her obsessions diminished in intensity and she became more able to understand their meaning: namely, her hostility toward her mother, which she had never before recognized. In this particular example, we see on one hand a diminution in the severity of the conscience and on the other hand the conscious expression of a certain amount of irritation which has been present in the unconscious. Thereafter, the expression of hostility becomes more a matter of conscious ego consideration than a pathological defense mechanism. This young girl's friendship with her mother and general ability to adjust improved remarkably. The mere fact that she could recognize and occasionally express resentment toward her mother did not mean that their relationship disintegrated, but rather that it improved. The gratification of the need to express some of her own feelings helped to make it possible to replace some of the hostility with love.

During the therapeutic process with an obsessive patient, his inherent obstinacy is a great barrier. While he is coming for the purpose of understanding his illness and is making sacrifices in terms of time and money, he nevertheless has an obstinate need to resist interpretations and suggestions made to him. His tendency is to deny the correctness of interpretations merely because the therapist has made them rather than because he has seriously considered their worth and weighed the factors involved. Again such a situation needs to be called to the patient's attention repeatedly before he begins to see the pattern of rebellion that is involved.

One does not see, early in the therapy of the typical obsessive patient, the clearly evident manifestations of positive transference, at least in terms of emotional expression, that one sees in people with a conversion or dissociative type of reaction. However, if we recognize that the obsessive patient, like all other neurotic individuals, projects his own conscience onto the therapist and reacts to the therapist as if he were a parent, we would expect that, at least under the surface, there would be a great deal of emotional turbulence including both positive and negative feelings. This is, in fact, true. The more infantile, anal, sadistic side of the patient is in a constant relationship with the therapist like that of the child with the original parent. In one sense the patient is demanding, obstinate, stingy, and sadomasochistic. On the other hand the mechanisms of defense hold these inner emotional reactions to an absolute minimum so that, even though they may become evident in the therapeutic process, it is often very difficult to get the patient to really feel them. He may intellectually agree that they must be present and yet not reveal overtly an emotionally convincing attitude.

PROGNOSIS

The prognosis in obsessive-compulsive reaction varies from one case to another but, in general, is not as good as in the other psychoneuroses. This stems from the fact that in this neurosis the basic fixation in psychosexual development is somewhat earlier than in the others. Characteristically there is a larger element of anality in these patients—although certainly there is some in the majority of psychoneurotics. Further, the prognosis is made worse by the nature of the defenses used by the obsessive patient. Isolation of his affect means that he may seek psychiatric help but will often be unable to form a warm or usefully emotional relationship with the therapist. The patient intellectualizes so adroitly that he is able to learn much about himself in treatment, yet have this knowledge mean little to him. One patient who had had much previous psychotherapy and who had read extensively in the field began his first interview by giving an accurate, dynamic evaluation of himself with a good formulation of the structure of his own neurosis. Unfortunately he still had most of the obsessions and compulsions with which he had originally begun treatment. The obsessive patient is not nearly as suggestible as the dissociative or conversion patient, and simple measures directed toward symptom removal are not usually very successful. Prolonged treatment of a psychoanalytically oriented type is usually required to rid these patients of their symptoms.

Case History: Obsessive-Compulsive Reaction

This twenty-four-year-old male was referred by a dermatologist whom he had consulted because of a rash on his hands. It had become evident that this rash was due to a compulsion to wash his hands innumerable times each day. The patient said that he had recognized for a long time that he should seek psychiatric help but had always avoided doing so for fear it would be found that nothing could be done for him. He then proceeded to give the examining physician a relatively complete history from notes which he had prepared and brought with him to the interview. He began by saying that ever since he was five or six years of age he had been concerned with what he considered to be obnoxious and dangerous thoughts which would come to his mind. He had even at that age begun the habit of "undoing" them by thinking thoughts of an opposite kind. He went on to say that during puberty he had been greatly disturbed by the possibility of dating girls or otherwise associating with them and had tended to withdraw from the majority of social functions.

At times, from early childhood, he had been concerned with antireligious thoughts which had been quite disturbing to him. He also mentioned that many of his "bad thoughts" had been about people who were close to him and it subsequently developed that they were primarily in relation to his parents. He was chronically concerned that either disease or injury would come to his parents. During late adolescence he had begun to wash his hands excessively and this compulsion had continued until the present time. He then said that he had made a list of things which he felt were wrong with him. It read: "(1) I get so I cannot see the forest for the trees. (2) I am always fearful that I am saying the wrong thing. (3) I am never certain that I've done something right. (4) I must do everything perfectionistically. (5) I am always overpolite and I am extremely uncomfortable if I have to accept anything from people. (6) I am overly clean."

This patient several years before had recognized the presence of emotional disturbances within himself and had sought out many psychiatric textbooks. By the time he reached the first interview, his intellectual acquaintance with psychiatric principles was rather extensive. He had correctly diagnosed himself as an obsessive-compulsive type of person.

He was familiar with the fact that he suffered from the typical obsessions and compulsions characteristic of the condition. He realized that he was doing these things for unconscious and symbolic reasons and yet admitted that this knowledge had been of little assistance to him.

His family consisted of his mother, father, and two older sisters who were twelve and fifteen years his senior. He, being a boy, had always been the favorite child of both parents and he had always been given everything that he desired. Great attention and "affection" had been lavished upon him and little, if anything, had ever been asked of him.

At the end of the first interview, the patient expressed considerable distrust of psychiatry, saying that after all he himself had become acquainted with the majority of the principles of this science and they had been of little use to him. He said that he failed to see how coming and talking over these things, which after all he already knew, would be of any benefit to him.

He was encouraged to continue psychotherapy and did so for a period of many months at frequencies of two to three times a week. The initial phases of his treatment consisted in his intellectual recitation of the many books which he had read. It was as if he were trying to prove his intellectual superiority to the therapist by quoting his extensive knowledge of various psychiatric and psychoanalytic writings. The therapist adopted the attitude of being uninterested in such discussions, pointing out to the patient that they were purely on an intellectual level and did not produce any benefits.

The therapist was constantly on the alert for evidences of emotional reactions in the patient, or at least situations which would be expected to cause such reactions. Whenever, for instance, one would expect hostility in the patient and it did not appear, it was called to his attention. Any situation reported by the patient from the ouside, during the therapeutic sessions, where there had been a lack of emotion but where a good deal of feeling could have been expected, was discussed. Gradually the patient began to realize more clearly how he had attempted to intellectualize the whole therapeutic process. A great deal of attention was paid by the therapist to the patient's emotional reactions to the therapist himself. The patient was encouraged to bring forth even the most minor feelings that he had about the therapeutic situation. Gradually he became better able to see his own emotional reactions to various important people in his environment, including his parents and the therapist. Slowly he began to express some of this emotion and, at least in the therapeutic situation, having found it safe, continued to bring forth more affect. Eventually this patient began to see more clearly how his emotional problems had arisen. His mother and father had never gotten along well with each other and both had been oversolicitous in their attentions to him as he grew up. His mother had overprotected him in a way that had kept him dependent upon her and extremely close to her. His father, on the other hand, had been invariably attentive, affectionate, and "good" to him. He had, it finally developed, originally had his negative thoughts toward his father. However, such thoughts seemed to him at the time extremely sinful, since his father had been so good to him. He therefore had attempted to have similar thoughts against his mother so neither parent would be better than the other. Then had come the "undoing thoughts." He attempted to undo the negative thoughts against both parents by positive thoughts. He had inwardly resented the oppressive type of overprotection that they had lavished upon him. They had literally forbidden any impulses toward independence or maturation and, although such a dependent situation was pleasurable, it robbed him of the many pleasures which other boys he knew were learning to have. It kept him tied within the small circuit of the home situation and forbade him to grow up. His growing resentment toward both father and mother could not be expressed because they were too good to him and therefore he built himself an extremely punitive and rigid conscience which forbade expression of the impulse and at the same time prevented him from achieving maturation.

This patient finally achieved a considerably improved adjustment wherein his overt symptomatology diminished to the point where he no longer suffered from obsessions or compulsions. He remained a somewhat rigid and generally perfectionistic sort of person who was not as spontaneous in his relationships with others as the mature person; nevertheless, his general level of emotional spontaneity improved and the patient was quite satisfied with the results of his therapy.

CHAPTER 11

Depressive Reaction

THE DEPRESSIVE reaction is a type of psychoneurosis in which the most prominent symptom is a chronic state of dejection or despondency accompanied by a tendency toward self-depreciation. This condition typically follows some environmental condition which might ordinarily be expected to produce a temporary unhappiness, but not to as severe a degree nor for as prolonged a period as is found in these patients. The death of a close relative, an economic failure, or some other unfortunate crisis in a patient's life often immediately predates the depressive reaction, but the patient's reaction is both more marked and more prolonged than would be expected in the reaction of a normal individual under similar circumstances. This condition was referred to in previous nomenclatures as "reactive depression."

The depressive reaction, as a type of psychoneurosis, is to be differentiated from more severe disturbances of a psychotic nature which occur in the depressed phases of manic depressive reaction or in involutional psychotic reaction. Even though the underlying psychopathology has some similarities to these more severe conditions, the disturbance in personality function is not nearly as marked and the ultimate prognosis is ordinarily much better. The depression of the affect is not as great in the neurotic condition and there is not as much concomitant physiological interference and slowup as occurs in the psychotic conditions. A tendency toward sincere suicidal attempts is less frequent in depressive reaction and the presence of hypochondriacal preoccupation is not as prominent.

The patient with a neurotic depression is essentially a chronically unhappy, complaining person. He withdraws from many of his previous activities yet is still more amenable to relationships with others and, consequently, to psychotherapy, than are the more disturbed patients who suffer from psychotic depressions. The patient with depressive reaction may still be able to carry on the more important of his daily activities. For instance, he may still be able to work and to relate on a limited scale to his family, but the joys ordinarily derived from these activities are greatly diminished. He no longer shows any zest or interest in the things which he does, but rather goes through them mechanically and almost automatically. In summary then, depressive reaction is a less severe form of depression somewhat like that seen in the psychotic depressions. It does not usually reach proportions which prevent the individual from engaging in everyday living. It rather removes the pleasure which he would normally obtain from these pursuits.

ETIOLOGY AND PSYCHOPATHOLOGY

Any depression, whether neurotic or psychotic in degree, represents the turning of hostility upon the self. There are several important prerequisites to depression, not the least of which is the possession of an extremely severe and punitive superego or conscience. An important cornerstone which lays the groundwork for the possible development of depression is the presence within a personality of marked ambivalence. This, of course, implies a mixture of love and hate in all relationships. It means that the patient cannot love anyone without there existing somewhere within him hostility toward the same person. It is with this hostility that the depressive patient gets into trouble and eventually becomes chronically unhappy. He has never learned to love freely.

From the standpoint of psychosexual development, there is a perpetuation within the depressed patient of many oral and anal features. Ambivalence itself is a prominent part of the anal phase of development. A severe conscience forbids expression of hostility, but because of the presence of ambivalence the hostility is an ever-present thing within the patient. Not only is it impossible for the depressive patient to love in a mature manner, but it is also impossible for him to feel secure about the love of those around him. He is quick to find evidences of rejection in every relationship. It is as if he feels that since he cannot love, others cannot love him, and since he cannot love freely, he does not feel he deserves the love of others. Such a patient usually expends great mental effort defending himself against feelings of rejection. He is apt to become ingratiating or self-effacing. He may extend himself to great lengths to "prove" that he loves others, rarely, if ever, revealing his hostility to them or to himself. There is, however, within him an inner insecurity about his relationships with other people. Therefore, even though such a patient may have been able to attain an adjustment which outwardly appears relatively good, it is nevertheless devoid of real joy in sharing or healthy depth and the whole situation may collapse if severely threatened by an unexpected, tragic environmental occurrence.

The ego of the reactive depressive is in a position to handle the difficulties with which it is beset in a somewhat better manner than is the ego of the psychotic depressive. The neurotically depressed ego, like the psychotically depressed ego, is beset with inner immaturities striving for expression from the id and is also under the sway of the harsh dictates of a punitive superego. It does not, however, lose its basic grasp on reality to the degree that the ego of a psychotic depressive does. In a depressive reaction an incident occurs in which the patient suffers the loss, or perhaps threatened loss, of some portion of his security—most often a love object such as a spouse, parent, or sibling. The relationship to this love object has been ambivalent and at the time of the loss the previously unconscious hostility is turned back against the ego by the conscience. At this point the patient is belabored by his own conscience, feeling inferior, self-critical, and unworthy. He has a tendency toward withdrawal of interest from all those about him. This interest has been previously maintained through considerable mental effort and the patient is quick to lose it.

A review of the life history of a patient with depressive reaction reveals that he has always been rather selfish, demanding, rigid, and unbending. These qualities may not be obvious on the surface, but extended inquiry usually reveals that they have been noticeable to those most close to the patient. The individual with depressive reaction has within his unconscious many exaggerated infantile demands and needs stemming from perpetuated orality. He wants and requires a great deal from those about him and yet has little basic impulse toward altruistic living. Alongside this unconscious childishness stands the ever-present rigid superego which forbids expression of the immature strivings. In other words, the patient wants a great deal and yet his conscience forbids him to realize, or even clearly strive for, his wants. As a result there is a constant state of frustrated bitterness within him which disturbs his relationship to others.

Such an adjustment is at best a tenuous one. The patient usually sets up many defenses against his infantile nature and may even appear superficially altruistic, ingratiating, and pleasant. Yet, upon further observation, these latter qualities are seen to be comparatively artificial, rigid, and without meaningful depth. The result of such an adjustment is a defensive, rigid psychic formation which is prone to collapse whenever the environmental situation is seriously upset by the death of a close relative or by some other crucial situation. There is an exaggeration of the hostility which is still forbidden expression by the conscience and much of the hostility is turned back upon the ego in terms of self-recrimination. As with the psychotic patient, many of these presumably self-accusatory remarks are really, in the most basic sense, meant for the lost love object. The ultimate result is an unhappy, depressed, uninterested individual who is living within himself with comparatively little interest in other people or anything going on in the outside world.

SYMPTOMATOLOGY

The symptoms of depressive reaction are primarily in the realm of the affect. Mood is stabilized at an unhappy state and the patient chronically feels life is meaningless and useless. He finds little interest in anything or anyone. His cares and worries are exaggerated to the point where each task seems almost too difficult to undertake. Any job completed does not produce the normal sense of gratification. The patient is prone to feel either that he did not do the job correctly or perhaps that he should not have attempted it at all.

Occasional social events or excessive attention by one or more friends or relatives may produce a temporary rise in the patient's spirits, but even this does not last. Most of these individuals are, if given an opportunity, willing to enumerate their numerous troubles to a good listener. They will go on at great length as to the hopelessness in which they are engulfed. They can be compared to a person who still eats but has lost his sense of taste. They realize that certain things must be done in order to meet minimum requirements and yet they no longer enjoy doing them. The symptoms of reactive depression vary in severity from comparatively minor diminution in spirits to a more severe depression which approaches a psychotic state.

Usually in these cases one finds a history of a crucial environmental situation immediately preceding the depression. It is, most frequently, of a type which would be expected to cause some temporary unhappiness. Yet, in these individuals, this unhappiness has continued far beyond normal expectations. In addition to this, the patient's entire life seems to have suffered from the precipitating event. His relationship to everyone is impaired and he seems unable to regain interest in even close friends or relatives. He criticizes himself in many ways which are not realistic but which contain a grain of truth. He does not behave as generously and kindly as his ego ideal tells him he should, and he reproaches himself for this without being able to find within himself the ego qualities which would bring about change. Insomnia is also a common symptom.

The patient with a typical psychoneurotic reactive depression is apt to claim a loss of interest in everything, yet is quite willing to enumerate his multitude of complaints. He states that he no longer is interested in his job, nor does he see any purpose to his life. He says that he is not able to "get going" as he had in the past. Everything seems more of an effort to him. Small frustrations or irritations seem too big to tackle. The most typical history includes a past tendency toward perfectionism, meticulousness, and other similar compulsive features. There is often a history of the patient having driven himself excessively, and many of these individuals accomplish quite a bit in terms of material gains. However, the patient now finds himself at a loss in that he is no longer interested in attaining his previous goals or even enjoying what he has accomplished. He frequently, during the psychiatric interview, will revert to a discussion of the crucial situation which he feels brought on his problem. He may state, for instance, that all of this has resulted from the death of his "beloved" relative, or the disappointment he feels over an expected promotion he did not receive, or because of a move from one city to another.

At times there may appear in the history a number of somatic complaints. Vague aches and pains, constipation, dizziness, difficulty with vision, are examples of such complaints. There is often a preoccupation with a particular body function, rather than a true painful somatic symptom. Such complaints do not reach the degree of intensity that is found in an involutional psychotic reaction or in a depressed manic depressive. However, the patient may seize upon his somatic complaints and try to make them the only illness present.

Typical in the history of these patients are the numerous attempts that have been made by members of the family, close friends, or perhaps even other physicians to stimulate the patient's interest in his surroundings. He may, for instance, have taken a trip or have changed his job as a means of recapturing what he considers to be his previous normal feelings about things. Many of these attempts may have been, at least initially, apparently successful, but the patient's newly awakened interest faded rapidly and he regained his depressive, morbid, unhappy outlook. Such an individual, if asked, will usually admit ruminations about suicide, although these rarely have approached the severity which leads to an actual attempt. He will tend to bemoan his fate and feel that life is not worth living and that the frustrations and difficulties of ordinary activities are too much to tolerate and that death offers rest and peace.

Throughout the interview the therapist gains the impression of a self-centered individual who is chronically wrapped up in his own problems which he has markedly exaggerated, and who is completely uninterested in and not actively participating in normal activities. The patient no longer loves anyone around him, nor is he able to think of much of anything other than his own unhappy plight and the difficulty in which he finds himself.

TREATMENT

One of the basic hurdles to be surmounted in the treatment of a neurotically depressed patient is the establishment of a sufficiently good relationship with the physician so that the treatment process becomes meaningful to the patient. Unfortunately, one of the cardinal symptoms in a depressed patient is a general lack of interest in other people. He is preoccupied with his own problem and has great difficulty in establishing anything approaching friendly, meaningful relationships with others. Such a patient often shows considerable interest in relating in some detail all of his unhappy feelings and multitude of complaints. He does not, however, accept and utilize advice, reassurance, or interpretations offered to him. Such a patient is struggling with a sort of "closed-circuit" type of psychological difficulty. His chronic inner resentment feeds the fires. He, in turn, turns the resentment against himself and punishes himself for it. He has lost track of and interest in much of what surrounds him and the prime therapeutic goal is to break into this cycle and establish a sufficiently good relationship to effect an improvement.

Many of these individuals, especially if not severely depressed, may respond after two or three interviews with a friendly, understanding therapist. They have retained enough ability to relate to others so that they are able to sense the potential usefulness of the therapeutic relationship and soon reveal their eagerness to understand more about themselves. The patient's premorbid life may reveal how well he will react to psychotherapy. If his life has been at least superficially well adjusted and has included some basically good relationships, the therapeutic outlook is reasonably favorable. If, however, there have been excessive rigidity, perfectionism, and other compulsive tendencies with few, if any, warm relationships, the outlook is less favorable.

As soon as the patient has allowed the physician to assume considerable emotional importance to him, the really necessary changes toward improvement begin to take place. The patient, as in any treatment situation, begins to endow the therapist with superego qualities. In other words, he begins to at least in some degree use

the therapist as a sort of conscience. The therapist's kind, understanding, and permissive attitude thus allows the patient to begin
to explore more thoroughly his own relationships with people. It
means that the patient can permit himself a dawning awareness of
his mixture of feelings toward even those whom he loves. As his
ambivalence comes more to the fore, he finds less need to keep it
locked up within him and turned upon himself. At the same time,
as the therapist's importance grows, the patient can slowly be made
aware of his own excessive demands upon the therapist and see how
these demands have been made in other relationships in a manner
of which he has hitherto been unaware. Gradually, as these processes
are worked through, the patient's tendency to bottle up or form a
"closed circuit" of his inner ambivalence becomes lessened and the
entire psychic structure becomes more flexible. The treatment of
the neurotically depressed patient has some similarities to that of the
psychotically depressed individual.

Of value in the treatment of some depressed patients are the
psychic energizing drugs which are discussed more thoroughly in
Chapter 22. These include certain amphetamines and amine-oxidase
inhibitors. Some patients who seem unable to respond to psychotherapy may respond sufficiently to these drugs that they can make
use of a therapeutic relationship. The drugs by themselves should
not be considered as replacements for solving the patient's inner
problems. It is unfortunately impossible to predict accurately which
patients will respond favorably to medication and those who will
not.

There are some severe neurotic depressions in which a reasonable
trial of psychotherapy and medication proves unsuccessful. In these
cases it becomes advisable to consider the usefulness of electroshock
treatment. Such a decision should not be made rapidly or without
an adequate trial of psychotherapy and drugs by an adept therapist.
Anywhere from three to twenty or more treatments may be required. In such cases as may require electroshock treatment the
purpose is to enhance the patient's ability to establish a relationship
with the therapist. Its purpose is not, as is so frequently assumed,
merely to "cure" the depression. In many of the cases treated in this
manner, it is found that a comparatively small number of shock

treatments, perhaps four to six, are sufficient to allow the patient to establish a useful treatment relationship.

It is an extremely common error of both physicians and patients' families to react with joy at the dramatic improvement produced by electroshock in the depressed patient, and yet fail to make any further plans for psychotherapeutic assistance. The patient who has improved as a result of electroshock still has his basic personality pattern which, of course, leaves him prone to another attack of depression. This personality structure can only be changed through further psychotherapeutic work.

PROGNOSIS

The prognosis of the depressive-reaction patient is generally good under a psychotherapeutic regimen. To ensure against future recurrences, it is wise to see that every depressive-reaction patient has a psychotherapeutic trial of at least a few weeks. Too often, however, family pressure and the results of drug treatment lull the patient into going back on the job without the continuing support of psychotherapy. If, however, psychotherapy of a probing, uncovering type is instituted the recovery rate in depressive reaction will be quite high. The future of such patients should be symptom-free as a result of their acquired insight.

Case History: Depressive Reaction

This thirty-two-year-old woman was referred to the psychiatrist by an internist. The latter had known her as a patient for a period of many years, but the complaints which led to her psychiatric referral had begun approximately nine months before. At that time the patient's mother had died. The expected ordinary period of mourning had become prolonged and intensified to the degree that the internist no longer felt time alone would be sufficient to cure the patient. The patient's chief complaints concerned her inability to enjoy her family or husband in the way that she had previously. She had begun in the past few months to consider her children an increasingly great responsibility and she no longer obtained any pleasure from spending time with them. Arguments had become more frequent with other members of her family, particularly with her three siblings. She had begun to feel that every household task was a burden. She felt constantly depressed and unhappy and had frequent crying spells. She had begun to have difficulty sleeping and her appetite was poor. All of these symptoms stemmed from the time of the death of her mother, and had gradually assumed a pattern which interfered with most of her ordinary pleasures and duties. She had occasionally entertained suicidal thoughts, but at the time of referral had never actually attempted suicide.

This patient's past history revealed that she had been brought up in a family which was ruled tyrannically by her father. He had made his children feel that they were unworthy of any democratic relationship with him and had totally discouraged any attempts on the part of his children to get closer to him. His philosophy markedly exaggerated the old saying that children are to be seen and not heard. He never spoke to them at mealtime. He never inquired about their work, friends, school, or anything else in which they were engaged. He considered his duties fulfilled when he supplied board, room, and education for his children. He felt that they should value these things highly and should be able to shape personalities for themselves from merely these basic provisions. Any love, affection, or concern about them or their future came only from the mother and this only when the father was not present. The mother, however, was overworked and chronically tired as well as discouraged with her marriage. She found it difficult to give the proper time and attention to her children. This was particularly true since her husband constantly reiterated his feeling that strictness and sternness were the elements which built character and that he would not condone any "softness" in his home.

One of the results of this upbringing was the patient's marriage to a very calm, easygoing man. However, even though her husband was in many ways the opposite of her father, she was unable to utilize any of the emotional possibilities of her marriage. She bore two children, but still felt that she had accomplished nothing and considered herself to be living a useless life. Her sense of self-esteem had never achieved its proper proportions and she was unable to concentrate on her job of being a mother and a wife.

Then came the death of her mother. The latter was the one person in her life toward whom she had had a reasonably close relationship. This, however, had still been a very mixed emotional relationship in which she entertained not only feelings of fondness and dependency toward her mother, but also resentment, because she had, from an early age, considered her mother partly responsible for her own plight. Following her mother's death the patient cried a great deal of the time. She would often call her husband at work, demanding that he give her some relief from her drudgery and provide her with more than he had in the past.

When she entered therapy, this patient was able to establish reasonably good rapport with the psychiatrist. She soon came to understand that she had much pent-up resentment within her toward many people close to her. However, at the same time, she understood that this resentment had never been expressed, nor had she ever clearly been aware of it. It developed that she had always been the type of child who absorbs a good deal of punitive rigidity without rebellion. She became aware during therapy that she was not only hostile toward her father, but also, to a degree, toward her mother and her siblings. The patient gradually understood the severity of her own conscience and how she was most critical toward herself outwardly, but within herself had many resentments and critical feelings toward those close to her. It required several weeks for her to learn that she could express some of this resentment and allow more freedom in the expression of her emotions. At the same time, as she began to be more aware of the childishness of her own inner feelings, she slowly demanded less of those around her and became more willing to make some efforts on her own part toward them. She had previously been resentful of having to do any "work" in order to improve herself. She had felt in her typical childish way that all efforts should come from others and she had remained basically dissatisfied, bitter, and discontented that others had not met her needs. At the same time, being unable to express this resentment, she had turned much of it upon herself, feeling that she was unworthy and life was useless.

In the beginning of her treatment this patient had many vague physical complaints. She was initially unable to accept the idea that previous physical examinations had revealed nothing abnormal. There still, for a time, remained within her the infantile hope that someone would give her some type of "magical" medicine which would remove the discomfort from which she suffered. As she began to understand more about herself, her willingness to accept the emotional origin of her problem increased. As the therapeutic situation continued, the patient became increasingly interested in understanding her own psychological development. She related well to the psychiatrist, although in many instances she made excessive demands on him. She gradually learned to feel her own resentment toward the psychiatrist and to express it. This was done in a friendly and understanding atmosphere so that she could learn from the experience. She was helped to vent her hostility wherever it was stirred up and helped at the same time to understand the guilt which had previously caused much of her difficulty. She was encouraged to understand her unreasonable demands on the environment stemming from her inner childishness and to seek a more workable relationship with others. She developed more appreciation for the interest, love, and friendship which were available to her. The patient's depression gradually lifted and she assumed a much more normal living pattern.

Personality Disorders

CHAPTER 12

Personality Disorders

PERSONALITY disorders form a large and heterogeneous group of emotional problems which are characterized primarily by abnormalities in the patient's mode of behavior or action. In the past, these entities have been classified under the heading "character disorders." Personality, defined broadly, encompasses the sum total of an individual's behavior which is peculiar to him. Each person creates certain impressions on others of how he will react to various situations. For instance, one individual becomes recognized by his associates as being aggressive and dominating, while another is soon labeled as shy and retiring. It is with the deviations from the normal behavior pattern that personality disorders are concerned.

In the process of growing up, when an individual perpetuates within himself inner immaturities and conflicts, thus leaving a certain deficiency within the over-all structure of his personality, he may reveal his emotional problems in any one of four general directions. He (1) becomes psychoneurotic (thus developing defenses against his immaturities and neurotic symptoms); or (2) becomes a personality problem (thus displacing his conflicts toward the outer world by acting them out in his pattern of behavior); or (3) develops psychophysiologic disorders (thus draining his chronic emotional tension off into autonomic channels and producing eventual organic pathology); or (4) becomes psychotic (thus suffering ego disintegration with loss of ability to face reality).

A real understanding of personality disorders is, of necessity, based on a knowledge of the ego and its functions. The ego, as discussed in Chapter 2, is that portion of the personality which mediates between the inner individual and his outer environment. It is through the ego that perceptions from the outer world are taken into the personality, and it is also through the ego that inner instinctual urges must either be denied or permitted access to the outer world. As the ego forms throughout the period of childhood, it slowly develops certain habitual methods for dealing with inner and outer pressures. As the child grows older, his ego must deal with the additional complicating factor of the superego and its requirements.

The essential point, then, in dealing with a patient with a personality disorder, is to accurately evaluate the ego's attitude toward and handling of inner instinctual drives. For instance, the ego may allow relatively free access of instinctual urges to the conscious mind and even to the voluntary musculature, with a subsequent expression of them toward the outer world. This is most apt to be true in the absence of a rigid or even firm conscience. The ego of another person may set up elaborate defenses to prevent the open expression of his own instincts, whether they be sexual or aggressive in nature. There are many possible variations. For example, the ego may allow expression of aggressive instincts and not sexual instincts, or certain elements of one or the other, or even both. However, it should be remembered that once the ego's pattern has been formed, it remains more or less constant, and a particular mode of behavior is the result.

No two individuals have exactly the same personality, any more than they have the same fingerprints. However, both personality and fingerprints can be subdivided into certain general categories. In terms of personality disorders, the primary concern is with the degree and manner in which the individual's pattern of behavior deviates from the normal. The mature individual develops a pattern of behavior which allows a reasonable expression of his sexual and aggressive drives in a manner that will not come into conflict with society. At the same time, he has successfully passed through his earlier, more immature psychosexual stages, and thus does not have immature childish drives within his unconscious which strive constantly for expression. The mature person has achieved a well-adjusted balance between his instinctual urges, his conscience, and his environment. He reacts efficiently, he loves comfortably, and he works with satisfaction. He is, above all, realistic and flexible, so that he can adjust his pattern of behavior not only to his inner needs, but in particular, to the environmental situation.

The patient with a personality disorder is comparatively inflexible in that he reacts the same way to almost every situation, regardless of the appropriateness of his pattern. If his personality formation involves a chronic exaggerated reaction against authority, he may repeatedly be in conflict with the law or other social standards. If, on the other hand, the patient has a predominantly passive type of personality, he may rarely, if ever, become antisocial, and yet may live an unhappy, inefficient, and unsocial life. Thus it may be seen that, for the psychiatrist, the term *personality disorder* implies variation from normality, realistic adjustment, and maturity.

The study of personality formation is fascinating. In an ordinary class of seventy-five students, there are to be found a certain number who are excessively shy, timid, and hesitant in expressing themselves. Another group, on the other end of the scale, are constantly expressing themselves to anyone who will listen, and they obviously take great pleasure in being the center of attention. They are not only aggressive with their own colleagues, but also with instructors in positions above their own. Then there is a certain group who are noted for their studiousness, have little in the way of social life, and spend most of their time buried in books. The opposite of these are those students who rarely spend more than a bare minimum of time studying. They prefer to absorb their knowledge parasitically in "bull sessions," into which they draw other students who have done the laborious reading.

While the members of the class can be divided into broad groups, it nevertheless remains true that each student differs somewhat from the others in his particular group, and we can predict reactive behavior only broadly. In the individual whose reactions are surprisingly few in number, we have little difficulty in prognosticating what he will do in a certain situation after we have known him for some time. He is, in that sense, inflexible. His ego has learned to deal with his inner urges, as stirred up by the environment, in only a few specific ways. Other students, who are more flexible and mature, are less limited in their available patterns of reaction. In summary, all of this that we see about a person we know as part of his personality, and if it departs in a pathological manner from normal behavior, we classify it under the heading "Personality Disorders."

NORMAL PERSONALITY

The well-adjusted personality, because it is so smooth-flowing, efficient, and lacking in marked idiosyncrasies, is more difficult to describe and to define than is the abnormal personality. In essence one might say that a person with a mature personality has worked out a harmonious relationship between his id, his superego, and the environment which enables him to make maximum use of his psychic energies in constructive work, heterosexual adjustment, and altruistic living. Of importance in the mature personality is a degree of flexibility which enables the individual to utilize a wide range of possible reactions. These reactions are based upon external reality rather than upon a rigidly constructed, pathological internal defense system. The ego of such an individual is strong and yet continues to grow through added experience. It is never rigid and inflexible.

The mature personality utilizes the mechanism of sublimation rather than pathological defenses. Sublimation does not require the additional expenditure of ego energy to defend the ego against residual infantile impulses. Instead, it utilizes such impulses in a constructive and socially acceptable way. The personality of the mature and "normal" person is not uninteresting because of its lack of idiosyncrasies. Certainly each mature person differs somewhat from the next mature person in that his background and his interests are not and have not been the same. Nevertheless all mature people have a healthy interest in what is going on about them. They meet each new problem with a desire to solve it, as well as to learn from it. The personality of the normal individual does not contain a rigid, punitive, authoritative superego which constantly warns against the expression of instinctual drives. Nor does it contain a large amount of residual childish instinctual needs striving for expression. In summary, the personality of the mature person is headed by a strong, flexible ego whose task is made easier because the person has successfully passed through his earlier stages of psychosexual development and because his superego is in reasonable accord with his ego and makes no excessive, impossible, and punitive demands.

ABNORMAL PERSONALITY

The individual with a personality disturbance either (1) sexually or aggressively behaves in such a way as to come into conflict with the mores of society, or (2) because of his pathological defensive dealings with his residual infantile striving, leads an inefficient or unhappy life. In other words, the individual either makes himself unhappy through his own rigid defensive mechanisms to the point where he cannot lead a pleasant, productive existence or he gives vent to his infantile strivings, in which case he runs into conflict with society. As an example, we may consider the person who has within his unconscious a strong homosexual tendency. He may either give full open expression to this tendency and become an overt homosexual or he may set up strong rigid defenses against this tendency and inhibit his life generally, thus warping his personality. In the latter case the homosexuality is said to be *egodystonic,* in that the ego refuses to accept or give expression to the perverted impulse. In the former example the perverted impulse is said to be *egosyntonic,* because the ego accepts it and provides avenues of overt expression for it. In the same way, a person who is inwardly seething with pent-up aggression may give full expression to this aggression and become an openly antisocial individual continually fighting with everyone, or he may set up rigid defenses in order to maintain his aggression within the limits of his unconscious and show no outward expression of it. In fact he will probably be too deferential, even obsequious—like Uriah Heep in *David Copperfield.*

As the child progresses through the successive levels of psychosexual development, it is possible for him to retain within his personality strong residuals of one or another phase. For instance, the youngster who is severely deprived during his oral period may thereafter carry within his growing personality strong oral characteristics. These then may be given free expression, or may be denied such expression by the developing ego because of environmental restrictions and similar subsequent restrictions of his severe conscience. Such events lead finally to the formation of the type of personality, or mode of behavior, which either gives expression to or denies expression to the residual infantile characteristics. Therefore, we may speak of certain oral characteristics or anal characteristics which appear in some people.

Oral characteristics, as we would expect, are those stemming from the persistence of strong dependent traits within a personality. If they are given free expression by the ego, they lead to open and obvious seeking for a dependent relationship. Oral individuals are not uncommon in our society. Their basic orientation seems to be that the world owes them a living; and they have no compunction about seeking what they feel is their just due. They find it difficult to give and are constantly trying to form relationships in which they will be able to take from others but will not have to give in return. Such a relationship, of course, is available only to infants and, since such adults cannot achieve it, they may turn, for instance, to alcohol in order to soften the blows of what they consider to be a "cruel world." They are generally grasping and demanding people. They contribute little and expect much.

If such a person cannot accept his oral characteristics because his superego would produce excessive guilt, dependent characteristics may be covered by a superficial attitude of extreme independence. In this case, he rigidly seeks to deny his dependency by forming a relationship of an independent type in which others have to come to him for aid. Frequently the superficial and external appearance of such a person belies his inner dependency. At such times it may be difficult to discover his inner oral needs and these may come to light only when he develops, as he certainly might, a gastric ulcer. The ulcer condition we would expect to stem from strong unsatisfied oral cravings for dependence. If such a patient comes into treatment in a situation where dynamic psychiatry and psychiatric thinking are part of the therapy, the dependency is likely to be made conscious and therefore more thoroughly understood, whereupon of course it is incapable of producing further psychophysiologic problems.

The so-called anal characteristics stem from that period of life when the child is ambivalent, hostile, self-centered, bisexual, interested in dirt and messiness, and is generally incapable of a true, warm, loving relationship. The anal-type person, if he gives expression to these traits, is a thoroughly obnoxious individual who is dominating, authoritative, capricious, and generally difficult to tolerate. He is messy, vulgar, easily stirred to hostility, and in general quite childish. If, as so often occurs, these traits and characteristics are relegated to the unconscious because of severe superego pressure, the patient then appears quite the opposite. He assumes perfectionistic, meticulous characteristics and is possibly even ingratiating. A description of this "compensated anal personality" has been given in Chapter 10 on the obsessive-compulsive reaction. The only difference between the "compensated anal personality" and the obsessive-compulsive reaction is that in the former there are no overt obsessions and compulsions or other such psychoneurotic symptoms. There are, however, the typically anal rigid, meticulous, cold attitudes which are defenses against the expression of unbridled primitive instinctual impulses.

In summary it is important to stress that the category of personality disorder is a heterogeneous one. Many of these people act out their immature impulses and do so with little remorse. Others are only slightly different from neurotics in that they try to ward off their immaturities, often through the use of the mechanism of reaction formation. They "escape" becoming psychoneurotics only as long as their psychic arrangement functions to the extent that they do not develop overt neurotic symptoms. Most patients with personality disorders, even the latter type, are not particularly uncomfortable and thus not particularly motivated to seek treatment. Neurotic symptoms such as anxiety, obsessions, or depression are painful and lead people to seek help. Character attitudes, whether hedonistic or rigid, are not necessarily distressing to the patient and do not ordinarily motivate him to change.

CLASSIFICATIONS OF PERSONALITY DISORDERS

The classification of personality disorders has undergone many changes with the growth of understanding and knowledge in psychiatry. The latest and probably best attempt in this direction is the classification of the American Psychiatric Association. In the *Diag-*

nostic and Statistical Manual (see Chapter 4) it is stated that personality disorders "are characterized by developmental defects or pathological trends in the personality with minimal subjective anxiety and little or no sense of distress. In most instances the disorder is manifested by a life-long pattern of action or behavior rather than by mental or emotional symptoms." The general category of personality disorders is then further subdivided into three main groups.

The first general category under personality disorders is "Personality Pattern Disturbances." These are the conditions which are considered to be deep-seated problems which are extremely difficult to deal with from a therapeutic standpoint. The second subgroup is "Personality Trait Disturbances." In this group are individuals who under minor or major stress situations reveal the degree of pathological behavior peculiar to their particular personalities. When not under stress they may make a reasonably good adjustment, at least from a superficial standpoint. The third subgroup is the "Sociopathic Personality Disturbances." Individuals falling within this group are characterized primarily by their lack of conformity to society and the rules and regulations of the prevailing cultural milieu. There is a final and fourth subgroup of personality disorders called "Special Symptom Reactions." This category is added primarily to give flexibility to the outline and is used where one particular symptom is of special importance and appears to be the single outstanding evidence of psychopathology.

We will discuss personality disorders, generally following the outline of the American Psychiatric Association.

PERSONALITY PATTERN DISTURBANCES

INADEQUATE PERSONALITY

The primary characteristic of this type of individual is his inadequate response to his outer world. Such a patient is not physically nor intellectually deficient and yet his social, emotional, intellectual, and physical responses are below par. Such patients have little real zest for living. They are unable to become excited or enthusiastic about things. They maintain interest over a relatively short period of time and a review of their life history shows a consistently poor response to almost every situation. They have never been able to tackle problems and see them through to a successful conclusion. They have never formed adequate goals in living. They are generally inept in most things they do and are prone to show poor judgment, poor adaptability, and a general lack of ambition. They relate in a rather insensitive manner to other people and show little regard for the rights and needs of others. They are usually drifters who never attain much status in their occupation. They change jobs frequently and have apparently little concern about their own failure to achieve anything. Generally they are rather dull, uninteresting, and unexciting people. This condition, although not dramatic, is certainly severe and an extremely difficult one with which to deal. There is little drive, or energy, or emotional stamina which can be used to achieve something in any phase of life, including therapy, if attempted. Ordinarily such patients are not apt to seek treatment themselves but may perhaps be urged or pushed into it by others.

Case History: Inadequate Personality

A single, thirty-eight-year-old male came to the psychiatric clinic at his sister's insistence. She had urged him to seek some advice about his inability to cope with life. He had always been shy and unable to take responsibility. He left school at the eighth grade because he was too incompetent socially to be expected to go to high school. The son of a farmer, he considered himself too inept to plan to learn farming with all its requirements for managing animals and machinery and other farm activity. He left these things to a farmhand who was far less intelligent than he but who had a native capacity for accomplishing things. In addition to the patient's incompetence, he was extremely shy with the opposite sex. He had never had a girl friend and was lacking in confidence and social poise so that he was unable to even consider himself as a suitable companion for a girl. His mother had been a timid person but a good housekeeper. She had had little confidence in herself and had lacked the poise to mix socially. His father was of similar caliber. He would go to town, accomplish his business, but never take part in any community activity, make friends with people, or otherwise join in any social activities.

The patient had been the only boy in a family of four, and it had never been assumed by his parents that he would learn to do the things that other boys and men did. It was as if everything the parents did in terms of effectual living was done at such a cost of anxiety to them that their consciences would not permit them to ask the boy to assume his responsibilities in these directions. He was permitted to grow up afraid of practically every aspect of life from the physical to the social and emotional. As a result he could truly be described as a very inadequate personality. He performed a few simple tasks around the farm under the direction of the hired hand. He did not ask for more to do, nor did he want more. He had no ambition, no envy, and no jealousy. When he was in his late twenties he joined the local peacetime military organization and one summer went on maneuvers for two weeks. This involved traveling two hundred miles away from his home and constituted the biggest event of his life. He continued to discuss it, with what was for him considerable animation, even ten years later.

He lived a simple existence, doing a few chores on the farm, eating his meals, and following the barest outline of current events. His I.Q., established by psychological testing, was in the high average group. In spite of this he was not quick at learning new things. He had a lack of physical and emotional stamina and was socially most inept. He had become so fixed in his pattern that it was decided he would not make a good candidate for therapy, even had he wished to undertake it. He had made it fairly clear that he saw no great reason for receiving treatment and that he was not dissatisfied with his own pattern of living. As far as he was concerned, his sister was unnecessarily upset and his own adjustment satisfied him. His sister therefore was advised against further urging him into therapy.

The prognosis of this patient is very guarded as far as improvement is concerned. In all probability he will continue to live out his life on the very limited, inadequate scale which he has set for himself. There is little probability that he will develop a definite mental illness unless he is forced into a traumatic situation with which he is unable to cope, or unless perhaps such changes come on with senility. The patient essentially has very little conflict and is making what he considers to be a satisfactory and acceptable adjustment, so that it is difficult to conceive of his developing sufficient conflict to precipitate a mental illness.

Treatment: Inadequate Personality

It should be remembered that very few of these patients actively seek therapeutic assistance, because they are not particularly uncomfortable and see no great reason for change. They are essentially satisfied with their own limited adjustment and do not feel the need for extending themselves further. The therapeutic outlook is guarded if they are urged into therapy by someone else, since they have little real motivation for improving their own status.

If, however, they are coerced into getting therapeutic help the treatment is most apt to be supportive, directive, and educational. When such patients can develop a dependent relationship with the therapist this sometimes allows treatment to continue and therapeutic suggestions to be utilized. In the average case however, the relationship is tenuous, the patient's motivation is lacking, and he drifts out of treatment unless some more responsible person or agency constantly urges his continuance. The positive accomplishments of such patients can be somewhat increased, insofar as therapy acts as a guide to some constructive actions, even though motivation is lacking and maturity is never reached.

SCHIZOID PERSONALITY

There are many individuals in our society today who possess some of the personality traits associated with the schizophrenic individual. They are by no means overtly psychotic, and yet on the other hand show tendencies toward withdrawal, difficulty in relating to others, and a general tendency to live in a world of their own without adequate emotional relationships. These people are generally cold, aloof, and emotionally detached. They create in a world of their own a richness of fantasy and daydreams and yet accomplish very little in the real environment. They go on for years never reaching a seriously psychotic state unless some internal or external struggle becomes sufficiently powerful to precipitate an overt schizophrenic reaction. Generally speaking, their emotional relationships are colorless. They cannot express healthy negative or positive feelings because they never become sufficiently close to anyone to do so. They find sufficient gratification in their own private worlds which they have created that they are disinterested and apathetic about the real world. They avoid competition, they show little drive, and if forced into a situation of social intercourse, become either more withdrawn or anxious. Most people who know them consider them odd or eccentric and find attempts to get to know them better useless.

These patients may or may not have paranoid coloring to their thinking. If this is present, they read hints, threats, or other painful discouraging remarks into ordinary conversation. They are extremely sensitive individuals who are easily hurt and this is one of the primary reasons they refrain from making close relationships. It is extremely difficult for this type of person to feel that he is genuinely liked and therefore it is equally difficult for him to like anyone. He figuratively holds everyone at arm's length, for fear he will be injured in a relationship. Efforts by others to make a friend of him or even to befriend him in some minor way are either rejected or perhaps passively accepted without reciprocation or positive emotion.

A certain number of these patients, when confronted with serious environmental situations which stir up their inner conflicts, are capable of becoming overt schizophrenics with all the symptomatology including delusions, hallucinations, and generally bizarre actions.

Case History: Schizoid Personality

A young man of nineteen complained that he was doing poorly in school, could not concentrate on his studies, could not make friends, and at times felt so discouraged that he had thoughts of suicide.

This patient's family background was that his father, like the patient, had been a shy, serious, hard-working man. The father had been fond of both the patient and his older brother but was not the kind of person who could show his feelings for anyone, even his children. The mother was a socially ambitious, overly sensitive person who wanted her children to excel in everything. Instead of helping them to do this and praising them in their learning experiences, she was much more likely to point out where they failed her and how difficult her life was because they were not measuring up to her ideal. She somehow felt that any child of hers should be far above the average and was continuously dissatisfied with her youngsters' own efforts. Her attitude was one of driving and nagging rather than helping and praising.

As the patient grew up he did not find it easy to mix with other children in school, but was always told by his mother that he should play more games, should go to more dances, and should have more children around to play. She continually nagged him to enter into more activities. These things only made him feel more inferior even in his own home, and, of course, inferior also on the outside. This state of affairs continued until he went to college where he was burdened by feelings of his own worthlessness and a deep conviction that he could not satisfy anyone and that he could not possibly measure up to what was expected of him. His overtures of friendliness were therefore so tentative and lacking in warmth and sincerity that he was not accepted and taken into any groups. He began to stay in his own room daydreaming about the social and athletic successes that he would prefer to have had and he began to fall behind in his work. As he contrasted his lonely life with that of others who were much more successful, his thoughts turned toward precipitating himself into some kind of accident so that it would appear to be merely a misfortune which had befallen him. His real intent was to end his life.

Treatment: Schizoid Personality

This young man, as do most patients with this disorder, required prolonged psychiatric therapy to overcome and undo the effects of his traumatic childhood and to learn how to form new relationships that he trusted. A great deal of effort had to be expended in order to give him confidence to feel that he was socially competent and acceptable.

This patient's therapy extended over a period of many months and was slow and tedious. He was easily disappointed, prone to feel that the therapist really did not understand him, expected too much of him, and could not deliver sufficiently gratifying results in a hurry. However, he did manage to improve his social relationships a good deal and found himself beginning to enjoy the company of other people. A trial of tranquilizer was only partially successful. The patient seemed to respond temporarily and to evince more interest in people, but he soon began forgetting to take the drug. Although he was encouraged to resume the medication, he did not respond as well and eventually either did not take the medication, or when he did, claimed little benefit from it. He still, however, even at the termination of his therapy, remained a rather sensitive person who was easily hurt by casual remarks of others and who as a result made friends rather slowly, tentatively, and hesitantly. He did rid himself of suicidal thoughts and began to get a somewhat more healthy view of the give-and-take of friendly relationships. A great deal of what this patient learned was accomplished in his relationship with the therapist, who remained kind and understanding and yet firmly required him to give something of himself in his everyday living.

CYCLOTHYMIC PERSONALITY

The individual who belongs in this category is a sort of conventional counterpart of the manic depressive psychotic without the overt signs of psychosis. Generally speaking, the person with a cyclo-thymic personality has relatively wide mood swings from hypo-manic elation to moderately severe depression. During the patient's elated moods all of his activities are increased. He thinks rapidly, he acts rapidly, and he makes decisions rapidly. He is quite com-petitive. Everything seems to be relatively easy for him. He works long hours and accomplishes a good deal. He is generally outgoing, enthusiastic, friendly, and, at least superficially, warm. Continued acquaintance with him gives one the feeling that his pseudo-friendly relationships do not achieve a deep or lasting level, and that he really does not have as deep and warm a feeling toward others as one might initially be led to believe.

During the depressive phase, these patients are generally slowed. Everything is difficult for them to accomplish. They find little joy in living. They relate poorly to other people and tend to be some-what irritable and grouchy. They are rather self-centered and de-manding during these phases but may also show a good deal of self-criticism, particularly for things which have taken place during their elated phases. They are prone to look back on these phases almost as if they had never really existed, and could never really see the world as a pleasant place any more.

Some of these patients remain for prolonged periods either in the depressed or the elated phase, but generally their instability is suffi-cient to produce at least some semblance of alternation between the two phases. Much of what is said about the manic depressive psy-chotic (see Chapter 15) is true to a lesser degree about the cyclothy-mic personality. Like the schizoid personality, the cyclothymic indi-vidual may occasionally swing beyond his usual mood variations and reach a psychotic stage, particularly if he is beset with severe conflicts in the outer world. In such a case the diagnosis usually becomes that of manic depressive reaction.

It is wise to mention here that there are certain limits of mood swing within which the ordinary individual is apt to stay. These must be widened by a few degrees to encompass the similar mood swings of the cyclothymic personality. If they are widened still further, they then encompass the beyond-reality mood swings of the manic depressive reaction.

Case History: Cyclothymic Personality

This patient, a businessman of forty-three, sought psychiatric help while during a depressed phase in which he felt his entire life was a miserable failure. As the history developed it became clear that all of his friends recognized him as being an extremely changeable individual who was apt to be either elated or depressed for periods of several weeks at a time. When "feeling good," as he put it, he preferred to play cards, entertain extensively, seek out all possible outside social contacts, and spend a great deal of energy on his business. Such a phase, however, would come to an end for no reason of which he was aware. He would then spend a few weeks in which his mood change was remarkable. He found going to work a drudgery. He felt that his thriving business could not possibly continue to be a success, he condemned himself for some of the business deals that he had made, and felt that his product was inferior and could not be made into anything acceptable. He gave up his social activities, snubbed his friends, and was generally irritable and cantankerous with his own family. It was difficult to draw him into a conversation and he seemed to be distant, withdrawn, and uninterested in social contacts.

Therapy with this patient primarily involved attempts to give him an understanding of some of the mechanisms which precipitated his wide mood changes. He had a rather severe superego from which he periodically escaped into an elated phase and which then caught up with him and again forced him into a self-depreciatory phase. As he gradually learned some of the unrealistic aspects of his rigid conscience, he began to blame himself less punitively for his activities. As a result it was possible for him to feel some renewed interest in his business, his friends, and his family. At the same time this made it unnecessary for him to "run" into his elated phase in order to escape his severe conscience. This patient essentially had many of the dynamics of a compulsive patient and his therapy was somewhat similar, although he presented no overt neurotic symptoms but instead a personality problem primarily illustrated by his remarkable mood swings.

Treatment: Cyclothymic Personality

The individual with a cyclothymic personality is most apt to seek psychiatric help during a depressive phase, particularly if he is acutely uncomfortable from self-depreciatory ideas. At such times one of the psychic energizers is often useful. It may lift the patient's mood to the point that he becomes more accessible to the therapy which is necessary for real improvement of a lasting kind. It is extremely rare that such a patient will feel the need of or seek help when he is in an elated phase, because as far as he is concerned he is not in need of any assistance. Unfortunately, the patient who is helped out of a depressive phase is prone to leave treatment as soon as he begins to feel better. Many of these patients, because their depressions never reach major proportions, do not seek therapy at all but become more or less "accustomed" to their mood swings and take them for granted, as do their families.

PARANOID PERSONALITY

A paranoid person is one who is extremely sensitive in all his relationships, with a tendency to be suspicious of the motivation of everyone. He relates much of what is said or what goes on about him to himself and attributes to other people a dislike of himself. Whenever anything happens his first concern is whether or not there is anything in the occurrence directed against him by someone else. These individuals are envious, jealous, stubborn, and quick to feel a lack of attention on the part of others. They seem to start on the basic assumption that no one likes them and everyone is out to do them harm, and subsequently they find in their environment innumerable "realistic" reasons to believe this. Such individuals are not the reserved, modest, self-critical people one finds in the schizoid personality group. Instead, they complain loudly and bitterly against all the imagined slights and rejections which they feel are thrust upon them. Their primary difficulty is an extensive use of the mechanism of projection. Basically they are bitter against the world but they project this bitterness and feel that the world is bitter against them. Unfortunately, the world usually does become bitter against them because of their tendency to be so suspicious and resentful. This, of course, makes it easier for them to find reasons to "prove" that they are disliked and maligned.

These patients have suffered great deprivation of affection during their early years. However, rather than return to an attitude of discouragement and defeat, they come out fighting at every possible occasion and feel that they have not been treated fairly. Their favorite phrase is "Nobody is going to push me around." They are often an extremely disturbing and antagonistic element of society. On many occasions they go further than fighting for themselves and take up arms against various social injustices so that they become "crusaders." They may take legal steps to protect their personal rights and to correct what they consider to be unfair circumstances directed against them. They have often, as a result, been referred to as "litigious personalities." They are quick to resort to lawsuits and other legal procedures, feeling that they will not be denied their "basic constitutional rights." The result of this is often a long series of lawsuits over relatively minor points. These people are usually of sufficient intelligence to have made themselves adequately aware of legal procedures so that their cases cannot be dismissed without expensive trials, suits, and so forth.

Such individuals do not reach the degree of unreality where they are truly mentally ill and require hospital care. However, many of these patients are regarded by others as obnoxious, queer, and difficult to deal with. Of course, some people refer to them at times as being mentally ill but such a label, although perhaps seriously meant, cannot be adequately substantiated as far as legal procedures are concerned. This is complicated by the fact that, should anyone make known to such an individual that he is considered mentally incompetent, it will only lead to further lawsuits which the patient is belligerently willing to fight. Essentially such people are extremely individualistic in their approach and therefore appear to be odd and disturbed. They have a great need for attention and consideration stemming from their early deprivation. They, in a way, plan to force everyone to give them their due consideration, attention, affection, and recognition.

Case History: Paranoid Personality

This patient, a woman of thirty-two, came to the psychiatrist complaining that her life was not a happy one. Her story revealed that her feeling of unhappiness and neglect had begun early in life. Her parents had been hard-working, serious farm people. She was the middle one of three children and felt that of all her siblings she had been given the least love and attention. As she proceeded to discuss her school life, she pointed out that other youngsters did not seem to like her. She said that there were "some of them who wanted to make my life pleasant." However, she felt that the majority of them disliked her and took pleasure in tormenting her. She had gone on to take a secretarial course after high school and had begun work in an office. There she had felt her employer, a young man, was interested in her, but "someone who is jealous of me and did not like me broke that up." She later married someone else. Her husband had tried valiantly to make her life happy but she felt that she saw in him negative, critical attitudes and that he "tried to be a good husband but he found out before long that I was not the right woman for him." Thus it went with every relationship which she formed. She was not happy because she did not feel accepted in her neighborhood. She enumerated many incidents of fancied or small slights from friends or neighbors. It was extremely difficult to evaluate adequately each incident which she related, and yet after many such incidents it was obvious that she herself was the primary cause of most of them. She eventually said, "I guess that neighborhood liked a different kind of person than I was—a person of different background maybe."

Many efforts were made by the therapist to show her that if she were able to put aside her suspicions and greet people with open friendly warmth and with the expectation of being accepted, she would find that her relationships could be much happier. Such efforts on the part of the therapist met with questionable success. When it was pointed out to her that it was easy for a child to feel that others are favored over him and that such an event must have happened early in her life, she reacted with only casual interest. She continued to feel that therapy directed toward a more thorough understanding of her earlier life was really misspent and the therapist should more clearly recognize how she was at the present time misunderstood and maligned by everyone.

Such a patient as this has a very questionable prognosis. This woman left therapy after about four or five months, having learned very little. She felt in the main that the therapist was not particularly understanding and was somewhat irritated with him because he did not side thoroughly with her in all of her complaints. She felt in a way that he missed seeing the essential point, namely her liability to be misunderstood by everyone else.

Treatment: Paranoid Personality

The paranoid personality not infrequently seeks medical help, but unfortunately such medical or even psychiatric assistance is sought by the patient for the purpose of proving his own veracity. Innumerable patients of this type have collected or attempted to collect medical data revealing their own maturity and sanity. This has often resulted from the patient having received open or veiled insinuations by others as to the possibility of some mental difficulty within himself. These patients are extremely aggressive and defensive. Any attempts on the part of the therapist to show them that perhaps they are out of step with the world are often met with further defensiveness and resentment. Generally speaking, the prognosis for these patients is extremely guarded. At times, under a severe environmental situation, they may suffer a further personality disintegration and become openly psychotic, usually in the direction of a schizophrenic reaction, paranoid type.

PERSONALITY TRAIT DISTURBANCES

EMOTIONALLY UNSTABLE PERSONALITY

People within this category probably can be best described as extremely childish. They are generally ineffective, volatile people whose emotional control is extremely poor. They are easily stirred to marked mood changes with little provocation. Such individuals upon the slightest pretext are stirred into unreasonable anger. They are just as easily precipitated into tearful or perhaps guilty spells by similar small provocations. Generally such people lack emotional equilibrium and even minor stress precipitates remarkable disturbances in emotional tone. These people were referred to in older classifications as "psychopathic personality with emotional instability." Obviously, they rarely achieve any particularly useful or contributory status in society because of their childishness and extreme emotional instability. They cannot remain at any one task long because they are so easily frustrated and stirred to anger. They quickly resent demands that are made on them and can live at peace only in extremely quiet, undemanding situations. They are prone to create difficulties in their family life, in their work, and among their associates.

Individuals who are of this particular type often reveal a history extending back to childhood of emotional instability, difficulty in tolerating frustration, and a strong persistence of very early childish traits. They have been given very little and have never been exposed to a mature, stable, consistent type of environment. They are generally self-centered, egocentric individuals who love themselves primarily and have little true concept of altruism or of giving to other people.

Case History: Emotionally Unstable Personality

A young woman of twenty-one who worked as a domestic came to the psychiatric clinic complaining that she was dissatisfied with her work and would like to undertake something else which would be more to her own liking and more suited to her particular talents. Her history revealed that she had been brought up by a self-centered, demanding mother and an alcoholic father who rarely worked for any length of time. She had, as a result, weak ties of loyalty and a marked inability to identify herself with her environment and the needs of her employers. While extremely critical of other people, she could not tolerate even the gentlest suggestion of what was required from her without pouting, crying, or threatening to quit. She was a physically attractive young woman and consequently did not lack male admirers. However, she quarreled with each one in turn at the slightest provocation. If her escort was even five minutes late for an appointment with her or showed the slightest interest in another female she flew into a tantrum and broke off her relationship with him.

At twenty-one years of age this young woman's emotional control was similar to that of a very small child. She would lose her temper frequently and say impolite and unkind things. Yet a few hours later she would be most contrite, or sometimes feel guilty. Nevertheless, she could not effect any improvement in this tendency, even though she could be happy and friendly in her more "normal" periods. Although her duties were explained to her carefully and repeatedly, she would frequently leave them undone and could not seem to accept the idea of responsibility or co-operation. Her employer worked with her patiently for a long time and yet there was no appreciable change. Obviously this girl's effort to seek a new vocational opportunity would not help her personality problem, which would be with her wherever she went. Her desire to seek new opportunities really represented a flight from her present environment, which was beginning to make more demands upon her and from which she seemed unable to learn new patterns.

Treatment: Emotionally Unstable Personality

The emotionally unstable personality, while listed under personality trait disturbances and being therefore more circumscribed and hence not as serious or incapacitating as the personality-pattern disturbances, is extremely difficult to treat. In the first place, like many other patients with personality disorders, these patients rarely of their own volition seek psychotherapy. They tolerate it poorly because it often involves a certain rise in tensions, guilt, and anxiety and therefore their reaction is to run away, rather than to stick to the process and work it through. Their childishness permits them to seek easier, smoother, more comfortable ways of dealing with their environment and, although they are frequently unhappy, they cannot persevere in anything, including psychotherapy, for a sufficient length of time to benefit greatly. They do not learn well by experience and their entire emotional instability is so diffused through their personality that it is difficult for the therapist to form the stable lasting relationship with them which is necessary for therapeutic success. Some of them, if not severely incapacitated by their problem, may benefit to a degree which will improve their life adjustment. Many, however, try therapy for a short time only to find it difficult and quit.

PASSIVE-AGGRESSIVE PERSONALITY

Individuals falling within this category are those who have a distortion in the passive and aggressive elements of their personality which makes them extremely immature, childish, and often obstinate. Passive and aggressive elements are normal in every individual of every age and of both sexes. However, at times because of early childhood trauma, there is a subsequent exaggeration and perpetuation of extremely immature passive and aggressive elements within the personality. If these reveal themselves in behavior, but not in the proportions of overt antisocial behavior, the individual then probably falls within this category. Actually there are three possible subdivisions of the passive-aggressive personality. These are frequently not clear-cut in the individual; some patients reveal all three types alternately.

The possible variations of the passive-aggressive personality are (1) the passive-dependent type, (2) the passive-aggressive type, and (3) the aggressive type. The passive-dependent individual is an extremely helpless, childish, clinging person who seems almost parasitic in his relationships with others. It is obvious that he still has, within the elements of his personality formation, many of the traits associated with very early childhood. The young child is normally dependent, clinging, and relatively helpless. He looks to others to meet his needs. He expects to give little in return and has no real ability to consider others altruistically. So it is with adults suffering from this passive-dependent type of personality disorder. They relate to other adults almost as if the latter were parent figures who are expected to supply everything and require little in return. There is a large oral element to the personality formation of these individuals. Such people do not have a conscience which forbids the clear, overt expression of such childish dependency. They seem to have accepted this as part of their existence and expect other people to accept it also. The oral dependency can be said to be egosyntonic in that such patients are not guilty about it, at least to any marked degree or for any period of time.

The passive-aggressive personality is manifested by a passive type of rebellious resistance. This is most clearly seen in a tendency to pout, to be obstinate, to be stubborn, to procrastinate. There is obviously a good deal of underlying resentment against what is required. Yet, such individuals do not dare, apparently, to rebel openly and refuse to follow orders. They merely follow orders in such a way as not to produce adequate results. This type of personality reminds us very much of the little child again. If he is constantly ordered and nagged by his parents to do this or do that, perhaps to come to meals or to take a bath or to clean his room, he may not have the strength and the ability, or perhaps even the courage, to rebel openly. Yet he is very slow in accomplishing these tasks, or perhaps he does them in such a way that they are not really efficiently accomplished. He may pout, he may be obstinate, saying very little and at the same time doing very little. He expresses his resentment, rebelliousness, and in a sense, his aggression and yet does so passively. It is essentially an obstructionistic pattern. In the adult such formation is not uncommon. There are many individuals who, although chronologically adults, nevertheless still pout, are still stubborn; they procrastinate; they inwardly resent what is asked of them and yet do not have the ability to refuse.

The aggressive personality within this category is characterized by a more open expression of inner resentment. This rebelliousness reaches its outward expression in terms of irritability, temper tantrums, and impulsive, destructive behavior on occasion. Neither these patients nor those in the previous two subcategories are actually antisocial. They usually do not conflict with the law or the rules of society outside their own homes. Nevertheless, they cannot by any means be described as mature, co-operative individuals. The aggressive type of person, again, acts very much like the small child who when required to do something may be stirred into open rebellion. This sort of behavior is found in the husband who, although dependent through most of his life, occasionally is stirred into childish temper outbursts during which he becomes extremely angry, perhaps breaking furniture or physically abusing his wife. The large dependent element in his personality is easily traced by thorough review of his day-to-day living. Again, reflected in this person's basic problem is his immaturity, requiring more of the world than he is prepared to give back. This builds within him a chronic resentment which periodically reaches the explosive point. After it is over he again resorts to his more passive dependent behavior.

Case History: Passive-Aggressive Personality

A thirty-five-year-old married woman came to the psychiatrist about her husband, complaining that he had, over the past five years, become increasingly irritable and had been showing more frequent temper reactions which at times amounted to destructive, openly hostile behavior. For instance, he would lose his temper if the children were too noisy and would deliver a tirade, occasionally beating the children. If his breakfast eggs were not cooked in the proper manner for him, he would throw the plate and eggs on the kitchen floor, leaving broken crockery and the mess to be cleaned up while he went off to work. If his wife did not show all the sexual ardor he felt he deserved, he would become angry, degrade her, threaten to leave home, and on one occasion did go out of the house and remain out most of the night. Life had become very difficult with him and his wife was hopeful that something could be done. Fortunately, in this particular case it was possible to arrange to have the husband seen. Obviously, little could be done in such a case if the husband was unwilling to co-operate—to come in and to join in a therapeutic endeavor. The family physician in this case was a fairly close friend of the patient and was able to convince him of the necessity of seeking help. He was able to put pressure upon the patient to at least come to see the psychiatrist in order to try to improve the marital situation.

The history of this patient's life revealed that he had been an only child of a doting mother who had catered to him throughout his child-hood. He had been a typical spoiled young man during his teens and, because he was attractive and intelligent, things had come easily to him without his having to make any great effort. When he married he expected the same kind of service from his wife that he had previously had from his mother. Actually, his wife gave him a great deal. However, he soon demanded more than she could give. The difficulty lay in the fact that, like anyone who has been overindulged during early life, he had never learned to identify with the kind of loving person who is willing to make sacrifices for others. As usual, instead of his demands decreasing as he grew older, they increased. Lacking the capacity to appreciate his wife and being unable to be satisfied by what she gave him, and at the same time being unable to give her much in return, caused him a great deal of inner resentment. He felt increasingly that he was justified in complaining and misbehaving, since he felt that he was being starved of attention and affection by his wife. It did not occur to him that his requirements were far beyond those any human being could meet.

During psychiatric treatment it was possible to arouse this man's will-ingness to try to grow up and to achieve some discipline within himself. In spite of his irritability and tantrums, he was not achieving happiness and therefore was more willing to listen to suggestions. He gradually developed a spirit of fair play and a give-and-take which was put to use in therapy. As his liking and respect for the therapist grew, he accepted new values and came to treat his wife with the love and consideration which she deserved.

This man's mother was like so many mothers who take too literally educational propaganda about "making the child happy." They think they make their children happy, but in reality prevent them from learn-ing some of the valuable lessons of independence as well as of give-and-take. They do not give such youngsters the ability to endure frustration or to respect those who co-operate with and serve them.

Treatment: Passive-Aggressive Personality

The treatment of the passive-aggressive patient depends first, of course, upon his willingness to realize that his own longings and require-ments are impossible to satisfy and that this is one of the main reasons why he is so unhappy. With this knowledge the therapeutic endeavor has begun. If, then, he can be helped to establish a firm, positive, useful relationship with the therapist, he becomes more willing to accept some of his shortcomings and begins, almost like a little child, to cure them, partly in order to please the therapist. He takes within himself the therapist as a part of his superego, much as the little child takes within himself the parent. He begins then to try to live up to a more mature standard of living. He is more willing to accept some of the values which the therapist is able to pass on to him.

COMPULSIVE PERSONALITY

The person with compulsive personality resembles closely the obsessive-compulsive psychoneurotic with the one exception that there is a lack of overt obsessions or compulsions. There is a typical concern toward "doing things right." This individual is perfectionistic, meticulous, and generally rigid. He requires of himself excessively high standards in almost every area of his life. He is scrupulous in house-cleaning, meticulous about appointments, and perfectionistic about his work. He is generally rather cold and "formal." He is unable to relax, to be flexible, warm, and changeable.

While it is perfectly reasonable for a person to be careful and thoughtful about his attire at an important dinner engagement, such standards would seem rather ridiculous on a hunting trip far from civilization. Nevertheless, the compulsive personality must retain his same perfectionistic, rigid, unbendable standards no matter what his surroundings. Such a person may create, at least initially, an excellent impression. A woman of this type keeps her house immaculate, but she nevertheless has a house rather than a home. A secretary of this type allows nothing to chance and performs an above-average job; nevertheless, she prefers and as a matter of fact even needs to keep everything in a routine, ritualistic schedule that never allows for changes. Such a compulsive personality prefers to plan things ahead so that he knows what is coming and when it is coming and therefore stands less of a chance of being disturbed in his equilibrium. As he rises in status he is often saddled with responsibility to a degree larger than he can manage entirely by himself, in accordance with his rigid standards. He is unable to delegate authority and therefore becomes subject to increasing anxiety.

Many an individual with a compulsive personality makes an extremely favorable impression, at least initially, because of his tendency to be "friendly," often to the point of ingratiation. However, when one spends time with him, one invariably realizes that this is artificial behavior. The compulsive person has difficulty revealing his real feelings and it soon becomes evident that his "friendliness" is not sincere and deep. Whenever such a person does give vent to his inner hostility, it is apt to be in an explosive outburst for which later he feels extremely guilty. Such a person is capable of becoming quite punitive, obnoxious, disagreeable, and sarcastic in his periodic releases of pent-up hostility. He is ordinarily a rather obstinate individual—who may again appear very amenable to suggestion in some areas of his life and yet extremely obstinate in others.

Such a patient has a truly "anal" personality in that, at least unconsciously, there is a large amount of obstinacy, tendency toward messiness and disorder, ambivalence, selfishness, and hostility. His personality structure has incorporated a large element of defensive formation by which these inner objectionable traits are, for the most part, reversed into their opposites, so that perfectionism, meticulousness, rigidity, and ingratiation are the result. It is only at times that there is a true breakthrough, almost explosively, of the inner characteristics. The compulsive person holds his emotions under such tight control that he is unable to express flexibly what he feels but instead must present to the world a rather rigid pattern which is wholly artificial. At times such a patient, particularly if involved in severe environmental pressures, resorts to the use of obsessions and compulsions, thereby becoming a true obsessive compulsive psychoneurotic.

Case History: Compulsive Personality

This thirty-five-year-old married man came to the physician complaining primarily of difficulty in his marital adjustment. He had been married only a few years at the time he consulted his physician. His visit had been mainly instigated by his wife.

As his history was pieced together through contributions of both the patient and his wife, it soon became evident that his rigidity was a primary problem. Instead of living enjoyably with her, as his wife had a right to expect, the patient seemed to focus his entire attention upon managing her. He felt that they must live on a budget which he himself dictated and over which he maintained a rigid control. He closely supervised every item she purchased. He would reprimand her if she did not buy as wisely as he expected. He disapproved of the fact that she talked too frequently on the telephone. He gave her suggestions about cleaning the house and even controlled the kind of flowers she planted in the garden. He criticized her grammar and the tone of her voice and advised her concerning the purchase of her own clothes. When she contracted a cold he would tell her how she could have avoided it, had she been sufficiently farsighted. While he constantly "worked" to improve her and to bring her behavior up to his perfectionistic standards, he was at the same time unable to take any suggestions at all from her or others about his own adaptation.

He acted as if he did not need any modification in his own personality and as if he were being the most kind and altruistic individual. He felt that to take this much time and effort to impart his "wisdom" to his wife was a great contribution. He could not understand why she was frustrated and angry rather than grateful to him about it. After a few warnings that she would leave him if he did not mend his ways, they separated and his wife threatened to divorce him. It was at this point that he grudgingly agreed to seek psychiatric help. He still felt misunderstood and had great difficulty in seeing that there was any reason for anyone to dislike his personality.

His history revealed that he had been brought up by an extremely strict mother and father who cared little about social life. The father worked to earn enough money to provide for his family and felt that this was the limit of his obligation. The mother was a worrisome, nagging person who required excessive conformity of him very early in life, generally beyond his ability. No matter what he did it was not sufficient. While he did not like this, he had no choice but to accept it. A good portion of this rigid strictness had been introjected and thus had become a part of his own personality. He did not realize how much he wanted to act toward others as his mother had acted toward him and how he had actually pleasurized this trait within himself, even though he disliked his mother and had tried to keep her out of his life. He felt, much as his mother did, that in working for order, punctuality, and meticulous attention to detail, he was really being kind.

The therapeutic endeavors for this patient were initially directed toward stimulating his tendency to admire his own intellect. He had, as many of these patients do, a reading acquaintance with psychiatry.

The physician deliberately stimulated his interest in this direction in order to challenge his desire to excel from an intellectual standpoint. This was done by engaging the patient in discussion, for instance, of his dreams. He was encouraged to produce all of his ideas about these dreams and subsequently became intrigued with the idea of understanding the mind. However, as he gradually became more involved in the therapy, it became possible to help him understand his lack of true emotional participation in relationships. He was helped to see how he was treating the entire therapeutic process as an intellectual exercise and was encouraged to participate in it emotionally. He also gradually came to see himself more objectively as an excessively demanding, rigid person who placed too extreme requirements upon himself and upon others. The intensity of his whole defensive pattern gradually diminished to the point where he could become more understanding and tolerant of both himself and of others. During this process he was reunited with his wife, who found him a more enjoyable person as a result of his increased flexibility. His treatment consumed many months, but nevertheless was sufficiently successful to re-establish his marriage on a more stable foundation and allow him to live a more useful and pleasant life.

Treatment: Compulsive Personality

The compulsive type of personality generally comes to treatment only when his environment becomes sufficiently demanding that his personality structure begins to cause him discomfort. Such patients are apt to have had an increase in anxiety, a development of obsessions or compulsions, or perhaps the onset of a depressive episode. Quite frequently they request help with the bothersome symptom from which they suffer, and at the same time resist efforts to make their whole living pattern more flexible. They seem to fear, as it were, that the physician will make them into sloppy, lazy, good-for-nothing characters, and, as a result, they are rather difficult to change. They are prone to defend their own meticulousness and perfectionism. The patient, for instance, who gives exaggerated attention to detail, if challenged about this, is apt to rise up in righteous indignation, inquiring whether the therapist expects him to be a sloppy, careless person who does not care about his work. In a sense he seems to fear that his defensive structure will be removed and that he will have only the inner childish anal characteristics.

Such patients can be reassured that, in spite of prolonged therapy, they will never become what they seem to fear, namely useless, lazy persons.

They can be helped to see slowly how some relaxation in their own rigid standards will increase their pleasure in living and their efficiency in work. One of the most difficult features of the treatment of compulsive-personality patients is to help them put true, sincere emotions into their interpersonal relationships. This is often accomplished primarily during the therapeutic process, where the patient is encouraged to vent his feelings toward the therapist and to do away with his artificial, defensive, ingratiating manner. Situations where anger would be expected but is not forthcoming are discussed, and the patient is helped to see how he is unable to show either this anger or any other emotion.

SOCIOPATHIC PERSONALITY DISTURBANCES

It seems wise here to say a few words about this general sub-division of personality disorders. We have discussed personality pattern disturbances which are quite far-reaching pathological prob-lems, and include such problems as the inadequate, the schizoid, the cyclothymic, and the paranoid personalities. We have then dis-cussed personality trait disturbances which are of a less diffuse structure in that they do not involve many areas of the individual's adjustment and are theoretically less incapacitating than the first type. These include such entities as the emotionally unstable, the passive-aggressive, and the compulsive personalities. Now there is a third group, the sociopathic personality, which is characterized primarily by the individual's conflict with the society and cultural milieu in which he lives. He frequently runs afoul of the law because he transgresses the rules society has laid down.

Sociopathic personality disorders are quite severe in terms of psy-chopathology and difficulty in therapy. Their severity and guarded prognosis is contributed to by the fact that the patient frequently is in difficulty with the law and therefore has a problem staying out of prison long enough to attain beneficial results from psycho-therapy. A factor which is evident in many personality disorders obtains here: that is, many of these people are not acutely uncom-fortable and do not seek psychiatric treatment themselves. The majority of them do not suffer from any strong sense of guilt or motivation for self-improvement. They represent a tremendous problem for society and one which unfortunately has not been satisfactorily dealt with to date. It must be remembered that some individuals react in an antisocial or nonconforming manner because of an underlying psychosis or neurosis, and thus run into conflict with the law. These individuals are not properly classified within this category. It is ordinarily not too difficult, upon interview, to ascertain the presence of a severe psychotic or neurotic pattern in some individuals who are in difficulty. When this is true, the patient is often willing to see the need for treatment or, if psychotic, can be hospitalized and given therapy.

ANTISOCIAL REACTION

There is a certain proportion of individuals within our society who are extremely self-centered, hedonistic, and live primarily upon the pleasure principle. They are callous people who have little regard for the rights and privileges of others. They want what they want when they want it and give no thought to the person from whom they are taking it. They lie, steal, fight, or use any other means which seem to gain them their own ends. They profit little from experience or punishment and form extremely weak relationships with others. They have no loyalty to anyone except themselves and primarily love only themselves. They reveal a remarkable lack of a sense of responsibility. They are inconsistent except in seeking for their own pleasures. Such individuals as this have been classified in the past as "constitutional psychopathic inferiors" or "psychopathic personalities." Most of them give a history dating back to very early childhood of an attitude which obviously does not take into account the feelings of others. They have never attained a real devotion or sincere relationship with anyone. They often have drifted, again seeking their own gratification.

Such patients, when confronted with a psychiatric interview, rationalize the greater part of their behavior. They admit only what they feel the interviewing physician already knows. They minimize or, if possible, deny other things which they feel may not be known. They attribute to themselves relatively high motives in many cases. If they are frustrated, which can happen during an interview, they become irritable and resentful. The emotional instability of these patients is notorious and they are easily stirred to anger. If they have sufficient courage, they will attack; otherwise they will quickly find other means out of their plight. Many of them are capable of making excellent initial impressions, only to be found later to have meant nothing of what they originally said. Such people as this have often achieved, by one means or another, relatively respectable standings, perhaps even in the professions. They then go about their business of hedonistic pleasure in such a way as to quickly run afoul of society's rules and mores. They may attempt to show guilt when punished but really do not feel it. Essentially the majority of them lack a stable conscience and do not learn from repeated difficulties in the same antisocial act. Their problem presumably stems from an extremely early and relatively severe lack of parental warmth, often combined with excessive parental punishment. They have been unable, early in their lives, to form a stable relationship with their parents. Their ego growth has been slight and has been distorted to the point that they are extremely narcissistic and egocentric.

Case History: Antisocial Reaction

This thirty-nine-year-old prisoner was interviewed in jail, where he was serving a life sentence for a fourth offense of armed robbery. He and one or two companions had, on several occasions, attempted bank robbery. The first three times he had been caught and had been sentenced to varying periods in jail. The interviewer asked him why, after having had three previous convictions, he had been willing to take a chance on the fourth. He replied that he felt he needed the money with which he could then buy a business and settle down and "go straight." He made a great attempt to convince the interviewer of his sincerity in wanting to go straight. He seemed at the same time to accept the idea that robbing a bank was a perfectly justifiable method of getting the money to accomplish this.

His history revealed that he was one of five children of a working man who had deserted the family when the patient was five years of age. The mother had had to go to work and had been away from home so much that the children had had little supervision except that provided by the older siblings. The patient attended school through the seventh grade, although he had frequently truanted prior to this. He sought jobs but was unable to hold one for any period of time. He soon fell into the company of others who were living a predatory life. His involvement in armed robbery began before he was out of his teens. He illustrated his defective judgment and his inability to learn from experience and punishment by his remark about his fourth offense.

As is typical of such patients, this particular man exerted every effort to gain the psychiatrist's confidence and—to the patient even more important—the psychiatrist's influence in the legal side of his difficulty. He obviously felt that if he could impress the psychiatrist with his sincerity, his honesty, and his goodness of purpose, he would attain what he was really seeking, namely his release from prison.

Treatment: Antisocial Reaction

It should be remembered that the majority of these individuals do not seek treatment actively. They come into the psychiatrist's hands, as a rule, only when forced to do so by someone in their environment or by their circumstances. Society's method of "treatment" is that of incarceration. However, this tends only to confirm the antisocial person's conviction that it is not worthwhile loving anyone. He is treated, in many instances, with cruelty and deprivation, which enhances his feeling that loyalty ties are useless. Such an individual really suffers a severe basic personality inadequacy. It is extremely difficult to establish a therapeutic relationship with him and this, of course, is necessary for any real maturation.

These patients are infantile in their emotional lives and relate on this basis to others about them, including psychiatrists. They are willing to listen, to agree, and to try to seek their own ends from the therapeutic relationship. However, the moment anything is asked of them or they are put under any pressure in the treatment situation, they are apt to pout and become irritable and even rebellious. If they are seen on an outpatient basis where they are responsible for their own lives, they frequently miss appointments, particularly if the material discussed has not been to their liking. Any small irritation produced by the psychiatrist results in their refusing to return. They have such a lack of superego that they suffer little guilt from their repeated transgressions toward other people. There is little that motivates them to continue therapy and they prefer to seek their own satisfactions by the infantile acting out which they have always used. The therapeutic prognosis for such people is extremely guarded. Sometimes limited gains can be made if they are treated on an inpatient basis where their daily activities can be controlled so they cannot get into trouble. However, innumerable patients of this type have begun therapy on an outpatient basis only to quit because of the anxiety produced or to commit some antisocial act for which they were subsequently incarcerated so that therapy could not proceed.

This category is represented by the individual who disregards the social rules and regulations and frequently runs into conflict with the law because he comes from an environment in which such practices are considered the normal and usual thing to do. There are certain isolated segments of our population in which behavior standards are a great deal different from those accepted by society in general. At times this variance is within a family and at times within a small group of society. The patient with the dyssocial reaction may have little conflict within himself and be a relatively mature individual from the standpoint of his own family or small segment of society. However, his values have been so distorted and disturbed that he is unable to live at peace with the rest of society. It is interesting to note that psychological testing of such an individual may reveal a relatively mature pattern because the relationship between id, ego, and superego seems to be free from conflict and there is little demonstrable immaturity present. However, this same "mature" person may, at the same time, be chronically involved in conflicts with the law.

Case History: Dyssocial Reaction

A young man of nineteen was arrested, convicted, and sent to jail for stealing supplies from the warehouse of his employer. He had subsequently been selling them to other people. While serving his sentence he revealed little guilt about the matter and was at a loss to explain why everyone seemed to feel that he had done wrong. He thought that he was merely unlucky to have been caught. His history revealed that this very practice had been common with many members of his family: not only his father but several of his uncles and cousins had been involved in the same type of behavior. He had literally grown up in an atmosphere where stealing from one's employer was the accepted and wise thing to do. One made a mistake only if one was caught. Having absorbed such superego ideals from important people in his environment, the patient felt that this kind of behavior was perfectly legitimate. His family considered that stealing from one's employer was not only acceptable, but that anyone who did not do it was not very smart. It was felt by the entire family that those who lived upon their own salaries were different and unusual and that their own family practices were the normal ones.

Treatment: Dyssocial Reaction

The slum areas and other underprivileged sectors of our population are fertile breeding grounds for dyssocial reactions. There, youngsters, particularly during their adolescence, often come into conflict with the law. The majority of their contemporaries are doing the same things as they are and for them to try to abide by the usual rules and regulations of our society would be extremely difficult. Their parents often talk freely about stealing or lying or cheating and these youngsters absorb the same qualities. A beneficial therapeutic milieu is one wherein they can learn some of the more stable, useful, and accepted social mores. It is for this reason that such places as Father Flanagan's Boys Town are extremely useful to this type of delinquent adolescent. Such youngsters are not emotionally sick in the true sense of the word, but simply have never been exposed to an environment which teaches them the proper modes of behavior. They are able to introject and take into themselves better methods of behavior if they are surrounded by the proper environment. They are loyal, capable of good relationships, and, if placed under the care of socially mature individuals, are capable of changing their behavior patterns to get along with society. These individuals have a much better prognosis in general, especially if they can be removed from their pathological environment, than do the antisocial-reaction types.

SEXUAL DEVIATION

The sexual deviate is an adult individual who does not prefer and seek as an object of his sexual instincts genital union with a member of the opposite sex. The child in the process of growing up passes through several stages of psychosexual development, and only eventually reaches mature heterosexual adjustment. The mature human seeks gratification for his sexual instincts through sexual intercourse with a person of the opposite sex. There are, however, many people who because of childhood emotional problems are never able to attain this mature goal and remain fixated at an earlier level. They may turn to members of their own sex for gratification or perhaps to some other object which falls short of the ordinary mature goal. Such individuals have been referred to as sexual perverts, in that their sexual practices do not fit within the mores of society, or even within the standards of maturity.

The child, if allowed and helped to grow up in a normal way, will eventually reach heterosexual maturity. However, if enough barriers are placed in his way he will stop short of this goal and prefer some other means of sexual outlet, because of fear or envy or some other reason. There are some children who, by virtue of their early surroundings, are unable to love the opposite sex and therefore love the same sex. There are other children who would like to love the opposite sex but, because of one reason or another, such as a feeling of danger or resentment, may prefer to love only an item of clothing of the opposite sex. There are still other individuals who are so fixated in an extremely early level of psychosexual development that they can love only while they hurt, and thus become sadists. Others may love only as they are being hurt and become overt masochists. The essential problem to be considered is that the individual deviates from the normal heterosexual adjustment by virtue of his earlier childhood problems.

Homosexuality

The homosexual, or invert, is an individual who has as the object of his sexual aim other individuals of the same sex, rather than those of the opposite sex. Homosexuality is an extremely important problem both from psychological and social standpoints, and is much more common than is ordinarily realized. There is a social stigma in present society attached to homosexuality; and little, if anything, constructive has been done toward dealing with this problem on a large or efficient scale.

The label of homosexuality as a real perversion should not be applied to an individual except where his preferred sexual object is a member of the same sex. According to Kinsey,[1] 37 per cent of the male population "has had some homosexual experience between the beginning of adolescence and old age." This, however, does not mean that approximately one-third of our male population can be

[1] Kinsey, Alfred et al. *Sexual Behavior in the Human Male.* Philadelphia, W. B. Saunders Co., 1948.

correctly labeled homosexual. Many of these individuals whom Kinsey includes have had perhaps one or two experiences which can be called homosexual. Such experiences may have been in the nature of an experiment or precipitated by circumstance and do not reveal a definite personality trend, and therefore these figures do not reflect the general trend and tendency of each individual. It may be pointed out here that, as Kinsey has shown, certain people have at their disposal four possible outlets for their sexuality. These outlets are: (1) heterosexuality, (2) homosexuality, (3)bestiality, and (4) nocturnal emissions or masturbation. If the environment or circumstances remove the first, primary outlet, the individual is apt to seek another from the remaining ones. Perhaps the best example of this situation is seen in prisons where heterosexual outlet is completely denied. The result is an increase in the incidence of homosexual practices. Many such prisoners, at least outside jail, could not be referred to as true homosexuals, since they would ordinarily lead active heterosexual lives. However, in the absence of members of the opposite sex, they will resort to homosexual outlets. Similar situations were occasionally seen in isolated outposts of the armed forces during World War II. Whatever tendencies of latent nature were present toward homosexuality came to the fore under circumstances lacking heterosexual but containing homosexual opportunities.

It is necessary to the understanding of homosexuality to review the psychic development of the child. The infant begins in the oral phase, during which his mouth apparatus is his chief source of pleasure. Following this comes the anal phase, where the anal area assumes the primary position as a source of pleasure. Then comes the genital phase, at which time the genitals begin to assume their importance as the principal locality providing pleasure through stimulation. The child, as he slowly moves from one of these levels into the next, is what has been described as "polymorphous perverse." This indicates that until the internal psychic apparatus has reached its proper level of mature adjustment, the youngster is capable of being led into various so-called perverted activities for pleasure without much difficulty. It is relatively easy for an adult to lead a youngster before the latency period into any type of perverted sexual activity and to have the youngster find pleasure in such activity. If, on the other hand, a child goes through the ordinary phases of development, he will eventually become a heterosexual person in whom the object of his sexual aims will be genital union with an individual of the opposite sex. If, however, environmental circumstances impinge upon his emotional growth and distort his psychic development, it is possible that there will be built into his personality an entirely different sexual structure. The sexual instinct still demands discharge, but the object may change because of these environmental and psychic circumstances. The latency period has been referred to as the "homosexual phase." It is during this period of life that boys normally prefer the company of other boys, and girls the company of other girls. The two sexes have very little in common and have very little respect for each other. It is only with puberty that a real interest in the opposite sex appears. It comes to the fore at this time only if previous personality development has been relatively normal and if there are no immature fixations which still forbid this type of development.

Generally speaking, the overt adult homosexual prefers his sexual contacts with an individual of the same sex. His outward behavior and mannerisms may or may not reveal characteristics of the opposite sex. It is possible, for instance, for the male homosexual to appear either extremely masculine or extremely feminine in his manner of speaking and behavior; while the female homosexual may have a thoroughly masculine or thoroughly feminine appearance in her type of dress and behavior. Ordinarily the overt homosexual shows a predilection for certain types of homosexual practice. For instance, one male homosexual may prefer to play the passive role in his relationships, assuming what appears to be the feminine role with other more aggressive male homosexuals. Some Lesbians play the feminine role but can do so only with other more masculine women. Homosexuals often tend to have what they refer to as "affairs" which are characterized by strong attachments between two people which subsequently are broken, only to be replaced by new attachments.

Etiology and Psychopathology—Homosexuality

It is impossible to outline in clear and simple form one cause of homosexuality, since ordinarily this condition results from a combination of factors. In the first place, in spite of increased knowledge of personality function, we cannot completely exclude the possibility of constitutional factors. In certain youngsters, beginning in early childhood, there is evident a clear homosexual orientation toward environmental situations which ordinarily would not be expected to produce this marked reaction. Such children's entire approach to life is homosexual. A boy, for instance, by the time he is seven or eight, may reveal obviously feminine characteristics and mannerisms in such a way that his difficulty appears to have diffused throughout his body and included all of his musculature. In other instances we find that childhood experiences with adult homosexuals have played a large role in the production of a patient's difficulty. The youngster who grows up constantly exposed to, and introduced from an early age into, homosexual practices stands a much greater chance of eventually showing this type of difficulty and having it imprinted indelibly into his fantasy life and perhaps his overt behavior.

From the standpoint of internal psychodynamics, the major contributing cause of homosexuality can be said to stem from the fact that the growing youngster has never learned to love, comfortably and by preference, and feel thoroughly warm toward a member of the opposite sex. The reasons for this are various. In the case of a boy, a strict, cold, domineering, authoritative mother may have closed the door to her son as far as future heterosexual relationships are concerned. On the other hand, a frightening, threatening father may so intimidate his boy that the youngster never feels comfortable in loving women but can only try to save himself by submitting passively to men. He is unable to seek the love of a woman if he has to compete with a man to do so.

In the case of a girl, there is often an extreme degree of inability to accept the feminine role. Such a woman, at least unconsciously, has great resentment toward what she considers to be the superior masculine role and thus refuses to accept the feminine role. She instead attempts to prove herself "the better man." It is also possible that a girl may not have had a truly feminine mother with whom she might identify, or that her father rejected her and her femininity, or that perhaps a combination of the two ensued. For whatever inner psychic reason in these cases, homosexuality results. The essential point is that the female homosexual finds assuming her feminine role in sexuality with a man both unpleasant and unacceptable.

Treatment—Homosexuality

The degree of success in psychiatric treatment of the homosexual depends upon several factors. Certainly not the least in importance is the sincere desire evinced by the individual toward being cured. There are many homosexuals who not only accept but seem to welcome their pathological orientation and who do not seek treatment for it. They would not co-operate actively in such treatment if it were forced upon them. They feel that the concept of learning to love a member of the opposite sex would be as difficult to understand as it would be for the normal individual to learn to love only members of his own sex. For such people, because of their inability to co-operate thoroughly in therapy, psychiatry has relatively little to offer. For the person who greatly desires to be rid of his homosexual tendencies, the outcome often depends upon the extent and degree of his homosexuality. It also may be determined by the amount of his libidinal investment in other aspects of life beyond sexuality. Treatment is ordinarily prolonged and tedious, but may, if the degree of pathology is not too severe, have favorable results. At the present time homosexuality is certainly not one of the conditions considered most amenable to psychiatric treatment.

Case History: Sexual Deviation (Homosexuality)

This thirty-six-year-old male patient came to the psychiatric clinic seeking some sort of advice about his homosexual activities. His immediate family, as well as a number of his friends, had become aware of his problem and he greatly feared that he might lose his job as a result. In his initial interview he said that he had, as far as he knew, been a homosexual "all my life." He had had numerous homosexual experiences during childhood which had involved a large number of boys. This type of activity had continued sporadically throughout his adolescence and the years following. He had twice, during his early twenties, come into conflict with the law because of his homosexual practices and had finally joined the Army to escape prosecution.

The patient had remained in the Army four years, serving two years overseas. He gave a history of many homosexual contacts, both active and passive, during his military service. These acts were finally discovered by the military authorities. The patient was hospitalized and subsequently received a discharge on the basis of homosexuality. He had resumed civilian life in a town some distance from his original home. There he had met a girl and married. He obtained a good job and, at least for a while, attained a fairly satisfactory social adjustment. Within about a year, however, after his marriage, he began a series of sporadic homosexual contacts. The patient had never been particularly satisfied with heterosexual relationships, either with his wife or with the few women with whom he had become involved. He was not impotent, however, to a degree which entirely prevented heterosexual intercourse.

The patient's homosexual activities were again discovered when he approached a man who reported his advances rather than accepting them.

The patient's early life revealed that he had come from an extremely psychopathological family. His mother had been a chronic alcoholic who had shown little interest in her children. She had been openly promiscuous during her married life, and the patient and his older sister had both known about it. The patient's father was a passive, ineffectual type of man who frequently flew into childish temper tantrums. Both parents had been extremely inconsistent with their children but not often severely punitive. The patient had finally graduated from high school, although he had always shown indifference toward his education. He was highly intelligent and obviously had a good deal of potential.

This patient unfortunately suffered little anxiety. He was mildly guilty about his homosexual experiences but was primarily concerned because these activities were a potential source of difficulty for him in society. He was seen only four times, during which attempts were made to help him understand more clearly the pattern of his early life as it related to his homosexuality. His difficulty in loving and accepting women was also a subject for discussion during these interviews. However, by the third interview it became clearly evident that the patient was not seriously motivated toward achieving a more mature type of sexual adjustment. He felt that the solution of his problem was a continuation of his homosexual activities with more efforts directed toward keeping them a secret. He readily accepted the idea that he had a pathological sexual orientation, but nevertheless felt that it would be impossible for him to change this and preferred to drop treatment.

Fetishism

This is a condition in which the essential element or object by which an individual attains sexual satisfaction is a certain article of clothing or portion of the body. This particular object, whether clothing or a body segment, is invested with a great deal of sexual interest. The fetishist may have as his own fetish feet, hands, hair, various articles of underclothing, and so forth. For this individual, his own particular object of sexual attraction holds far more interest and sexual excitement than anything else, including heterosexual intercourse. The typical male fetishist is apt, for instance, to obtain his own libidinized special article of feminine underclothing and to utilize it to stimulate masturbatory activity. Fetishism essentially is the replacement of adult sexual genital union by a substitute object onto which the entire sexual feelings can be transferred. It stems, as do all sexual perversions, from an inability of the individual to reach a level of mature heterosexual development. Ordinarily the individual is fearful of attaining sexual union in the usual way and therefore he picks some object which he can substitute and thereby avoid anxiety. Once again, the cure is often difficult and in great measure depends upon the patient's motivation toward co-operation and his desire to be cured.

Transvestitism

This is a condition in which the individual prefers to wear the clothes and live the life of the opposite sex. It may or may not be associated with overt homosexuality, although usually it is. Even if it is not, the internal dynamics closely approximate those of homosexuality and the prognosis and treatment are very similar. Transvestitism in clinical practice is so often seen as a corollary of overt homosexuality that the latter usually forms the primary process and the transvestitism is only an offshoot of this homosexuality.

Exhibitionism and Voyeurism

Exhibitionism is, in the male, characterized by repeated episodes in which the individual displays his genitalia to someone of the opposite sex, usually a person unknown to him. In the female, exhibitionism is characterized by the exhibition of the entire nude body. To explain simply, the male exhibitionist is attempting to reassure his inner doubts about his masculinity by displaying his genitalia to women who he feels will obviously react rather violently and will thereby reassure him that he is truly a man. Voyeurism is the active element of exhibitionism and represents a tendency to look at rather than to be looked at. Such people are commonly referred to as "Peeping Toms." Both the exhibitionist and the voyeur feel a compulsive and sexualized need to look at or to be looked at, but are ordinarily quite fearful about actually indulging in sexual experiences. There is in these conditions a continued heightened importance attached to the childish desire to look at and be looked at which is present in every youngster. Such desires are ordinarily present in the adult as a part of ordinary sexual activity and play a secondary role to mature heterosexual intercourse which remains the primary end goal of the sexual life. In the exhibitionist or voyeur, this role of looking at or being looked at plays a primary role and displaces and even rules out eventual adult heterosexual intercourse, at least in many cases.

The treatment of the exhibitionist and voyeur depends primarily, again, upon the real motivation of the individual toward achieving a cure. If such patients are willing to undertake a rather prolonged course of psychotherapy, they can often be rid of their infantile fixations and can be freed to progress toward a more mature heterosexual adjustment. However, many of them do not suffer greatly because of their perversion and therefore do not seek assistance. The exhibitionist is more prone to get into difficulties from a legal standpoint and be coerced into psychiatric treatment. This alone does not suffice as adequate motivation for complete psychotherapy. If the individual truly recognizes his difficulty and is anxious to be rid of it, the prognosis is a great deal better.

Sadism and Masochism

The sadist is a person who characteristically derives his sexual pleasure from inflicting physical pain and punishment upon his sexual partner. The masochist is the reverse, a person who derives his sexual pleasure from having punishment inflicted upon him. These two perversions are again holdovers of early childish tendencies. Every youngster, particularly during the anal phase, is sadomasochistic, and if his tendencies, through early environmental trauma, are fixated within the personality and subsequently welded together with the sexual impulses, overt sadism and masochism are possible results. Such individuals have been unable to achieve mature love relationships so that love making, if it may be called such, becomes a matter of either hurting or being hurt rather than displaying the genuine warmth which normally would be present. The relationships of these people lack tenderness, while pleasure is derived from the kind of violent impact which is indentified with uninhibited conquering or killing. Differentiations should be made between the true sadist and masochist, who are sexual perverts, and the moral sadist and masochist. The latter are much more common and are differentiated by the fact that although they enjoy inflicting pain and being hurt, they have "desexualized" these attitudes. The real sadist gains sexual and even orgastic pleasure from physical abuse of his partner. The moral masochist may in fact abuse the other person, either physically or verbally, but does not feel conscious sexual pleasure. The "cruel husband" and the "long-suffering wife" are examples of moral sadomasochism. Of course, in all human relationships and particularly in the sexual relationship, there is an identification of the lover with the beloved and vice versa. Hence the sadist has latent masochism and the masochist has latent sadism, so that where one of each get together they may work out a completely satisfactory relationship. However, this is the exception rather than the rule. Hence, the sadistic personality can be a great burden to another individual who is not sadomasochistic in nature. The masochistic personality, who enjoys "taking a beating" from life, likewise can be very exasperating to one who is not similarly inclined. Some men will repeatedly accept exploitation in business opportunities and some women will accept excessive exploitation in their work and love lives, to the exasperation of family and friends. However, the individual who is cruel or self-destructively passive does not change readily. Such a person may say he wishes to be different but there is a subtle gratification with it all that helps to keep his behavior in motion and any changes usually call for the therapeutic discipline involved in Freudian psychoanalysis.

Rape and sexual assault are phenomena of the hostile personality —that is the personality with limited conscience reactions, which lacks tenderness and affection in the sexual sphere. The sadist and masochist rarely seek therapy unless forced to do so or unless they finally become involved in a sadomasochistic orgy which is beyond their ability to tolerate. Then, like other patients with personality disorders, they often do not remain in therapy for a sufficient length of time to attain an adequately mature heterosexual adjustment. The prognosis of these individuals from a psychiatric standpoint is guarded and once again depends upon their motivation toward cure.

ADDICTION

Human beings may become addicted to a variety of drugs, including alcohol. Such drugs have in common the fact that they induce a false sense of well-being and, at least temporarily, minimize the stresses and strains of the world and also lower the level of inner anxiety. The addict has become extremely dependent upon the repeated and chronic use of drugs. At times, with certain of the drugs, there are physiological changes which produce severe symptoms when the drug is withdrawn. Other drugs do not have painful physical withdrawal symptoms, but nevertheless are difficult for the addict to leave alone. Almost everyone who becomes an addict does so because of underlying personality difficulties. Addicts are unable to tolerate the tensions and frustrations of ordinary living and resort to the use of a drug in order to escape. Since removal of the drug only places them again in the difficult anxiety-ridden state present before the addiction, such patients are extremely difficult to cure.

Alcohol is discussed in Chapter 18 ("Acute Brain Disorders").

Some of the other common drugs which are of importance are discussed here.

Morphine and Opium

Morphine enjoys the reputation of being an extremely valuable drug in the practice of medicine. Unfortunately, however, it must also be branded as a dangerous drug because of the malignancy of the addiction which it is capable of producing under certain circumstances in certain individuals. This is also true of several other related drugs, such as opium, heroin, and some of the newer synthetic preparations such as demerol and dilaudid. These drugs are capable of producing a euphoric state, removing all the worries and cares of reality. So attractive is this state of being to certain people that they repeatedly resort to the use of drugs in order to attain it. In some cases the initial administration of the drug is given by a reputable physician and is directed toward the amelioration of some type of physical pain. The individual because of his inner psychological difficulties remains chronically in need of further doses of the drug even though the root of the pain has been removed. Other patients begin the use of the drug through association with addicts. Often the drug habit begins insidiously with the individual taking small doses occasionally in order to produce the longed-for feeling of well-being. There is an increase of the dose ultimately and the patient tends to become more tolerant of it so that larger doses become necessary in order to produce the desired effect. Many addicts reach a daily dose that would be fatal to a nonaddict. The person who becomes addicted to morphine or one of the related drugs has many similarities to the alcoholic from a psychological standpoint. There is a deep oral craving which the patient attempts to satisfy by using the drug. The ordinary frustrations, disappointments, and difficulties of routine living are too difficult for such people and they resort to the creation of an artificial world of their own in which they are not beset by all of these problems. Unfortunately, in the morphine addict, as the required dosage increases, the patient has more and more difficulty obtaining his supply. This often results in the patient becoming completely untrustworthy and getting himself involved in various nefarious schemes in order to obtain the drug.

These patients often try in every way to conceal their addiction from all but their fellow addicts. Many become experts at feigning physical illness of a type that would ordinarily require morphine. They put on such a convincing show that the physician prescribes morphine for them without recognizing the true nature of the difficulty. It is exceedingly rare that a true psychotic picture results from the use of morphine or any of its related substances. It is true, however, that sufficient doses of these drugs are capable of producing hallucinations, at least temporarily. The most obvious personality disturbance which is seen is the gradual disintegration of a sense of responsibility, duty, and obligation. These patients reach a stage where their primary aim in life is to insure their daily dosage of the drug and they become willing to go to almost any lengths to meet this need. Contrary to popular belief, the use of morphine and the allied drugs does not lead to an increase in criminal activity other than as a secondary result of the patient's attempts to insure his daily drug supply.

The stopping of a drug in an addict, particularly if he has been taking moderate or heavy dosages, results in severe withdrawal symptoms. These symptoms come on during the first day and terminate, as a rule, after about a week or ten days. The patient becomes increasingly agitated and there is apparent a remarkably heightened sensitivity to temperature, both hot and cold. There are gastrointestinal disturbances, especially nausea and vomiting, as well as diarrhea. All of these symptoms are accompanied by severe abdominal cramps. There is increased irritability, and fits of crying and temper reactions are not uncommon. Patients in the throes of withdrawal symptoms suffer a great deal and often plead for a dose of their drug or try to utilize any means at hand to obtain a fresh supply. In weakened, emaciated patients with malnutrition or other physical difficulties, it is not impossible for death to occur from exhaustion during this period. The symptoms are thought to be an aftermath of morphine's inhibitory action on the sympathetic nervous system, there being a compensatory heightened activity of that system coincidental with the withdrawal. This heightened activity following the removal of morphine is thought to be the basis of withdrawal symptoms.

The treatment of morphine addiction is an extremely difficult problem and even under the best circumstances is not successful in many cases. The most extensive experience is that of the group who are working at the United States Public Health Service Hospital in Lexington, Kentucky. Many types of therapy have been proposed but the biggest difficulty still remains that of insuring the patient's freedom from relapse in the future. The drug may be withdrawn abruptly, rapidly, or gradually. Generally speaking, abrupt withdrawal may be utilized only in those individuals in good physical health who have been taking relatively small doses. Rapid withdrawal is the most popular method and is accomplished ordinarily in a period of one to two weeks. The patient is given initially a daily divided dose of three to four grains of morphine and this is gradually cut so that at the end of one to two weeks he is taking no drugs at all. He is not told the amount of the drug that he is getting during the withdrawal period. Gradual withdrawal involves five to six weeks during which the dosage is more slowly diminished. Some workers feel that the administration of daily small doses of insulin is of benefit in reducing the severity of the withdrawal symptoms, but this is somewhat questionable. Physical means such as tub baths and packs have some value, especially in that they result in the patient's receiving more attention, which is beneficial. Any other measures of a similar type are obviously useful in most cases.

It is obvious that the successful treatment of morphine addiction must take place within the confines of an institution. Addicts are extremely adept at obtaining supplies of the drug and they may do so even in a well-guarded and -maintained institution. Psychiatric workup and psychotherapy form a cornerstone in the successful treatment of morphine addiction. Addicts need an extensive follow-up. They require help in rearranging their living and also prolonged therapeutic efforts directed toward furthering their insight into their own personalities.

Case History (1): Drug Addiction, Heroin

This twenty-two-year-old male was admitted to the psychiatric ward from jail. He had developed, while in jail, what appeared to be an acute and violent psychotic episode. He had begun reading the Bible continuously for as much as fifteen or more hours a day. He had wet and soiled himself, had visions, apparently heard voices, and gave every appearance of being out of contact with reality. When he had been transferred to the hospital, this "psychotic behavior" ceased rather abruptly. He became talkative in an apparent effort to gain favor with the physicians and nurses who were caring for him. The following long and somewhat complicated story was gradually pieced together.

This patient had had an exceedingly pathological and traumatic life which had finally culminated in his incarceration in jail prior to his hospital admission. He had come from a family of father, mother, and an older sister. He had gone to school through the seventh grade, having repeated several grades as a result of failing. He had truanted for two years before his parents discovered that he was not going to school. During this period he had spent his time going to the movies and getting into various minor difficulties with a group of delinquent boys who were somewhat older than himself. As a child he had suffered from enuresis until the age of ten. Somnambulism had become a prominent symptom during his adolescence. He had often been beaten with a belt or an ironing cord by his mother until he was six years of age, at which time a physician suggested to his parents that they stop this severe treatment because of his nightmares and enuresis. He had a history of having had a violent temper as a youngster and at times would chase his sister with a butcher knife. He had for a long time had the idea that people were trying to make some kind of a fool of him. He said that his mother used to put feminine clothes on him trying to make him look like a girl, again, as far as he was concerned, in order to have people laugh at him.

He learned about the differences between the sexes at the age of about six. He had attempted intercourse with girls at this same age. There were only two rooms in his parents' apartment and the patient was used to hearing parental intercourse. When he was twelve or thirteen he slept in the same bed with his parents and on at least one occasion tried to have intercourse with his mother. His first successful sexual intercourse was at the age of fourteen with a girl in the neighborhood. Sexual activity had been frequent and promiscuous. As far as the patient was concerned, it had been satisfactory. He developed gonorrhea at the age of eighteen and attempted to cure himself by increasing the frequency of intercourse.

He had begun drinking beer at the age of fourteen. Shortly after this he took up wine and whisky and "reefers." When he was seventeen he began "snorting" cocaine and taking heroin occasionally. At the age of eighteen he began taking heroin regularly. This, like all the other drugs, was introduced to him by a group of older men with whom he associated. The heroin, he said, at first made him "feel warm all over my body." Subsequently he would develop a drowsy feeling of complete supremacy over every person and every obstacle. He usually took his first dose immediately after arising in the morning and consequently had little interest in food. He soon began to lose weight. He stated, at the time of hospitalization, that he had progressively lost interest in his appearance and often went about dirty and unkempt. His parents and his girl friends had complained about this but he said that his only interest had been in acquiring and taking heroin, and that the remonstrations of others meant little to him. He was so sleepy and fatigued during the day that he was discharged from his job in a factory. This made little difference to him and he shortly obtained another position in another factory. He would go to work in the morning, punch his time card, go home, and then return in time to punch his card at the quitting hour. When this was discovered he was warned to show up at work regularly, but when he refused to do so he was fired. His next source of income was from selling narcotics. His entire earnings by this time were utilized to purchase heroin. He eventually had to give up this work because he was consuming too much of his own product and could not adequately pay for it. Thereafter, he obtained money by stealing. This was accomplished while he was "high," that is, under the influence of heroin. The patient said that at such times he felt brave enough to steal from any of the prominent stores. Occasionally he would sell baking powder as heroin and would use the money to buy further heroin for his own use.

He had never married but had had six children by three different women. The welfare society had finally had him arrested for nonsupport of these children and had had him sent to jail. It was during this incarceration, when he was visited by two detectives, that he formulated his plan to get out of jail. The detectives had tried to question him about a robbery in which the patient had taken part with a couple of other people. He did not want to inform on these friends and so he refused to answer the questions which the detectives put to him. One of them made a remark about the fact that if he was going crazy, they might as well send him to the hospital. This idea appealed to the patient, so he began his "psychotic" behavior.

This patient was subsequently transferred back to jail when it was discovered that he was not psychotic. A medical report was sent with him to the proper authorities indicating the patient's severe degree of psychopathology and also including recommendations for further treatment, if possible, in a hospital especially designed for the care of narcotics addicts.

Case History (2): Drug Addiction, Morphine, Demerol

This twenty-seven-year-old married woman was admitted to the hospital at the request of her family. Her husband and brother accompanied her to the hospital and both were quite upset, having recently discovered that she had secretly been taking morphine. Her brother was a physician and it had been discovered that she had forged his name to several prescription blanks when it had proven otherwise impossible for her to get morphine.

The majority of the history was given by the husband, who was also a professional man, although not in medicine. He said that their marriage of seven years had been a chronic state of unrest, emotional upheavals, and deceit on the part of his wife. She had, he discovered, lied to him during their courtship, not only about her age but also in several other important matters in regard to her family. Following their marriage, she had proven herself to be an extremely poor housekeeper. She had subsequently had one child; during pregnancy she had suffered an extreme emotional upheaval, frequently complaining of severe distress. Thinking back on it later, the husband remembered that on several occasions she had received "shots" from the various attending physicians and, on a few occasions, even from her brother. According to her husband, she had always been a fearful, highstrung person, easily irritated and also easily depressed. She had often complained of aches and pains and had often sought the advice of numerous physicians. Yet, as far as her husband knew, no definite organic diagnosis had ever been forthcoming. Many instances had come to light where she had lied to both her husband and her brother regarding her activities.

The patient came from a family in which there had been little warmth or love. Both her mother and father were busy, active, prominent individuals with little time for their children. She had one sister who had made two unsuccessful marriages and had led a generally unproductive life. The patient had apparently never carried anything through to completion. She had tried several jobs, none of which had lasted over six months, prior to her marriage. In her earlier life she had been given every possible opportunity to learn art and music but had made little of her chances. She had always made an initially good impression wherever she went but had never been able to keep friends over a long period of time.

The patient herself was a fairly attractive, although not particularly well-groomed woman who was obviously tense, anxious, and defensive. She went to great pains during the interview to impress the examiner with the degree of suffering which she was undergoing. She tried to impress him with the tremendous guilt which she felt at having taken demerol. Whenever possible she did not admit any gross misdemeanors in the past unless she had reason to feel the examiner already knew about them. She vehemently denied that she was a morphine addict, claiming that she had occasionally taken this drug only to alleviate her numerous pains, and on rare occasions to alleviate her anxiety. She cried several times during the initial interview, again in a somewhat histrionic way which had little real depth or meaning to it. She felt that this was because she had come from an unhappy home and that no one had loved her. She felt in general that most of life was quite difficult and that everything made her too nervous, so that she had on occasion resorted to the use of opiates. The guilt which she expressed seemed relatively superficial and the examiner had the over-all impression that there was little real emotional rapport between the patient and himself.

This woman remained in the hospital for approximately two weeks. During this time it was necessary to prescribe barbiturate sedatives for her in the evenings as she would otherwise be unable to sleep. From time to time she became excessively anxious, restless, and difficult to control. A regimen had to be instituted shortly after her admission whereby small doses of one or two cubic centimeters of demerol were administered twice daily. She had, previous to admission, not had any specific level of demerol intake, although on some days she had taken as much as thirty cubic centimeters. At the end of two weeks and many psychotherapeutic interviews, it became obvious that this patient was unable, at least for the time being, to maintain an adjustment in her own home. She oscillated markedly between attempts at a more mature attitude and learning how to cope with her own problems and an extremely immature, childish attitude of irritation and bitterness whenever she did not receive her "rightful" dose of demerol. Eventually it was necessary to transfer her to a more suitable institution where long-range plans could be made for a thorough approach to her addiction.

Cocaine

Cocaine is not resorted to by drug addicts nearly as often as morphine and its related drugs. Many of the features of addiction are similar, with one exception: the prolonged use of cocaine has more deleterious effects and may more often produce a psychotic picture. At times certain addicts alternate between the use of cocaine and morphine. Initially, cocaine produces a feeling of euphoria, an increased psychomotor activity, and a sense of well-being. As its effects pass, the patient is left with a "hangover" which involves weakness, irritability, and restlessness. Commonly found in the prolonged use of cocaine are paresthesias which give the patient the sensation of bugs crawling under his skin. There is a progressive deterioration seen in cocainism where the patient at times becomes hallucinated, agitated, and terrified. There is a loss of social and moral responsibility and the patient becomes oriented primarily around attempts to obtain additional supplies of his drug.

The withdrawal of cocaine does not lead to the violent symptoms seen in morphine withdrawal. Treatment, however, must obviously be undertaken in an institution where it can be assured that the patient cannot obtain further supplies of his drug. Successful treatment must also be accompanied by psychotherapeutic interviews similar to those described in the section on morphinism.

Marijuana

The use of marijuana has become more common in recent years and is exceedingly difficult to control because of the relatively widespread growth of the plant. The leaves of this plant, which can be grown in a wild state or cultivated, can be dried and made into cigarettes which are often called "reefers." Marijuana is much less malignant than morphine, cocaine, or any of the other related drugs. Smoking marijuana produces a feeling of euphoria, a distortion of time in which time itself seems actually to be "stretched," and an increased sense of well-being, of power, and of ability. Fortunately the prolonged use of marijuana does not result in the mental deterioration so commonly seen with cocaine. The effects of inhalation of marijuana are not essentially different from those of alcohol and certain individuals prefer marijuana because of the ease with which it can be obtained and the fact that it is often less expensive than alcohol. The treatment of a patient using marijuana revolves essentially around the psychotherapeutic approach. Many of these individuals have personalities similar to that of the chronic alcoholic and the treatment is essentially similar.

Barbiturates

The various members of the barbiturate group have achieved an unhealthy popularity, particularly in the United States. While it is true that the abuse of this group of drugs does not lead to the malignant problems which follow the abuse of the various opium derivatives, it is also true that the vast consumption of barbiturates offsets this lower malignancy. There has been a false sense of safety associated with the use of barbiturates on the part of the medical profession and the laity. The physician may with ease prescribe all sizes and colors of capsules and pills containing barbiturates. Such prescriptions may temporarily smother anxiety and, if given in sufficient doses, induce sleep. To the tense neurotic patient suffering from insomnia they appear to be a boon. To the prescribing physician they represent a quick and easy method of calming the complaints of his neurotic patients. Frequent visits, a few moments of conversation, and a renewed prescription are all that are apparently required to mask the symptoms of many such individuals.

Unfortunately, the widespread use of and popularity of barbiturates has often led to their choice as a method of suicide. These factors, combined with the relative ease with which such drugs can be obtained, require that every physician be alerted to the dangers of indiscriminate barbiturate prescriptions and also that each physician be adept at recognizing the signs and symptoms of acute barbiturate poisoning as well as its treatment.

It has been our impression that the majority of people suffering from the abuse of barbiturates are essentially neurotic individuals seeking an escape from insomnia or anxiety. There is no increased tolerance of the barbiturates with their prolonged use, as is found in the opium derivatives. The beginning of the average barbiturate habituation occurs when a patient consults a physician because of an inability to sleep. A prescription for one of these drugs is provided and the patient subsequently becomes aware of the state of relaxation produced and the disappearance of anxiety. He may then mention to his physician the periods of diurnal anxiety which he suffers and receive a prescription for smaller doses of another barbiturate. Soon such a patient is relying heavily upon repeated small doses of such drugs in order to reduce his tension during the daytime and upon larger doses during the night in order to induce sleep. There is a sort of vicious cycle created in which the patient becomes increasingly fearful that should he refrain from taking these drugs he will either suffer severe anxiety during the daytime or be unable to sleep at night.

Depending upon the degree of anxiety from which the patient suffers and also upon the amount of immaturity and neurotic difficulties present, the patient continues to increase his dose of daily barbiturates until his ordinary life activities are severely distorted. He becomes chronically irritable, tired, and intellectually dulled. He is progressively less interested in maintaining his family and occupational adjustments. If relatively undisturbed emotionally, such a patient may continue for years taking moderate to heavy doses of barbiturates without showing obvious signs of maladjustment.

Acute barbiturate poisoning has become increasingly common during the last few years. Individuals suffering from various types of depressive reactions, as well as other emotional problems, may save up what they consider to be a lethal dose of barbiturate, wait until they feel their act will not be discovered, and then take all of the accumulated capsules. Following ingestion such patients sink into a deep comatose state from which they cannot be aroused. A frequent aid in diagnosis is the report by some member of the family of an empty bottle of barbiturates found near the patient.

Treatment: Barbiturates

The treatment of these patients, whether suffering from acute or chronic barbiturate intoxication, is first directed toward removing the toxic factors. In chronic barbiturate cases, there is ordinarily little danger in abrupt removal of the drug. If the patient, however, is taking excessive doses, convulsions have been known to occur in the event of rapid withdrawal. Where such a situation threatens, doses of sodium dilantin may be prescribed as an anticonvulsive.

Acute barbiturate poisoning is often a medical emergency. The patient may be brought to the hospital in a comatose state, unresponsive to external stimuli, with a weak, rapid pulse, low blood pressure, shallow, slow respiration, and rapidly developing cyanosis. Various therapeutic agents have been advised in acute barbiturate poisoning. Slow intravenous administration of a 0.3 per cent solution of picrotoxin is advisable. A stomach lavage with a solution containing magnesium sulfate is of benefit if there is a residual still present in the stomach. Amphetamine has proven to be a useful intravenous stimulant in these cases. One of the latest and perhaps most useful therapeutic devices is that of electrostimulation utilizing the machine by which electronarcosis is administered. As yet this treatment has not had wide use, but in the cases which have been reported its efficacy seems promising. One of the difficulties, of course, is that in the ordinary general hospital such a machine is not always available.

The recognition and treatment of the underlying psychological factors is of extreme importance in both acute and chronic barbiturate poisoning. In the chronic variety, the majority of patients must be helped to understand how continual reliance on barbiturates is an unwise crutch and how a more thorough understanding of the symptoms about which they complain is of even greater importance. Ordinary psychotherapeutic measures, as explained in Chapter 21 ("Principles of Psychotherapy"), are useful. The acute barbiturate patients are often still bent upon self-destruction, so that considerable care must be expended to obviate this possibility. These patients are often adept at covering up their inner feelings and postponing future suicidal attempts until they are released from the hospital. At other times one finds that an unsuccessful suicidal attempt seems to assuage much of the patient's guilt and leaves him in a state of mind which is no longer potentially suicidal.

Case History: Acute Barbitural Poisoning

This thirty-three-year-old female was admitted to the hospital in a comatose condition. There was a history given by her husband that sometime during the night she had apparently taken an indeterminate number of barbiturate capsules. The exact number was uncertain, but it was probably between seven and twenty capsules. The husband said that on two previous occasions similar incidents had occurred, but his wife had taken smaller doses at those times. He had, on both occasions, taken her to hospitals where she had been revived within a twenty-four-hour period and had been subsequently returned to her home. The husband was greatly concerned that each time she had awakened quite distressed to find herself in a hospital.

At the time of admission the patient's coma was of moderate degree. She was unresponsive to physical stimuli and had a fever of 100.5°. Her pulse was rapid, as were her respirations. Reflexes, however, were present and active. Breath sounds were increased and there were a few rales in the bases of both lungs. Breathing was primarily abdominal.

The patient was given oxygen and precautionary penicillin to prevent the development of pneumonia. Blood studies revealed a slight leucocytosis. This patient was also given several doses of amphetamine. Her condition slowly improved so that by the end of her day of admission she had regained consciousness. Her blood pressure and respirations improved and her temperature gradually returned to normal.

The following morning the patient appeared quite depressed. She would not eat and complained bitterly about her plight. She was particularly depressed at having again awakened in a hospital after an overdose of barbiturates. She was also extremely fearful that she would be given electroshock therapy during her hospitalization. She related poorly to the physicians who visited her and seemed to have relatively little desire to return to her family or to make attempts to improve her own life situation. A decision was made to administer electroshock therapy on the third day of her hospital admission. She was subsequently given a course of three electroshock treatments, during which time improvement was rather remarkable. Subsequent history revealed that she had always been plagued with emotional problems. She described her childhood as having been "very sad." She came from a broken home in which the children were placed either in foster homes or in homes of disinterested relatives. She had married at an early age in order to escape the drudgery of the work required of her in an aunt's home.

Her marital choice had been quite poor. She had married a man who was completely passive, unable to hold a job, and generally inadequate in the role of husband. He did, however, enjoy the limelight which he felt was thrown upon him each time his wife attempted suicide. On such occasions he childishly refused to listen to or heed medical advice and acceded to his wife's demands that she be taken home. At the time of the present admission, it was found possible to delay her discharge for a period of nine days but, by this time, both the patient and her husband were unwilling for her to remain any longer in the hospital. She had regained her previous personality pattern in that she was rather color-less, depressed, and determined to maintain her own way of life. She had a poor ability to relate to others, but her depression was no longer present to a degree that prevented discharge. She seemed unwilling to accept any accommodation for future psychotherapy and was discharged against advice.

TRANSIENT SITUATIONAL PERSONALITY DISORDERS

Classified under this heading are certain personality responses of a more or less acute nature which occur in a relatively well-integrated individual under situations of acute stress or strain. In order to qualify in this category the patient must have a reasonably well-developed personality with a good adaptive capacity and revert to his original normal adjustment with the passage of the stressful situation.

GROSS STRESS REACTION

It is generally agreed among those who have studied human personality under various conditions that every individual has his limits of endurance. Every personality has its limits in adjusting continuously to a particularly threatening or dangerous situation. Such situations are seen both in war- and peacetime. They are more numerous during wartime and, as a result, gross stress reactions are more common then. However, during certain peacetime civilian catastrophes these reactions are also seen. In combat they are caused by a constant threat of death by bullets, bombing, fire, ship sinking, plane crashing, or other such violent situations. They arise from such threats as mutilation, capture, noise, and death, especially when in combination with other such factors as lack of sleep, poor or insufficient food, poor leadership, excessive heat or cold, bad news from home, or friction with comrades or superiors.

Any one of these factors or a combination of them can in a varying length of time produce great anxiety, hostility, resentment, fear, depression, grossly disturbed physiology, and even transient symptoms of a psychosis. The same thing can happen in peacetime civilian situations, although not as often. Severe prolonged fires, loss of property or home, inadequate food or water supply, the necessity of living in strange and crowded quarters, and at times the threat of disease can cause gross stress reactions. Deeply emotional situations, such as the loss of relatives, can provoke serious symptoms of a temporary nature in a relatively well-integrated personality. Earthquakes or explosions, plane wrecks, train wrecks, and auto crashes may precipitate a stress upon people which can bring about any one of the symptoms of psychogenic disturbance which have been described.

Case History: Gross Stress Reaction

This twenty-seven-year-old lieutenant was admitted to the station hospital after having been evacuated from the front. At the time of admission he was essentially mute. He refused to answer questions and responded very little to outside stimuli, even painful ones. His admission note gave a history of his having been in steady combat for a period of approximately 150 days. His particular unit had been subjected to repeated bombings and strafings and had often been involved in extremely dangerous missions. This officer had proven himself an audacious leader, had frequently volunteered for dangerous missions, and had often subjected himself unnecessarily to risks.

The patient remained in his mute condition for approximately twenty-four hours after admission. Physical examination was essentially negative, except for some degree of malnutrition and dehydration. The patient was given approximately five grains of sodium amytal slowly, intravenously, at which time he apparently experienced a hypnotic type of trance wherein he was again with his unit at the front lines undergoing his battle experiences. He proceeded to give many commands in a loud and excited voice. He helped lay a telephone wire up and down the hall, excitedly giving commands to various hallucinated subordinates. His behavior was excited and highly emotional, punctuated by outbursts of crying and obvious signs of fear. Within about fifteen minutes he quieted down and fell into a deep sleep, and when he awakened, responded to questioning and to his environment. He improved rapidly during the next few days.

His history revealed that he had an essentially normal background, had always made a good adjustment, and had had a relatively good family situation in his childhood. He was an example of an individual whose well-integrated personality had finally given way under the extreme gross stress situation of 150 days of steady combat assignment.

ADULT SITUATIONAL REACTION

This is a clinical picture characterized by maladjustment in a difficult situation or in a new environmental experience of a type which occurs in everyday life. In such individuals there has been no previous evidence of serious underlying personality difficulty. This reaction is apt to occur, for instance, in a college student who is away from home for the first time. It may occur as a result of an individual's attempt to adjust to marriage, in response to a new type of work, or a new and additional responsibility on his regular job. Some of the symptoms which are seen in this reaction are anxiety, asthenia, reduced efficiency, low morale, and unconventional behavior. These symptoms are produced by the increased tension resulting from the new situation and the personality's temporary difficulty in adjusting to it. Even though these symptoms occur in people who have otherwise been well adjusted, they may, if untreated, become quite chronic in nature. This possibility clearly points up the need for such services as those rendered by psychiatrists and personnel counselors in industry, in colleges, and in the armed forces. In other words, almost everywhere where people are dealing with new responsibilities in life some of these conditions will arise, and adequate, prompt treatment is needed in order to prevent a more chronic disability. Nurses in training, new school teachers beginning to work, and fresh recruits in the armed forces are examples of individuals prone to show this adult situational reaction. If an individual with this diagnosis remains untreated he may have a difficult time and be anxious and physically uncomfortable for a period of days or weeks. He may, in fact, become psychoneurotic or develop a personality disorder. However, as he solves his particular emotional problem his symptoms will diminish quickly and he will suffer a relatively small amount of discomfort.

It must be remembered that there are many individuals in our society today who have what might be called latent psychoneuroses or personality disorders. This merely indicates that such a person has some predisposition in the direction of certain emotional problems and these problems will be brought to the fore if the person is placed under a new environmental strain. It is wise in assessing the personality of an individual to determine accurately the amount of latent psychopathology present prior to the outbreak of symptoms. As we have mentioned previously, there is a limit to the tolerance of every personality. In order to be diagnosed as adult situational reaction, the individual's personality must be relatively healthy and reveal an essentially good adjustment except for the temporary difficulty encountered in a new situation. It also must be a relatively flexible personality capable of adjusting to difficulty, perhaps with a minimum of guidance or psychiatric help, or even perhaps without such help.

Case History: Adult Situational Reaction

This patient was a twenty-year-old senior student nurse referred for psychiatric consultation by an internist whom she had consulted. Her history revealed that she had been born in a small town, the third child in a family of four. Both her parents were school teachers. Her family, from the history, seemed well adjusted in every respect. She had always been an above-average student. She had been active in sports and popular with both boys and girls. She had decided to become a nurse while still in junior high school. She had worked part-time in order to save money for her tuition in nursing school. Her social life was normal as far as could be determined and she had become engaged to a boy from her own home town. She had intentions of being married after the completion of her training. During her two-and-a-half years of training she was regarded as a "Class A" nurse both from practical and academic points of view. She had been popular with all of her roommates, as well as with most of the other nurses in her class.

All had gone well until she was placed in a particular job which had previously been filled by a skilled graduate nurse. She averaged fourteen hours of work each day and, in addition to this, had been on call four nights during the week. The tension in this position was particularly high and the pressure from her supervisors became greater as the shortage of nurses increased. She was constantly being checked, corrected, and criticized, until she began to feel that she was failing in a job for the first time in her life. Symptoms of nervousness, tensions, fatigue, insomnia, lack of ambition, nightmares, and poor school work began to occur. Finally one night, after twelve hours of assiduous work, the patient went home and had a severe attack of vomiting and diarrhea which required hospitalization.

The internist whom she consulted realized quite soon that her entire problem was an emotional one and referred her for psychiatric consultation. She was seen for two visits. During these visits her life history and nursing situation were reviewed with her. As she talked she revealed a remarkably good ability to see the tension and undue stress to which she was subjected and also her great concern lest she not measure up. She began to realize that more responsibility had been placed upon her than she was able to carry because of her student status and began to see more clearly how she had been striving for an impossible goal. The psychiatrist assisted in obtaining her transfer to another section of the hospital where her duties were commensurate with her stage of training. This resulted in immediate improvement and she was able to return to work within a period of twenty-four hours.

A follow-up revealed that she continued to adjust very well. She was quite happy and efficient and was subsequently elected to an executive position in the student body. She led a satisfactory social life and was getting along so well that, to her at least, the above experience seemed like a nightmare of the forgotten past.

PART V

Psychophysiologic Disorders

Psychophysiologic Disorders

CHAPTER 13

Psychophysiologic Autonomic and Visceral Disorders

THE TERM *psychophysiologic* refers to those conditions caused by the physiological expression of chronic and exaggerated emotion, much of which is unconscious. It seems wiser, in accordance with the official classification of the American Psychiatric Association, to use the term *psychophysiologic* rather than *psychosomatic*. The latter word has come to indicate so many different ideas that it lacks the specificity required in a scientific classification. On the one hand, the term *psychosomatic* indicates an approach to the patient which is as old as medicine itself and implies the consideration of man as a unit rather than as separate psyche and soma. On the other hand, *psychosomatic* has more recently been used to indicate a certain group of physiological disorders whose etiology often stems from psychological problems.

Many terms have been proposed for these and related conditions. Such terms as *organ neurosis, cardiac neurosis,* and *gastric neurosis* are examples. It is advisable here to recall the broader implication of the old term *psychosomatic*. It indicates that each man possesses a psyche and soma, and what occurs in one system influences the other. Man reacts, in other words, as a unit, and it is basically impossible to consider one system without considering the other. When a man is angry this is not purely a psychological state. There are equally important somatic components which are easily measurable and demonstrable. Similarly, one cannot consider a cirrhotic liver without taking into account the fact that it belongs to a man with a wife, three children, and a mortgage, and that the man's emotional state depends upon his physical well-being and ability to meet the demands which his environment places upon him. In other words we do not find a specific disease, but rather a human being who is suffering from some pathology.

While it is true that astute practitioners of the art and science of medicine have always approached their patients from a psychosomatic viewpoint, it nevertheless remains true that many of the most important advances in understanding relationships between mind and body have come relatively recently. In the past many physicians excelled in their ability to produce improvement, particularly in certain patients, because of their intuitive understanding of the great importance of the emotional elements in such patients' illnesses. Particularly within the last few decades, however, our increased understanding of these matters and improved techniques of research have added a firm scientific foundation to what originally was part of the art of medicine. Of course, measurement of the emotional factor in disease must to a large degree include the changes wrought by psychotherapeutic improvement. This is complex and requires the highest kind of collaboration on the part of the clinician, physiologist, and psychotherapist.

The psychophysiologic conditions, then, as we use the term here, refer to those conditions in which physiological, or eventually even pathological, dysfunction is brought about by a chronic emotional state present in the individual. We know that there is a close interrelationship between the autonomic system, the endocrines, and the psyche. This is an extremely complicated relationship but it is recognized that a disturbance in one of these systems is capable of producing changes in the other two. What we are concerned with particularly are chronic disturbances of the psyche which subsequently produce changes through the autonomic or endocrine systems and thus eventually lead to physiological and possibly pathological bodily disturbances. When a normal individual becomes angry, his sympathetic system becomes more active, his adrenals increase their output of adrenalin, and the body makes preparations for either fight or flight. In the normal individual as soon as the danger situation is past the physiological activities return to normal. However, there are certain people who, by virtue of psychological problems, remain at least unconsciously angry all the time. In such a situation the physiological functions remain in a constant state of preparation for fight or flight. Blood pressure is elevated, sympathetics are hyperactive, and other such mechanisms are constantly alerted. If this situation continues over a period of days, weeks, months, and years, certain physiological changes eventually become pathological and tissue damage becomes apparent. Eventually the entire process reaches a stage of irreversibility because of the organic damage that has ensued. At this point, although we have a truly organic condition, it is nevertheless mainly psychophysiologic in its origin.

Such conditions are to be differentiated, at least according to most observers, from the physiological changes which accrue in conversion reaction. In the latter condition the physiological change is symbolic of the inner psychic conflict. In addition to this, it most frequently involves voluntary systems such as the voluntary musculature. The paralysis of an arm, for instance, in the conversion reaction may represent a conflict between the desire to, and the prohibition against, masturbation, or perhaps the impulse toward and prohibition against an aggressive impulse. The symptom in a psychophysiologic disorder, on the other hand, represents merely the "normal" concomitant of a certain emotional state and has no symbolic significance, as, for example, when an individual is angry, one of the normal results of this anger is a heightened blood pressure. The main problem of a patient suffering from a psychophysiologic condition is that he, at least unconsciously, remains constantly angry and therefore his blood pressure remains higher than normal. In reality it is not always easy to differentiate between the conversion reaction and psychophysiologic conditions, since, at least on a primitive level, some psychophysiologic symptoms do have a certain symbolic meaning. It is possible, for instance, to attach symbolic meanings in some patients to the colitis symptoms which they acquire.

Of primary importance is the concept that a sick man is not either organically or psychologically ill but rather that his illness is a total reaction of the total person. In certain diseases the organic plays a major role with the psychic reaction being secondary. In others the psyche plays the predominant role and organic disturbances follow. It would appear, however, that in the vast majority of patients there is a combination of the two factors, both of which are extremely important in the etiology. With the recent popular growth in the concept of "psychosomatic" medicine, some physicians have facetiously remarked that soon even fractures will be considered to fall within this realm. Such facetious prognostications have been long since shown to be true by insurance and industrial physicians. They have pointed out how certain individuals are accident-prone and, because of inner psychological problems, are more apt to have accidents and thus are poor insurance or occupational risks.

METHODS OF STUDY

Modern psychophysiologic medicine has come to rest on a firm scientific foundation as a result of advances and researches in the various branches of medicine. Psychoanalysis, through its ability to bring to light the unconscious dynamics of personality function, has been one of the major contributors to this field. Advances in our knowledge of physiology, endocrinology, and autonomic nervous system function have also brought valuable knowledge to the science dealing with the interrelationships between the psyche and the soma.

Scientific studies contributing to our knowledge of the psychophysiologic elements of various human illnesses have used several approaches. Some investigators, such as Alexander and French,[1] have concentrated on a relatively thorough study of a small number of patients, both those suffering from the particular illness under consideration and those either normal or suffering from other ill-

[1] Alexander, Franz: "The Influence of Psychologic Factors Upon Gastro-Intestinal Disturbance; A Symposium." *Psychoanalytic Quarterly*, III, 1934; Alexander, Franz and French, Thomas et al. *Studies in Psychosomatic Medicine.* New York, Ronald Press, 1948.

nesses. Such patients have undergone psychotherapy or psychoanalysis and the findings from the patients with the particular illness in question have been compared to findings from the others. This method has the advantage that, as the patient's emotional problems are worked through and a resolution achieved, the concomitant effect upon the physiological symptom can be determined. Still other investigators of psychophysiological disorders, like Binger,[2] have undertaken to study large groups of individuals who suffer from those conditions which presumably have an emotional component. They have made attempts to determine by psychological and psychiatric evaluation the personality structure involved. Such findings have then been compared to those of a similarly large group of individuals who either were normal or who suffered from some other pathology. Certain other investigators, such as Dunbar,[3] have constructed what they refer to as a "personality profile." This is a sort of graphical representation of the major dynamics of the human personality. It lends itself relatively well to comparative study, particularly when two different groups are involved. For instance, one group of patients may score relatively high in aggressive areas, while others seem to have a far lower average. Interestingly enough, as more of these studies have accumulated, there have resulted certain unexpected findings. For instance, some conditions which were not assumed to have had an emotional etiology surprisingly enough showed certain characteristic personality profiles. Finally, as another method of study, Wolff and others[4] have tried to correlate physiological, endocrinological, and autonomic responses with certain trial situations. For instance, individuals may be measured under emotional stress and their various responses charted. Patients suffering from one particular type of illness may be compared in these responses to other patients who are either normal or who suffer from other conditions.

[2] Binger, Carl et al. *Personality in Arterial Hypertension.* Psychosomatic Medicine Monographs. New York, 1945.

[3] Dunbar, Flanders. *Psychosomatic Diagnosis.* New York, Paul B. Hoeber, Inc., 1945.

[4] Wolff, Harold G. et al. *Stress and Disease.* Springfield, Illinois, Charles C. Thomas, 1953.

PSYCHOPHYSIOLOGIC REACTIONS

We will discuss in this chapter only those conditions which are widely accepted as having a large emotional component.

PSYCHOPHYSIOLOGIC SKIN REACTIONS

The skin is an organ of the body which readily and visibly betrays many variations in feeling tone. A person may blanch with fright, redden with embarrassment, or even become livid with anger. The ruddy liveliness of the hypomanic has often been commented upon. Similarly, the sallow, dull skin of the depressed patient is well known. Common everyday sayings reveal how emotions are often reflected in the skin. People may "itch" to get at a certain job. Other times we speak of an irritating person as "getting under our skin." At still other times an eerie noise in the darkness of the night may produce "goose flesh." A typical symptom of anxiety is hyperhydrosis, particularly of the palmar area. All of these common occurrences make us more aware of the degree to which the skin is affected by emotional changes. It is not difficult, therefore, to realize that certain chronic emotional states are capable of producing visible and measurable changes in the skin.

It is not within the scope of this book to discuss thoroughly all of the contributions which have been made in the area of psychophysiologic skin disorders. While many psychological problems have been shown to contribute to the development of skin disease, two of the more prominent ones will be mentioned here. These are sexual and aggressive difficulties. The skin has a sexual significance in that stroking it produces a pleasurable sensation. There are certain areas of skin characterized by a rich supply of nerve endings which are particularly erotic in nature, that is, capable of producing more pleasure if stimulated. The lips and genitals are two excellent examples, but it is also necessary to include a third, the anal area. The skin also contains another sexual significance in that looking at and being looked at are pleasurable contributing elements to sexual pleasure. We may therefore postulate that difficulties within an individual in the sexual sphere are capable of producing psychophysiologic skin disorders.

Pruritus ani is a not uncommon condition characterized by incessant itching of the anal region, often without demonstrable organic etiology. It is often complicated by the secondary results of repeated scratching and infection. While patients bitterly complain of the incessant discomfort of the itching, they nevertheless usually are agreed that the scratching is a somewhat pleasurable activity. There is a sort of admixture of pain and pleasure at the same time, but after the condition has persisted to the point of secondary infection, it is possible for the pain element to far surpass the pleasure element. However, the initial foundation of this condition is often rooted in a psychologically anal orientation held over in the personality from the anal stage in life. Many of these people, in other words, have never adequately attained a truly genital personality, wherein the genital area assumes supremacy as an erotic area. Instead they are still fixated in the earlier anal phase where stimulation of the anal area is more erotic. The situation is often complicated by other personality factors, particularly of the superego, which prohibit open, conscious, purposeful anal stimulation. The result is a frequent itch in the area of the anus with subsequent scratching resulting in pleasure and yet to a degree also in punishment by virtue of the ensuing organic problem which arises. Pruritus vulvae again can easily be seen to have a potentially psychological etiology. A patient may well be in conflict about stimulation of the vulva with again the vicious cycle of itching, scratching, infection, and hence punishment. Such patients at times are relatively easily relieved of their symptoms through psychotherapy but it is not infrequent to find some of them extremely refractive to this approach because of the depth and severity of their emotional problems.

Case History: Psychophysiologic Skin Reaction (Pruritus)

A forty-five-year-old male was referred to the psychiatrist by a dermatologist with a diagnosis of pruritus ani. He was a passive and somewhat effeminate man who had married an aggressive, dominating woman. She did not love him and had rejected him to an increasing degree during their marriage. This rejection had been most noticeable in the sexual area. The patient quite openly admitted that he derived about the same amount of pleasure from scratching his anal area as he had ever attained through sexual intercourse. In fact, he said that he got more excitement and pleasure on most occasions from anal stimulation, but that what was lacking was a climax to his excitement. Gradually in his treatment he came to see more clearly that he was identifying himself more in a feminine way than in a masculine way and that he had given up his masculine role to his wife. She was also seen by the psychiatrist on a few occasions and, as her understanding of the situation improved, she was able to co-operate in the therapeutic endeavor and allow and encourage her husband to reassert himself in a masculine role. She also gave him more opportunity for genital gratification. The psychotherapeutic endeavor was supplemented by giving the patient a medication to diminish the itching. It was explained to him that (1) he needed to exert some conscious effort toward controlling his scratching, (2) he needed to verbalize, and thereby dissipate the psychic energy bound up with his fantasies of femininity, and (3) he needed to practice a more masculine role, particularly in the area of sexual gratification with his wife. After approximately six interviews, the patient reported marked improvement in his pruritus ani. Undoubtedly the local applications were of some benefit in his recovery but the majority of it was due to a redistribution of his libido, both through his own increased understanding and through his wife's co-operation and assistance.

Quite a number of studies have revealed the importance of aggression and hostility in certain psychophysiologic skin disorders. In an oversimplified way, one may say that the patient often unconsciously would like to scratch someone else but, because of his own conscience, finds expression of this hostility impossible and therefore takes it out upon himself. Such patients are obviously quite masochistic and self-punitive and in many instances this difficulty increases the problems of treatment.

PSYCHOPHYSIOLOGIC MUSCULOSKELETAL REACTIONS

Emotional tension may express itself in the musculoskeletal system in a variety of ways. Some of the more common examples are "rheumatism," backache, cramps, myalgia, and certain types of headache. The majority of these individuals are "keyed up." They have a considerable degree of pent-up emotion which is draining off into their voluntary muscular system producing the various disturbances. It is sometimes difficult to realize how emotional tension is capable of producing such a clearly somatic symptom as backache. However, a simple example may suffice to clarify this relationship. If a person clenches his fist tightly for a period of five minutes, his entire lower arm will begin to ache through this overexertion. If he clenched his fist just half this tightly, the same physical discomfort would result in a somewhat longer time. If, however, we assume that the increase in muscular tension was only slightly over the normal but continued for a long period of time it is not unreasonable to assume that pain would result. In many respects this is what happens in quite a number of these musculoskeletal reactions. There is a slight but nevertheless constant increase in voluntary muscular tension in a particular part of the body which subsequently begins to become uncomfortable, and finally painful.

There are certain individuals whose inner tension, through frustration or some other means, is constantly above the average. We remember one particular patient who, when she awoke in the morning, found her fist tightly clenched to the point that her fingernails had made deep indentations in the skin of the palms of her hands. She was acutely aware of painful feelings in the joints of her arms. She was an extremely anxious, tense individual who, even though asleep, continued to suffer from this increased muscular tension. It is no wonder that her primary complaints were those of joint pains and muscular aches.

It is advisable here to mention the common "tension headache" which occurs so frequently. As a rule it results from some type of frustration and is the outgrowth of a situation in which the individual is angered and yet at the same time unable to solve his frustrating situation. A simple example is found in the person who sees a poor movie and who leaves the theater with a headache. Such tension headaches are to be differentiated from the migrainous type of headache. The latter type is also psychosomatic but belongs with the cardiovascular-reaction psychophysiologic conditions. A tension headache may result, for instance, when the boss gives a subordinate criticism and the subordinate is unable to vent his resultant anger.

Case History: Psychophysiologic Musculoskeletal Reaction
(Backache)

This nineteen-year-old soldier was sent to the station hospital for further study with a chief complaint of low back pain. The latter had come on during calisthenic drills several weeks previously and had resisted all attempts at treatment. X rays had been negative and nothing orthopedically pathological could be demonstrated from the outpatient studies. The history revealed that upon entering service, this boy had found the surroundings and rigorous training to be a difficult change from what he had been used to in his own home. He was the younger of two children and had always been coddled by his parents, who found it difficult to discipline themselves or their children to the responsibilities of everyday life. The patient had found the change from this dependent, protected atmosphere to the rigors of military life an impossible one. Attempts at psychotherapeutic interviews were essentially unsuccessful in the station hospital and the patient was finally given a medical discharge with a diagnosis of psychoneurosis.

Upon returning home, this patient's parents had the feeling that he could and should recover from his disability. They had him re-examined by an internist and an orthopedist, both of whom pronounced him free of organic pathology. He was referred for further psychiatric help and in his interview with the psychiatrist, he reluctantly admitted his extreme dislike for the service. However, it was difficult for him to see how he could have developed "such terribly severe back pains" from emotional tension alone. He felt that such an assumption on the part of the psychiatrist was a serious indictment of his home training, of his loyalty to his fellow soldiers and to his country. The physician assured him that such things were not uncommon and that his problem was one of accepting this possibility not with guilt and self-criticism but with a constructive attitude of attempting to solve his problems and improving his understanding of himself. This, he was shown, could help him lead a healthy civilian life and possibly allow him to re-enter military service at a subsequent date and perform the tasks which he felt were a part of his duty. At the latter statement he showed great consternation and said, "Oh, to go back in the service would break my back for sure." Here he was shown how clearly he had, without realizing it, verbalized what he really felt inside and how it was connected with his back pain. He was reassured that, at least for quite some time, it was very unlikely that he would be called back into the service.

As his psychiatric interviews continued, the patient gradually accepted the symbolic nature of his symptom formation and began to see more clearly the degree of dependency which had been fostered within him by his parents. He recognized that he had very sincerely wanted to do his full share in the war in which his country was engaged, yet his own immature dependent strivings had been overwhelming to the point of producing chronic tension and consequent backache. His improved insight soon provided him with a much healthier adjustment both toward his parents and his civilian life. Within a period of approximately six months he was able to mature sufficiently to request re-examination for military service and was successful in re-entering the service and subsequently proved a useful soldier.

PSYCHOPHYSIOLOGIC RESPIRATORY REACTIONS

This category includes various psychophysiologic disturbances of the breathing apparatus. Bronchial spasm, certain hyperventilation syndromes, sighing respirations, hiccoughs, and asthma are examples of this category.

Some of the effects of emotion upon the breathing function are well known to everyone through personal experience. In a sudden fright a person "catches" his breath. A person may feel that he "has a weight on his chest" when saddled with many worries. Perhaps the most noticeable example of emotional influence upon breathing is to be found in young infants in whom respiration is normally somewhat irregular. In such a youngster a sudden fright throws respiration into an irregular pattern for a long period of time. As a person grows older, such frights do not disturb respiration for so long a period, but nevertheless have a remarkable influence upon it. Also of major importance in the area of the respiratory system is the entire vocal apparatus through which an individual communicates with others from infancy onward. The phrase "involuntary cry" has been used so often that it is a standard phrase in much of the literature. The respiratory system is partly controlled by autonomic function but in part may be controlled by voluntary methods. This fact, of course, adds further complications to the physiological effects of emotions upon this system.

The condition within this category which has received the most attention is asthma. While it has been clearly shown that many cases of bronchial asthma are directly attributable to a high allergic situation, it is also true that many asthmatics do not show strong reactions to allergy tests. Many of these patients have been revealed to have certain personality problems which, if successfully eradicated, lead to a remarkable improvement in the asthma if the latter has not reached a degree of actual destruction of bronchial rings and thus become irreversible. As Thomas French [5] has stated, "Throughout the lives of patients subject to psychogenic asthma attacks, there seems to run as a continuous undercurrent, more or less deeply repressed, a fear of estrangement from the mother. The cause of this fear is usually the patient's own forbidden impulses which he thinks will offend the mother." In other words, people with a latent affectionate need for the mother which remained ungratified during infancy may continue to feel unconsciously this influence quite strongly. This particular emotional constellation, "I need Mother," has been clearly shown to have a strong effect upon the breathing mechanism. Just how this reaction takes place is not too well understood. It must certainly be tied up in a way with the infant's earliest cries which bring the mother. Moreover, crying of any intensity forces an altered respiratory activity. People who "cry all night" are as exhausted in the morning as an asthmatic who has gone through a nocturnal attack. When a child is closely but ambivalently tied to the mother, he is constantly worried lest his own hostile impulses result in a rejection by her. Yet, on the other hand, his own strong dependent needs make her presence essential. It should be stressed here that, as with all other psychophysiologic reaction, asthma represents relatively severe emotional problems, if it falls within this category.

Case History: Psychophysiologic Respiratory Reaction (Asthma)

This thirty-eight-year-old female sought psychiatric treatment, complaining of intense personal unhappiness. This unhappiness was almost as marked as that seen in depression and it had lasted quite a number of years. With this depression her marked feelings of inferiority were

[5] French, Thomas: "Psychotherapy in Bronchial Asthma. Psychosomatic Medicine." Part II of the *Proceedings of the Second Brief Psychotherapy Council,* 1944. Chicago, Institute for Psychoanalysis.

evident and at times her working ability was impaired. She said that her marriage was not happy and that her functioning as a mother was not satisfying to her. She went on to mention that in addition she had suffered since childhood from asthma and eczema. She had sought extensive allergic and dermatological treatment for both of these conditions but had never been satisfied with the results. Both the asthma and the eczema had waxed and waned, and it was rather difficult for her to determine how much benefit had been obtained by the various treatments prescribed for each condition. At times they seemed to improve as a result of a particular allergic or dermatological therapy, but at other times they had improved without such treatment.

The eczema had been at its height during her adolescence but in recent years had become less noticeable; however, the asthma attacks became more frequent. The patient said that she hoped she might gain some relief from her asthma through psychiatric treatment, although this had not been her primary purpose in undertaking such therapy.

The history revealed that this patient had been brought up by a mother who appeared outwardly fairly well adjusted and conscientious, but who had certainly lacked a basic warmth and knowledge of the emotional needs of children. The patient had not known mothering in the usual sense of the word, although she had been given good hygienic care. Her father was described as a high-tempered, self-centered man who was alternately seductive and neglectful of his children's emotional needs. He had apparently had relatively little true understanding of the role of the father in the family unit. The result of this situation was that the patient had found great difficulty in developing close relationships to other people. She had never been able to form warm friendships with others of either sex, but instead had found recognition through scholastic performance and the exercise of her artistic talent.

As therapy proceeded this patient proved herself relatively adept at verbalizing the inner feelings of which she had been dimly aware. An example which clearly reveals her relationships with others is her remark, "I guess I have always been too arrogant to talk to anybody about the problems of my children. I didn't want to admit that I didn't know it all. I couldn't let any other woman or even man tell me anything and really allow whatever they said to sink in." She went on to say, "When you have asthma you feel good, noble, virtuous, and brave. When I have asthma I feel placid, serene, and good instead of bitter, rebellious, and unhappy as I do at most other times." During another interview the patient said, "If my emotions had not gone into asthma and eczema I know I would have gone crazy. I'm afraid to love people. It does such awful things to me. It's like a raging fever. It tears me to pieces."

During her rather prolonged treatment this patient came to understand her unsatisfactory relationships with her family and she gradually developed an ability to love others without such emotional distress as she had previously known. She became a much more relaxed person and established a comfortable relationship both with herself and with other people.

During the two years following her treatment she has been free of asthma and has had only occasional mild symptoms of eczema. Her personality still reveals a great "neediness." She has a great hunger to be loved, to be accepted and praised, literally to be enfolded within the intense good will of everyone whom she likes. However, by being aware of this tendency she is able to maintain a fairly stable equilibrium. Her capacity to enjoy her husband, children, friends, and work has been enhanced through treatment and the personality changes which she achieved through psychotherapy have reduced her tension to the point where her psychophysiologic symptoms no longer occur.

PSYCHOPHYSIOLOGIC CARDIOVASCULAR REACTIONS

This category includes the various entities which involve physiological malfunction of the cardiovascular system through emotional etiology. Such conditions as migraine, hypertension, paroxysmal tachycardia, and vascular spasm are included here.

Of all the psychophysiologic conditions, those within this category are probably the most plausible to the average individual. Everyone is, from personal experience, aware of the remarkably close relationship between the emotions and the cardiovascular system. For instance, if one were to count the number of times the word *heart* is used in writing and speaking today, one would probably find that more than half the time this usage refers to emotions rather than to the organ of the body. Such phrases as "she gave him her heart," "heartbroken," or "with his whole heart in it" are examples of the emotional connotation of the word. The rapid heartbeat which results from sudden fright or anger is an experience which everyone has had and which makes the psychosomatic aspects of cardiovascular function much easier for the average person to accept. In addition to this, the effect of emotions upon blood vessels is also well known. Blushing and blanching are two very common examples.

At this point it seems wise to stress certain points concerning cardiology which are not ordinarily stressed in books on internal medicine or cardiology. It is one thing to examine and diagnose accurately the cardiovascular status of an individual; it is entirely different to impart the results of one's examination to the owner of this cardiovascular system. As far as the first part is concerned, medical students are ordinarily well-trained and confident. Unfortunately, however, after they have ascertained the condition of the patient's heart and blood vessels, their method of imparting this information to the patient is apt to be one which only accentuates whatever emotional problems are already present. The ordinary person in our society today is at least superficially aware of the frequency of cerebrovascular accidents, coronary occlusion, and hypertensive heart diseases. He recognizes these conditions as extremely serious and, particularly if he is insecure and neurotic, is extremely sensitive to the method and attitude of the physician who examines him.

The word *iatrogenic* refers to those ailments which are physician-produced—in other words, those conditions which are caused or exaggerated by ill-chosen or improper words of advice given by the physician. Probably in no other area are iatrogenic illnesses as frequent as in the realm of cardiac difficulties. Many people suffer from functional heart murmurs. Unfortunately a fair percentage of such people have been informed of this fact in a manner that leads them to focus whatever anxiety they may possess upon their hearts. Once an element of doubt has been injected about the healthy status of their cardiac function by even one physician, it requires a great deal of effort to eradicate this preoccupation. Patients have an ability to warp and distort through unconscious means the advice and knowledge that is given them to fit their own neurotic needs. Almost every physician has encountered the patient who quotes a previous physician as having made certain statements. When such statements are checked it is found that, although containing a grain of truth, they have been markedly distorted by the patient to fit his own unconscious needs. Whenever any physician informs any patient of a cardiac condition, he needs to evaluate not only the heart but also the personality. This obviously holds true in all areas of organic medicine, but is most evident and necessary in cardiology.

It has been often noted that the anxious, tense, insecure, hypochondriacal individual can easily become aware of his cardiac function. As he does so, he is apt to become more anxious, whereupon his pulse rate increases. This obviously furthers his anxiety, which begins a vicious circle. Palpitations are often a result, whereupon the patient is even more convinced that he has cardiac disease. An unwise word at this point by the physician will only solidify in the patient's mind the conclusion that his heart is damaged. A great deal of time and effort are often necessary in order to eradicate such a conviction within a patient. Even the individual who suffers from mild or moderate cardiac damage, if also neurotic, can be made a great deal worse as far as his general living condition is concerned by unwise, pessimistic, unnecessarily limiting advice on the part of the physician. Another frequently seen example of iatrogenic difficulty is the statement by a physician, "You have low blood pressure." The neurotic individual is prone to seize upon such a statement and attribute all his aches and pains, depression, apathy, and other problems to "low blood pressure." The ordinary physician would be gratified to have such a diagnosis made of himself, yet he unthinkingly gives the layman the feeling that such a condition is pathological and responsible for many serious problems, rather than that it promotes longevity.

It has long been known that charges of emotional energy moving over nerve pathways influence the caliber of the blood vessels as well as the pacemaking mechanism of the heart. As far as we know, this phenomenon of vascular dilatation and contraction can (1) take place anywhere in the body or (2) be highly selective in its location, as in blushing or migraine. It is inevitable that many of the transient aches and pains of psychophysiologic illness are on the basis of local fluctuation in vascular activity.

Paroxysmal Tachycardia

In psychophysiologic paroxysmal tachycardia the overactivity of the heart occurs in a setting of anxiety. It has been fairly well shown that patients of this type frequently suffer from a difficulty in competitive situations. They are moved to competition but at the same time afraid of actual, worth-while, efficient exertion toward the competitive situation, and so express exertion in overactivity of the heart. The first attack often appears when the individual has gradually lost, over a period of years, the security and emotional strength which have given his cardiovascular system its stability. As his experiences gradually pile up and reach a certain level, his ability to deal with them becomes inadequate and there is a "spillover" into the autonomic system, with tachycardia ensuing. Respiratory difficulty and emotional distress of the usual anxiety type with weakness, faintness, and loss of voluntary muscular control are associated with the palpitations. Such attacks may come on at any hour or any place. If the patient discovers such attacks are most apt to occur in certain situations, such as a crowded room, he will thenceforth try to avoid the situations, thus developing a phobic structure in order to attempt to control his uncomfortable sensations.

Case History: Psychophysiologic Cardiovascular Reaction (Paroxysmal Tachycardia)

This thirty-eight-year-old married man was referred to the psychiatrist by a cardiologist. He had come to the latter complaining of paroxysmal tachycardia, which had begun while he was at work in the grocery store which he owned. He had been examined and found free of organic disease. The patient's history revealed that his father had been a cold, taciturn, punitive, and negative individual. His mother had been a quiet, obedient, undynamic person, more or less subservient to the father. The patient had grown up without close, warm ties to either parent. He had had difficulties in relating closely to others and remained more or less ambivalent and self-centered. He had married but had had no children. He relegated his wife to the same unimportant place in his life that his father had given to his mother. He had no friends, no social life, and no recreation other than an annual brief fishing trip. Once his symptoms had begun he sought an answer through reading books on psychiatry and psychology. He became discouraged with this, since it gave him little relief in his symptoms. He sought the advice of his family physician, who referred him to the cardiologist. Fortunately the latter convinced the patient that his cardiovascular system was all right and that his problems were emotional and would require the help of someone trained in such matters before improvement could be expected.

In its initial phases this patient's psychotherapy was mainly concerned with his recitation of the various intellectual theories which he had built up for himself concerning the origin of his neurosis. Most of these theories he had put together as a result of his extensive reading of psychological literature. He revealed relatively little warmth, friendliness, or other emotion. Even anxiety did not show itself clearly. However, as the patient's psychotherapeutic interviews continued, he began to recognize more clearly his inner discontent with the life which he had made for himself. He was a remarkably constricted individual who showed little interest in or understanding of other people. His relationship with his wife lacked the normal emotional gratifications that should be present in married life. He slowly became aware of the fact that he resented the work in his own store and was irritated at having to "wait on other people." He had never been able to express resentment, nor, on the other hand, had he been able to show his positive feelings. He was a compulsive type of person in that he had drained most of the emotion from his everyday activities and interpersonal relationships. He had always attempted to reduce everything to an intellectual procedure and, in so doing, had become increasingly embittered at the lack of satisfactions in his life. As he learned in his therapy to recognize his own constricted pattern and slowly to become more thoroughly acquainted with his emotional needs, his anxiety decreased and with it his tachycardia. This patient was seen a total of eighteen visits, by which time he no longer suffered from his paroxysmal tachycardia. He had become much more comfortable and relaxed in his home life as well as his work. He remained somewhat less flexible and warm than the average person, but had nevertheless achieved a much better level of adjustment.

Migraine

The migrainous patient has been shown to be ordinarily of an intellectual type, more than usually conscientious and with a need to be independent. Such people are ambitious, sensitive to criticism, and often reveal sexual problems. With such a rigid personality structure, they obviously operate under severe difficulties in attempting to adjust to their environment. The characteristic results, for reasons which we do not understand thoroughly, involve the onset of severe headaches of a migrainous type.

Case History: Migraine

A professional woman, single, age thirty-one, sought treatment for migraine with the hope that psychotherapy might help her to achieve greater flexibility in work. An only child, she grew up in a home with a quiet, depressive, ungiving mother and a distant, hardworking, cold father. The patient's educational years were not remarkable for any real sense of achievement and, as might be expected, her inner resentment grew as the years passed. The patient may have possessed some special physiological or anatomical predisposition but in her twenty-third year, without obvious crisis in her life, migraine began. Drug therapy did nothing curative, and she sometimes questioned whether it was alleviative. The attacks were typical: preceded by "light-headedness" and belching, then one-sided head pain and nausea for about twenty-four hours.

This woman's presenting personality was shy and inhibited in seeking the recognition and attention she craved from others. As psychotherapy proceeded twice weekly, aggression came to the surface, first around her parents and the social handicap they had given her. Next her aggression began to show itself against her contemporaries and the therapist. As this aggression was abreacted, the patient could be more boldly friendly to get the attention she wanted and needed from colleagues and friends. It took approximately 150 hours of psychotherapy to relieve the migraine and to give this patient the social and professional ease and competence she wanted. By an odd coincidence in a case of migraine, this individual (twenty years after psychotherapy and a much more successful application of herself in her career) developed a rapidly growing brain tumor and died in less than a year. With an intervening twenty years of symptom-free health, there could have been no anatomical connection, but there may be some reason we do not yet understand as to why disease of any type will single out one particular area of the body.

Hypertension

Hypertension is an extremely common condition within our society today. It often begins in a relatively insidious manner with only occasional blood-pressure readings above normal and gradually progresses to a point where chronic hypertensive findings are present and where rest and even sedation are relatively inefficient in lowering the blood pressure. Psychophysiologic hypertension is one of the most easily understood of all the conditions under the psycho-physiologic heading.

Anger normally produces a rise in blood pressure. It is a mechanism whereby the individual prepares himself for fight or flight through an increased activity of the cardiovascular system. The normal individual when angered finds some constructive means of dealing with his frustrating situation, thereby alleviating his anger and making it a temporary matter. There are, however, many individuals who by virtue of emotional problems are chronically angered by most situations in which they are placed in ordinary living. Yet, at the same time, this anger is veiled by defenses and only explodes when stimulated to a considerable degree. At such times the explosion of overt anger is apt to be excessive. The point, however, is that there is a chronic "drainage" of this anger into the autonomic system constantly producing a rise in blood pressure, which over a period of time produces pathological changes in the blood vessels and eventually irreversible hypertension. It is a recognized fact that medical and even surgical treatment of hypertension leaves much to be desired in many cases. The mere fact that there are so many suggested therapies for hypertension can only mean that none is the true answer. It is an extremely common, although certainly oversimplified, recommendation on the part of physicians to tell hypertensive patients to "take it easy." Such advice to an emotionally disturbed individual whose entire personality is maladjusted is not sufficient to change the individual's living pattern to a degree that will alleviate his emotional problems and hence his hypertension.

Case History: Hypertension

A married man of thirty-nine with two children (both under the age of twelve) was referred because of high blood pressure. This condition had been present since his college days. The patient reported that he had never worried about it and some sympathetic colleagues in the Armed Services had "slipped me by" because they realized how much he wanted to be in the Service. The hypertension was no problem while in the Service and it was several years later when it seemed to complicate other pathology in him. The patient underwent weight reduction at this point and then studied the relationship of his emotions to the elevations of blood pressure and noted that they seemed to occur when he was very dependent upon the opinions of people in authority around him. When he could free himself of this, the blood pressure would drop as much as fifty points systolic. Hence, he tried both to avoid any such harassing situation as well as to equip himself emotionally to meet these tests of acceptance by others. Attention to both of these factors has kept this patient's blood pressure down to reasonable limits.

PSYCHOPHYSIOLOGIC GASTROINTESTINAL REACTIONS

There are a variety of syndromes within this category affecting both upper and lower areas of the gastrointestinal system. They include such syndromes as gastric ulcer, obesity, "dyspepsia," flatulence, belching, hyperacidity, postprandial discomfort, pylorospasm, mucous colitis, ulcerative colitis, and anorexia nervosa.

Everyone has experienced the effect of emotions upon the gastrointestinal tract. Common phrases describe such conditions. For instance, "He makes me sick to my stomach," or "I just can't stomach that" are examples of such psychophysiologic interrelationships. The student who has "butterflies in his stomach" or diarrhea prior to an examination is a further example.

In order to understand more thoroughly the more intimate relationship between psyche and soma in the area of the gastrointestinal tract it is helpful to review the first two phases of psychosexual development. During the oral phase, as we have seen, the child relates to the world chiefly through his mouth. This is the most highly sensitized area of his entire anatomy and the one through which he receives the majority of his pleasure. Feeding, to him, is the activity through which he forms his first relationship with his mother and thus with the outside world. The infant readily develops disturbances of function of his gastrointestinal tract if the emotional atmosphere of his feeding situation is pathological. Also, it is important to remember that the primary characteristic of the infant's psychological apparatus is dependency. As he grows older and enters the anal phase there is a heightened interest in the function of elimination, particularly in regard to the choice of retention or elimination. The baby looks upon his bowel movements as being valuable and gives or retains them depending upon the emotional atmosphere surrounding him and the relationship to the person who is asking him to conform in matters of toilet training. He cannot help but heighten the importance of his bowel movements because of the concomitant pleasure he receives in having them and also because of the obvious importance which his mother places upon his bowel habits. It is important as far as this phase is concerned to remember the characteristically ambivalent psychological approach which all youngsters present. In a sense they are both in favor of and against conformity at one and the same time. With these factors in mind we will discuss a few of the more common psychophysiologic disturbances of the gastrointestinal tract.

Gastric Ulcer

Gastric ulcer has become an increasingly prevalent disorder in our modern world. It has been shown that the average and typical peptic ulcer patient presents certain definite attitudes and personality. He is usually a hard-working, seemingly independent, ambitious person who seeks responsibility and appears to carry it well. He enjoys the fact that others depend upon him and generally gives the impression of being a self-sufficient, competent, and industrious individual. It has been shown with equal clarity, however, that underneath this external independent attitude is an equally strong dependent oral type of craving stemming, as one would suspect, from the oral phase of psychosexual development. However, this individual has developed a superego which forbids the expression and gratification of his inner dependent attitude. Therefore, he literally overcompensates in the opposite direction, hiding from himself and the world his infantile orality which is really the core of his personality. Each inner dependent striving only brings forth its opposite in the way of independent activity. The result is a large element of inner dependency which remains chronically unsatisfied. Such inner and unexpressed cravings influence, just as they do in the child, the activity of the upper gastrointestinal tract. Such individuals are unconsciously "hungry" for dependency and security and yet refuse themselves the very thing for which they long. The result is a malfunctioning of the stomach which eventually, through disturbances in tonus, secretion, and blood supply, causes ulcer formation.

It is well known how the medical treatment of ulcer patients often goes awry because of such patients' seeming unwillingness to conform to diets and prescribed limited activity. They often become asymptomatic after a short period of hospitalization and enforced rest. However, they are often prone to return to work too quickly and to become so engrossed again in their ambitious programs that they ignore medical advice and have a recurrence of their ulcer. They are, in other words, unwilling and unable to reveal over any period of time their dependent strivings in the form of catering to their illness, limiting their work, and depending upon other people.

Obesity

Obesity is an exceedingly common condition and plays a tremendously important role in our society. From a medical standpoint it is notable for its deleterious effect upon longevity. From a social standpoint it is a source of concern and frustration to the obese individual. Medical science has long sought an efficient and practical treatment for overweight. At the present time the existence of numerous therapeutic approaches only serves to prove the lack of efficiency of any one single method. It is true that advances in medical science have brought about an increase in the understanding of the etiology of various types of obesity. A few cases—they are a relatively small percentage—have been shown to be endocrinological in origin and their therapy has proceeded satisfactorily along this line. However, the ordinary individual suffering from obesity runs the gamut of various therapeutic measures, manages to lose a few pounds, but over a short period of time gains them back. It has been shown that in the usual case of this type the problem is relatively simple. The patient eats too much. Exercise, of course, plays a role but a surprisingly small one in the control of obesity.

Why is it then that although most obese people realize overeating is the cause of obesity they do not eat less? Sporadically, they adhere to diets, often of a nutritious and attractive nature, which have been prescribed by their physicians and yet eventually, through one rationalization or another, they manage to regain their previous excessive food intake and therefore regain whatever weight they have lost. It appears, even superficially, that such people have an inordinate need to eat and require an excessive amount of food to satiate this need.

Once again, in order to understand adequately the problem of obesity, we need to return to the first psychosexual phase of personality development, the oral phase. Here, as we have mentioned, is a period of life when the mouth and eating are of great importance to the infant. At this time the baby is extremely dependent upon his mother for gratification. At this period of life eating and emotional satisfactions are *anaclitic,* that is, the emotional needs of the infant literally lean on and are satisfied at the same time as are the nutritional needs. It is relatively easy to understand how one refers to the obese person as an "oral" individual. This refers to the fact that such a person's mouth and eating are overly important to him and that there is a heightened emotional satisfaction in eating which is absent in the average adult. Valuable psychiatric studies, particularly those made by Hilde Bruch,[6] have shown the typical family pattern which often produces obese children. First of all, the mother finds it difficult to love her children in a mature way. There is a general overvaluation of food on her part and a tendency to substitute food for love. The child, unable to gratify his needs for maternal affection and finding instead the repeated offering of food, tends to seek the latter as a substitute for love. Such a pattern becomes progressively ingrained into his personality. There is perpetuated a strong oral tendency, a dependent craving for satisfaction which the person has learned to satiate by means of food. Food, in other words, stands for love, security, and satisfaction as well as an emotional tie to parents. Such youngsters have been shown by Bruch often to be youngest or only children. They are generally immature, and surprisingly the obesity is rarely the chief complaint either of the child or of the parents.

Such patients are sensitive in their relationships to others both as children and as adults. They easily turn to food as a substitute for gratifications which they feel they are not receiving. Superficially

---

[6] Bruch, Hilde. "Psychiatric Aspects of Obesity in Children." *American Journal of Psychiatry,* XCIX, 1943; also Bruch, Hilde, *The Importance of Overweight,* New York, W. W. Norton & Company, 1957.

they often fret and worry about their excessive weight and the limitations which such a condition imposes upon them. Yet their concern seems insufficient to stem their insatiable demands upon the environment which they satisfy through excessive food intake. One particularly obese woman who complained bitterly about her weight remarked that she had from time to time gone on diets. However, she added that whenever her husband was unaffectionate, cool, or critical toward her she felt hurt and could only find solace in eating. She said that even when she was able to maintain her diet she had to chew at least two to three packages of gum a day. Extensive medical and laboratory studies did not reveal any demonstrable pathology to account for her obesity. She herself was superficially, as are most of such individuals, a jolly and seemingly likable person. However, it soon became obvious how sensitive, childish, and truly self-centered she was. She made great demands upon her environment even while she was in the hospital and expected complete attention and affection from her husband in spite of the fact that her physical appearance was most repulsive due to her obesity.

Case History: Obesity

A thirty-three-year-old housewife, married quite happily to an engineer, suffered obesity from the age of puberty onward. She was the oldest in a family of three siblings—a younger brother and a younger sister. Her parents had been aloof, distant people and while good to their children in material ways, neither parent had any sort of intimate devotion to the children. As a result, the siblings were all envious of each other and reacted jealously if one was favored over the other. The patient enjoyed eating more than anything else, and while she wanted to have a slimmer figure, she could not find the necessary impetus to adopt a satisfactory reducing regimen and stick to it. She was seen in psychotherapy two times a week during the first year and then reduced her sessions to an hour weekly, since her father (who was paying for therapy) threatened to withdraw support completely. He preferred purchasing a car for her rather than spending money for the intangibles of psychotherapy. But on a once-a-week basis the patient pushed toward a more meaningful relationship with her psychotherapist and finally decided that if she could feel that he cared if she disciplined herself to a dietary regimen, she would join forces with him and endure the hunger distress. From then on, this patient felt some closeness of interest which she had never felt at home and went on to achieve a normal weight.

Case History: Psychophysiologic Gastrointestinal Reaction (Dyspepsia)

This twenty-seven-year-old single man came to the physician complaining of marked gastric distress following meals. A thorough physical examination along with X rays and further gastric studies proved essentially negative. Various dietary changes and antispasmodics had been unable to provide any relief. The patient was an irritable, truculent person who had previously been married but had fought with his wife and had finally divorced her. He quarreled with almost everyone in his life. He was unable to get along with his coworkers and even with department-store clerks where he shopped. He had a tremendously exaggerated need for love and attention which, as far as he was concerned, had to be provided on his own terms. He was fortunately easily able to understand the probable emotional origin of his gastric discomfort. He originally had felt that the world was an unreasonably frustrating place but nevertheless was soon able to grasp the idea that he himself had been particularly unreasonable. His past history revealed that he had come from an extremely conscientious and rather rigid home. His mother and father had given little concern to their children, primarily because of their excessive preoccupation with making money. As the patient began to understand more thoroughly his excessive demands upon the world and his craving for attention and affection, he also more clearly saw how his own behavior had prevented him from attaining even an ordinary amount of affection and attention. As he continued to discuss his own problems and increase his own insight, his behavior became much more pleasant and friendly and as a consequence he received much more attention and a reasonable amount of love from those around him. His symptoms subsided rather rapidly.

PSYCHOPHYSIOLOGIC GENITOURINARY REACTIONS

This category includes some types of menstrual disturbances, dysuria, and other malfunctioning of the genitourinary system which stem from emotional problems.

Menstruation

The menstrual cycle can be affected in a variety of ways by emotional problems. Such problems are often closely interrelated with endocrinological malfunction. There may be a temporary cessation of menses, as is often found in the unmarried girl who violently fears herself to be pregnant. There may likewise be a cessation of menses in the adolescent girl who is having a great deal of difficulty accepting her femininity and increased sexuality. Menstruation, coming as it does from the pelvic area, often inherits some of the emotional problems which have been built up around the functions of excretion. Such problems combined with similar difficulties encountered in the area of sexuality by the growing girl are often sufficient to provide ample groundwork for painful and difficult menstruation. Many mothers unfortunately pass on to their adolescent daughters an attitude that menstruation involves something dirty, toxic, or unclean and that it is an unfortunate blight with which the feminine population is saddled. Once menstruation begins it cannot be controlled as the girl has been admonished to control other excretions from this area. Psychotherapy is often beneficial in cases of dysmenorrhea or other menstrual malfunctions. In the woman suffering from painful menstruation one often finds that as she accepts her femininity to an increasing degree she suffers less markedly from painful menstruation and develops an increased understanding and acceptance of her own sexual and excretory functions.

Sexual function is extremely complicated by virtue of the interrelationship between its endocrine, autonomic, and psychological components. A disturbance in any one of these spheres is capable of distorting the entire pattern of sexual activity. Successful sexual activity is an integral part of mature living. As such it requires the attainment of the optimal level of personality adjustment. Psychological immaturities may reveal themselves in this area even though all other elements of an individual's life may appear to be relatively satisfactory. Sexual activity has properly been called a barometer of emotional adjustment.

Impotence and Frigidity

We have dealt in Chapter 12 ("Personality Disorders") with the various sexual deviations. Here we are considering primarily some of the other difficulties in genital functioning, particularly impotence and frigidity. To understand these difficulties properly it is necessary to consider for a moment the growing child. The youngster is curious about everything and anything and is anxious to learn. He questions his parents as to the meaning and reason for everything in the world about him. The child invariably becomes curious about the reasons for sexual differences, where babies come from, and numerous other questions in this area. Unfortunately, in many homes such questions are either forbidden or answered in an obviously distorted, uncomfortable, or embarrassed way by the parents. Such a condition leads the child to assume that there is something wrong with his curiosity in this direction and he seeks his information elsewhere and builds within himself an exaggerated and distorted concept of sexuality. The parents' ability to answer sexual questions as they should be answered, truthfully and honestly and on a level which the child can understand, depends primarily upon these parents' own mature sexual outlook and adjustment. Another important element contributing to eventual sexual adjustment is the acceptance or nonacceptance of one's own sexuality. Generally speaking, the boy runs into difficulty from an emotional standpoint when he becomes fearful of accepting the masculine role because of the competition and aggression involved and thus retreats to a passive, feminine role. On the other hand, one of the primary sources of difficulty from the sexual standpoint in the girl is that of continued unresolved envy of the masculine role and a feeling that the feminine role is inferior.

Impotence is the term used to indicate an inability on the part of a man to perform adequately and enjoy the act of sexual intercourse. *Frigidity* is the term used to indicate a similar condition in the woman. We are here concerned primarily with the types of impotence and frigidity deriving from psychological causes. It is also possible for various organic and toxic difficulties to produce these conditions. Impotence and frigidity vary in intensity from extremely severe to relatively mild and it is often, although not always, possible to correlate the degree of psychological difficulty with the degree of the severity of sexual incapacitation. Impotence, for instance, may vary from an inability to attain an erection under any conditions to the more mild occasional inability to attain orgasm. Frigidity, on the other hand, varies from severe pain during intercourse, called *vaginismus,* a painful contraction of the vaginal muscles, to the mild, occasional inability to attain orgasm, although in the latter case the act of intercourse may be accompanied by pleasure.

Generally speaking, the psychological etiology of these two conditions can be discussed under four different headings. The first is that of sexual inhibition in which the man or woman is afraid of criticism either from the environment or from the conscience. The young unmarried couple indulging in clandestine sexual activities and constantly fearful of detection will often suffer from impotence or frigidity. After marriage a severe conscience which has long condemned all sexual activity with disgust may often also result in impotence or frigidity. Such a man or woman may have felt premaritally that marriage itself would entirely remove sexual inhibitions and allow him to participate comfortably in sexuality. However, being faced with the actual performance of the sexual act renews all the original and long-standing taboos which have been present in this area and provides a distinct barrier to actual sexual gratification.

The second possible cause for impotence or frigidity lies in an inability to love a person of the opposite sex, or as a matter of fact, to love anyone other than oneself. This results where there is a markedly heightened self-love or narcissistic condition. Such individuals have always gained their principal sexual satisfaction through the autoerotic habit of masturbation. They literally are unable to spare sufficient love from their own reservoir because they place so much of it upon themselves. Following marriage, they find themselves unable really to love anyone else to a sufficient degree to enable them to attain sexual gratification with another individual. The sexual gratification of the partner is relatively unimportant to them. For instance, a man of this type may be able apparently to have successful intercourse. However, intercourse is truly a substitute for masturbation and his partner's presence during the act is of relatively little importance to him.

A third difficulty which may lead to impotence and frigidity is hostility and fear directed toward members of the opposite sex. One thinks, for instance, of the woman who remains envious of the masculine sex because of what she considers to be their supposed superiority. She finds herself unable to accept a passive receptive type of role in sexual intercourse with a member of this envied sex. While her attitude may be thoroughly unconscious and she therefore may be totally unaware of it, it is sufficient to make achievement of orgasm impossible. The man, for instance, who has been raised by a dominating, authoritative, punitive mother may be uncomfortable, at least unconsciously, with members of the opposite sex. His relationships with them are guarded and when he is faced with the prospect of intimate sexual relationship with a member of this feared sex, he finds himself impotent to a varying degree.

The fourth possible cause for psychological impotence is homosexuality. In this condition, of course, a person is capable of loving only a member of the same sex and is, as we have explained in Chapter 12, unable to love an individual of the opposite sex adequately or thoroughly. Homosexuality is frequently a latent condition in that the individual seemingly, as far as his behavior is concerned, is attracted to and congenial with members of the opposite sex. This particular behavior is capable of maintaining itself until the final epitome of heterosexual relationships, namely that of intercourse. At this time such a person finds himself unable to adequately perform the act or a least unable to enjoy it thoroughly to the point of orgasm.

A word should be mentioned here concerning the aforementioned difficulty, namely the inability of a man to be thoroughly masculine and of a woman to be thoroughly feminine. In the boy who learns to compete with his father and with other boys of his own age there gradually comes to be, if he is normal, an ability to enter into competition with a normal and healthy amount of well-directed aggression. However, there are certain boys who because of punitive, critical, and inconsistent treatment from their own fathers feel unable and unwilling to assume the masculine, competitive, and somewhat aggressive role and who tend to retreat to a more passive, feminine type of identification. Other boys may seek this same passive, feminine type of role because of a feared or overly aggressive mother. They feel that they are unwilling to grow up and fulfill the masculine role if it means marriage to a woman as dangerous as they inwardly have assumed their mother, and therefore all women, to be. In the girl, on the other hand, there is the reverse of this problem, namely envy of boys. Girls often in their earlier years come to feel that members of the opposite sex have marked advantages and that they themselves have been cheated by having been born into the female sex. The roots of some of this difficulty in the girl lie in the small youngster's observation of the anatomical difference between boys and girls and the feeling on the girl's part that she has been cheated out of an obviously useful and visible portion of anatomy. Such an initial conclusion may be heightened and exaggerated by her observations of family life. If, for instance, her mother is overworked and maltreated by a dictatorial husband it will only serve to enhance her original conclusions. She may then be unwilling or fearful of accepting this passive, feminine role and seek to outdo or compete with men in a pseudo-masculine or aggressive manner.

Case History: Psychophysiologic Genitourinary
Reaction (Urinary Urgency)

This thirty-five-year-old married woman came into psychiatric treatment with a variety of symptoms, among which was a complaint of urinary urgency, particularly when she was in crowds, when she was traveling, or whenever she was in a situation such that a lavatory was not immediately available. Her past history revealed that she had spent her childhood years in a most strict, rigid environment as dictated by her meticulous mother and grandmother. These two women who dominated her early years had placed a great deal of attention upon her performance rather than providing a genuine affectionate relationship between themselves and the patient. As a result, this woman grew up having literally internalized many of the rigidities of her early life. She became overconscientious, partly frigid, and quite fearful of all authority. She said, "I'm as comfortable as anybody when I'm relaxed but when I go into a crowd I'm afraid I'll have to go to the toilet. I'm afraid when I go on an auto trip I may have to go and there won't be an opportunity and I won't be able to hold it." During treatment this patient began to more clearly see that she still considered all people as unfriendly and unbending about matters of urination as had been her grandmother and mother. She also recognized that really she still felt no more confidence in her urinary control than she had when she was a mere toddler of eighteen months. She was able to see that others were actually unconcerned about her toilet habits and that they would not scold her for her need to urinate. As these, as well as other factors about her personality, became more clear to her, she was able to increase her own level of self-confidence and her feeling that she could control her urination. As is typical of such women, this patient had been very sensitive at the beginning of treatment and could not, as she put it, "hold back my tears." She cried frequently in her initial interviews, but as she achieved greater understanding and insight and confidence, she was able to get "more things under control."

PSYCHOPHYSIOLOGIC ENDOCRINE REACTION

This category includes various endocrine disturbances in which emotional factors play an etiological role. As we have mentioned previously, there is a close interrelationship between the psyche, the endocrines, and the autonomic system; disturbances in one are frequently followed by reverberations in at least one of the others. Some of the most recent research has revealed the complexity of the various interrelationships between these three systems. The introduction of ACTH into the medical armamentarium has provided a stimulus to further research in this area. There has been a great deal of work, both past and present, done in attempts to show more specifically how endocrines affect the psyche and vice versa. Particularly noticeable is the work, for instance, of Hoskins [7] at Worcester State Hospital, much of which is published in his book, *The Biology of Schizophrenia*. It is only natural that as a result of all of this research various attempts have been made to treat apparently psychological conditions by means of hormonal preparations. As far as we are concerned to date such therapeutic measures remain in the experimental stage and are, at least for the general group of functional psychoses and psychoneuroses, relatively inefficient.

Certain endocrine malfunctions, however, seem to have been

[7] Hoskins, Roy G. *The Biology of Schizophrenia*. New York, W. W. Norton & Company, 1946.

proven to result at times from highly charged emotional situations. For instance, in many cases it has been shown that emotional shock in a certain type of individual is capable of precipitating the onset of hyperthyroidism. Another extremely important area in which the endocrines and the psyche are shown to have a definite close interrelationship is that of fertility. Many women who have been childless for years for no demonstrable organic reason, have conceived and borne a child after intensive psychotherapeutic measures. The latter have usually been undertaken for some other condition rather than for the infertility. It is also well known that women occasionally, upon assuming sterility after many years of lack of conception, adopt a child only to find themselves subsequently pregnant presumably because of a stirring of what must be called "the maternal instinct" within them. The degree to which this is psychological and endocrinological is debatable, of course, but it certainly would appear that there are strong psychological factors involved.

There are innumerable other endocrinological problems which undoubtedly have a psychological factor associated with them. This is one area in which a great deal more observation and research must be done in order to clarify these conditions.

Case History: Psychophysiologic Endocrine Reaction (Infertility)

This thirty-two-year-old married woman sought psychiatric treatment because of the presence of constant anxiety. She was uneasy in relationships with her fellow workers, unable to concentrate, and constantly bothered by a feeling that her life was totally lacking in constructiveness. She came to treatment with a reasonable understanding of what psychotherapy involved and willingly entered an intensive treatment program.

Her history revealed that she had been married for eight years and, in spite of a relatively great desire to do so, had never been able to become pregnant. She had never used a contraceptive at any time since marriage. As her treatment proceeded it became evident that her wish to become pregnant was only a halfhearted one and she clung to it in the hope that having a child would give her life some purpose. She had never felt that there was any emotional reason for her apparent sterility and she had not entered psychotherapy with any assumption that this would enhance her procreative ability.

Further history revealed that the patient had been brought up by an extremely tyrannical mother. The latter had ignored her, exploited her, mistreated her, had generally abused her father, and had been deceitful and predatory toward the entire community. The patient's father, on the other hand, had been a gentle, kind, devoted person, particularly fond of his daughter, and the patient had taken over many of the characteristics of her father. However, as might be expected from such a history, she had made an inadequate identification with femininity because of her total lack of experience with a truly maternal figure. Mothers, in her mind, were hostile, exploitive, and cruel. She feared lest she become the same sort of person.

It required several months of therapy for this patient to realize she did not have to be like her mother, but could be a gentle and affectionate woman. She gave up her halfhearted pursuit of professional interests and felt herself subsequently much more "married." She was no longer ambivalent or halfhearted about her ability or capacity to become a good mother. She already possessed some intellectual understanding of children's psychological life and began to add an emotional conviction to this knowledge. As a result her desire to become a mother became much more wholehearted. It was during this period in treatment that she became pregnant.

It is impossible, of course, to prove that this patient's pregnancy resulted from her altered psychological structure. However, it is felt that it would be a reasonable assumption, since no other changes had occurred in her life and she had had equal opportunities for pregnancy during the previous eight years. In such cases as this it is difficult to ascertain the changes which occur within the psychological as well as physiological and endocrinological apparatuses, but nevertheless the remarkable emotional changes in this patient immediately preceded her pregnancy. There is a great need for further research into such cases as this and much more must be known about the relationship between the psyche and the endocrines before any final answer can be given.

PSYCHOPHYSIOLOGIC NERVOUS SYSTEM REACTIONS

This category includes various disturbances of the nervous system, including the autonomic, which have an emotional etiology. Of particular importance is the so-called "asthenic reaction" which in older terminology was often referred to as "neurasthenia." It is characterized by fatigue, lassitude, multiple vague somatic complaints, and a general lack of adequate emotional participation in everyday activities. It is in this syndrome that the complicated interrelationship between sympathetic, parasympathetic, endocrine, and emotional forces is seen. There is in these patients a difficulty in adequate sympathetic response. Such patients are prone to go on for years with varied complaints which are rarely of an acute variety. They often change physicians in an attempt to find some form of treatment which will relieve their chronic lassitude and lack of pep. Such patients become adept at giving long, detailed histories of various difficulties. If the physician asks such a patient about an area of the body which the latter neglected to mention in his history, this particular area will usually be found to have presented some problems, according to the patient. One soon gets the impression that these individuals are investing a great deal more of their mental energy on their inner physiological processes than they are in the world about them.

Also included in this category are certain convulsive conditions with an emotional etiology which are not classified elsewhere. It is of importance to differentiate convulsions due to conversion reaction from those which belong in this particular category.

Case History: Psychophysiologic Nervous System Reaction (Asthenia)

A sixty-one-year-old married woman presented a multitude of complaints, the most prominent of which was chronic fatigue. She also complained of generalized body tenderness, stating that every part of her body was "as sore as a boil." She became extremely tired after minimal exertion. She would have to rest for two to three hours after performing even small tasks. She found some relief by exposing her body to a heat lamp and taking ten grains of aspirin every four hours. She gave a long and detailed history of the many illnesses of a vague type that she had had. She was most contented when she could relate at length the malfunctions of each system of her body. She also launched into a long description of the trials and tribulations which she had suffered in rearing her eight children. She complained of having been married to an indecisive man who was of little help to her and only made matters worse. In reality, her husband had worked all the time and had supported the family adequately, but the patient had never found the performance of any of the family members satisfactory to her. One child did not finish his education; others made wrong marriages; still others did not handle their businesses properly; her grandchildren were too noisy and disrespectful; her husband was thoughtless and inconsiderate. She felt that all of these people were a drain upon her and only increased her burdens in life. She felt none of them made any positive contribution to her. She was definite in her statement, "My family put me where I am."

This patient presented rather clearly the typical attitude of the individual with an asthenic reaction. She had never been a zestful, enthusiastic person. Her basic problem lay in the area of an inability to love and derive pleasure from being loved. As a result she became "tired" of giving and doing for others, and experienced a sense of fatigue. She had added a further fallacy to her thinking by assuming that doing things would actually result in bodily harm, as if she would literally deplete herself.

Treatment of such a patient as this is long, tedious, and difficult. Frequently, as in this woman's case, the secondary gain of the illness has reached rather large proportions and it is essential to have complete family co-operation so that the patient cannot again retreat into her numerous complaints. This woman was helped to understand the difficulties which she had had in loving and being loved. She was encouraged and even urged to participate in more activities with, at the same time, an effort toward deriving pleasure and satisfaction from such relationships and activities. Encouragement to do more things personally enjoyable to her and *insisting* that she verbalize her enjoyment from them gave this patient a much healthier living pattern with relief from the asthenia in three months

PSYCHOPHYSIOLOGIC REACTIONS OF ORGANS OF SPECIAL SENSE

Any of the organs of special sense may be disturbed in their function by emotional problems. Sight and hearing are much more commonly affected than are taste, touch, or smell. People who are under tension and particularly those who are doing close work requiring the use of their eyes may develop difficulty in focusing upon the material. They at times describe "halos," "crosses," and other patterns around lights.

Also included within this group are certain cases of apparently impaired hearing which do not fall within the conversion-reaction type. Some patients, by virtue of their inner emotional turbulence and difficulty in relating to those about them, hear only a small portion of what is said.

It is not uncommon for emotional tension to produce symptoms such as "dizziness" or "ringing in the ears." These are often mistaken for an atypical Meniére's syndrome and treated as such, when the symptom actually arises because of emotional difficulties. The tension state induces excitability in the midbrain which is then transmitted to the vestibular nucleus of the eighth nerve.

Case History: Psychophysiologic Reaction of Organs of Special Sense (Dizziness)

This forty-three-year-old married man had many complaints stemming from a chronic anxiety reaction. One of the most bothersome to him was that of "dizzy spells." Upon inquiry the patient said that at such times he felt shaky and unsteady and in danger of losing his equilibrium. This particular symptom became most evident when he quarreled with his wife, had business difficulties, or had problems with his large family of sisters, brother, and mother. In short, his symptoms became worse when anything occurred to threaten his security and increase his anxiety. As he learned to know his own need for approval and also as he learned to deal more maturely and adequately with his problems, his tension diminished and his giddiness disappeared.

PROGNOSIS

The prognosis in psychophysiologic illness is variable. In the main it is better than in most psychoses, alcoholism, and drug addiction. It may be poorer than in some of the psychoneuroses. However, just as in any psychiatric condition the prognosis must depend upon several variables:

(a) the original personality structure and its capacity for responding to therapy
(b) the length of time symptoms have been present
(c) the environmental situation in which symptoms have developed
(d) the type of treatment instituted and whether hospital or ambulatory in type

(e) the opportunities for operation of secondary gain

(f) the current and future life situation which patient faces, and

(g) skill and resourcefulness of therapeutic milieu.

As with disease in any part of the organism the doctor may understand the psychophysiologic pathology but be unable to modify it appreciably. In the main, however, the prognosis is good in that some patients, if the right treatment principles are applied in the most desirable settings, will be cured, others will be helped, and relatively few will derive no benefit whatsoever.

TREATMENT

It has been said that psychotherapy begins with the first contact of the doctor with the patient. The expectation of help from a parental figure with knowledge of the cure of disease predisposes the patient to make therapeutic use of everything which follows. A careful history, including history of personality, starts the patient off with the feeling that the doctor considers him and his emotions important in the search for the cause of his symptoms. A careful physical and laboratory study is then made in order to ascertain the presence or absence of organic disease. When organic disease is absent treatment should, with few exceptions, be entirely psychotherapeutic. If organic disease is present this does not preclude the need for psychotherapeutic treatment for a disease condition which has more than one etiological factor. When the illness is due to both organic and emotional factors it is well to try to give some estimate as to the relative importance of both. If more than one physician is treating the case it is important that they agree on this point. Disagreement on the part of the attending physicians will confuse the patient and enhance his resistance to psychotherapy.

In some cases treatment of the somatic symptoms may take precedence over the psychotherapy and also, in some cases, the uncovering of emotional material will produce exacerbation of the somatic symptoms. In some cases—colitis, for example—the removal of the somatic symptom may upset the inner psychic equilibrium so that a psychotic episode will be produced unless adequate psychotherapy is utilized. The working out of the secondary gain may be difficult in some cases and will require the fullest co-operation of those in the environment. For example, if dependency is a large factor in the personality structure it may give gratification to a relative on whom the patient depends as well as the patient, and the relative will have to undergo emotional change too if he is to provide the proper atmosphere and co-operation for the patient's recovery.

Chronic cases may need, ideally, to be in a hospital setting, preferably in a section devoted to the treatment of psychophysiologic conditions. Here they are separated from medical and surgical treatment and the atmosphere is focused around self-knowledge and the development of new attitudes toward life. Morbid concepts and destructive attitudes may be so ingrained that they need the counteraction of repeated impact with nurses, doctors, occupational therapists, art therapists, and social workers in order to bring insight and set new patterns of thinking and feeling into operation. Lacking a hospital setting the physician must function with a patient as well as he can on an ambulatory basis using a plan of treatment, of which the following is a sample.

TYPICAL CASE PRESENTATION

PSYCHOPHYSIOLOGIC GASTROINTESTINAL REACTION

*Social and Psychological
History*

Infancy: Age 1–2

Mother pampered him. Father ignored him.

Childhood: Age 2–6

Timid, shy. No special interests.

Grade School: Age 6–13

Fearful and tried to hide this by limited participation in play.

High School: Age 13–18

A poor mixer. Participated in a few sports. Little interest in studies.

*Social and Psychological
History* (continued)

Adulthood: Age 21

Married a gentle, competent woman in early twenties.

Went to work in a small industrial plant where father had worked. Felt like "the kid," unaccepted; did not know how to make friends. Could not share in camaraderie of the men.

Parenthood: Age 25

Son born. While he was deriving so little emotional satisfaction from work, he was also ignoring the potential pleasures in enjoyment of his wife and child. His psyche was becoming impoverished and empty and life was more burdensome, formidable and anxiety-producing.

The unfulfillment of emotional needs necessary for security resulted in anxiety, became more and more disturbing to body physiology.

Careful physical examinations, X ray, and laboratory studies were negative. But the distress he suffered made him feel that something toxic or "sick-producing" was being overlooked. After eighteen months of suffering, he stopped work and this event caused the treatment to be changed from antiacids and sedation to psychotherapy.

Symptomatology

Began to have anorexia in the morning; nausea after trying to eat. This was followed by distress after lunch and dinner; alternating constipation and diarrhea. A few weeks later he developed griping pain in abdomen. After two months of symptomatic treatment he developed fatigue so that work became an additional burden. One month later he began to sleep poorly. Six weeks later he began to feel that the griping pains meant ulcer or cancer. He worked under great anxiety, saw many doctors, and tried various self-medications, to no avail.

Psychotherapeutic Process

1. Kept in foreground the examinations which revealed no tissue pathology.

2. Used charts to show autonomic nerve distribution to glands, blood vessels, muscle tissues, and organs.

3. Called attention to emotions which disturb organ functions.

4. Pointed out his need for friendship and interest but also how he was missing it by fear of people and not knowing how to be friendly.

5. Gave him specific formulations of dynamics as learned from history as follows: "To get strength for healthy body-functioning again, you need security through better human relations. The men at work are willing to accept you if you accept them. Your wife and child need a cheerful man who will notice and appreciate them rather than one who worries about his digestion. Let your physician have the responsibility of deciding whether your body is sick or well. You relinquish that responsibility into trained hands while you do what you can learn to do; namely, to offer yourself to people in such a way that they can help cure you."

6. "Your body's distresses are secondary to your mind's need for love and good will and the sense of physical well-being which comes

Effects on Symptomatology

Some reduction of anxiety began when he received tangible explanation for symptoms. Doubts would creep in and he would ask, "Are you explaining the cause of all my trouble, as I feel 'wrecked' in my bowels?"

He would be reassured and then able to turn his mind a little more in the direction of personality self-improvement. He slept better. He began golf with a little less fatigue. He protested, however, at the idea of increased social activity. His wife liked dancing while he did not, so he needed encouragement to learn. He had never played cards so he learned—reluctantly, but he learned. He needed to be shown and convinced that a more altruistic and well-rounded personality would be productive of better health.

Improvement in symptoms is always convincing and one of the physician's best allies in psychotherapy.

*Psychotherapeutic
Process* (continued)

from good social relations. Take your wife and child out, go to the movies, invite your friends in. Begin that golf playing you have wanted to do. You do not need to suffer if you will begin new habits of thinking and acting."

7. "You need to live in friendly relations with people so that you make up to yourself for some of the lack of love and interest denied you by your father during your childhood. You should accept the fact that for health you need a wider range of interests and personal contacts for healthy living than either your mother or father required."

His upper and lower bowel quieted down: the griping pain stopped, appetite returned, and digestion became comfortable. Three weeks after treatment began he was back at work, albeit with some residual symptoms, but in three months he was symptom-free.

Functional Psychotic Disorders

PART VI

Functional Psychotic
Disorders

CHAPTER 14

Schizophrenic Reactions

SCHIZOPHRENIC reactions are characterized by a marked difficulty in interpersonal relationships and usually involve a strong tendency to withdraw from reality and a fundamental disturbance of personality organization. To varying degrees the affect is blunted and there may or may not be hallucinations (usually of an auditory nature) or delusions. The schizophrenic person is one whose difficulties in adjustment have become more serious and far-reaching than is true of the psychoneurotic person. He has, slowly or rapidly, begun to weaken, and finally break, his ties with reality and with those around him. He retreats into a world of his own making, since to him the real world is no longer tenable. He suffers a disorganization of his thought processes so that to the normal person he seems odd and bizarre. It is difficult to be with him without sensing the peculiarity of his emotional and ideational relationships. The idea and the emotion are not synchronized in him as they are in the normal, but seem disjointed. He is apt to laugh when there is nothing humorous or become irritated when there is seemingly no reason for it. If he is paranoid he seems to find hidden meanings in every action or expression of others. Attempts to build up a relationship with him often meet with failure since he seems to retreat before every approach. He may be merely cold and withdrawn or he may be obviously suspicious and irritable. He may be hallucinated and delusional or even catatonic but essentially there is the element of oddness, bizarreness, and strangeness that is apt to mystify and make one feel vaguely uncomfortable when around him.

Schizophrenia, or *split personality,* was the name given by Bleuler [1] to a group of conditions which had previously been gathered under the heading of "dementia praecox" by Kraepelin.[2] Certainly Kraepelin had simplified psychiatric thinking when he brought together the various syndromes under one title. He included a condition that had previously been described as "hebephrenia" by Hecker and the syndrome of catatonia described by Kahlbaum. "Dementia praecox," as a name for these conditions, however, had the disadvantage of indicating a progressive dementia of the young and thus lent a poor prognosis to the condition. Bleuler tried to imply with his term, *schizophrenia,* something of the dynamics of the condition. While both of these men and many others since have contributed to our grouping and understanding of these related syndromes, the final answer as to etiology is still disagreed upon in medical circles.

There is even considerable doubt as to whether all the conditions now known as schizophrenic reactions should be considered manifestations of one entity. However, psychiatric writings have so long grouped these phenomena in this particular way that it seems wise, at least for the present, to continue to do so even though future research may reveal some basic differences between them. The important consideration in each individual case is an attempt to understand how and why a particular patient has resorted to this type of mental disorganization as a result of his past and present stresses. *Schizophrenic reaction* is the name given to a psychosis occurring from early to middle life, without demonstrable organic pathology, and in which the basic symptoms are a general dissociation in the thinking process, inappropriateness of affect, and a deterioration of ability to test reality.

Schizophrenic reactions are more prevalent than mental-hospital statistics would imply, since only the more disturbed patients with this condition are admitted to mental institutions. About one-quarter of all first admissions to mental hospitals are schizophrenic. Since the disorder is chronic, almost one-half of all patients in these hospitals are ill with this syndrome. Many schizophrenic patients are

[1] Bleuler, Eugen. *Textbook of Psychiatry.* Translated by A. A. Brill. New York, Macmillan, 1924 (Dover Publications reissue, 1951).

[2] Kraepelin, E. *Psychiatrie.* Eighth edition. 1913.

suffering from chronic, insidious forms of the disease which do not reach proportions that force their families to resort to hospitalization. Of great importance is the fact that many of these schizophrenic patients are young, still in the prime of life, and without adequate treatment may remain hospitalized for years. It is commonplace to find so-called deteriorated schizophrenics in the disturbed wards of our mental hospitals. They have been there for years and have settled into a vegetative existence that bears little similarity to ordinary human life.

SYMPTOMATOLOGY

Because of the diversity of the syndromes grouped under the heading of schizophrenic reactions it is difficult to describe a set of symptoms which will suffice for all. Actually, schizophrenic reactions may begin at any age. It is probably better to consider them as personality reactions rather than as a single disease entity. Certainly it is very difficult to compare the three-year-old autistic child who is definitely showing a schizophrenic reaction with a forty-five-year-old paranoid schizophrenic. They are both having marked difficulties in adjustment and in forming relationships with other people on a normal level. We now know much more about personality dynamics and underlying psychopathology than we did when Bleuler used the term *schizophrenia* in 1911, and as a result the seemingly incomprehensible productions of patients begin to be understandable and the intrapsychic processes become separable into their various components.

A schizophrenic reaction becomes more understandable when we realize that inherent in the process is a disintegration of the ego and consequent break with reality. Since the ego has as one of its most important functions that of reality testing, the loss of this faculty makes possible many of the bizarre symptoms of the condition. The ego in its attempts to mediate between the instinctual drives and the conscience, in fact, between the id, the superego, and the environment, has failed and reality is no longer considered. There is consequently an emergence of unconscious material which has previously been held in repression by the ego. Such material seems disconnected and bizarre to us as we first attempt to understand the patient.

Although the onset of the psychosis may seem to have been very acute, it is usually possible to uncover a history of gradual changes in the patient for months or even years prior to the most obvious symptoms. It is not unusual to find that the patient has always been "schizoid" in that he has never socialized well, has been rather shy and retiring, cold and moody, and at times irritable, and has led a limited social existence. Gradually these characteristics have increased in intensity until he has become more asocial, withdrawn, irritable, and given to temper outbursts if frustrated. He has become careless in appearance, sloppy in his work habits, lacking in his sense of responsibility, careless and obscene in his language at times, and increasingly suspicious of everyone. He cares less and less what family and friends think about what he does and says. When the final break with reality becomes complete, delusions and hallucinations make their appearance and emotions and thoughts tend to become more unrelated and speech more irrelevant and illogical.

A general mental status outline follows for some of the more common symptoms seen in schizophrenic reaction patients.

GENERAL APPEARANCE

The schizophrenic tends to become, as his psychosis develops, less and less careful about his appearance. His clothes are unkempt and he is often disheveled. Some disturbed patients are unwilling to wear clothes at all. Occasionally the schizophrenic dresses in a ludicrous manner utilizing various articles which obviously do not fit in with the ordinary mode of dress.

The schizophrenic's behavior varies markedly from one patient to another. Some are completely catatonic and sit motionless for hours. At times one sees the phenomenon known as *waxy flexibility* in which if a limb is raised to an unnatural position the patient will leave it there for extended periods of time. Then there is the more agitated schizophrenic who is constantly rushing about and producing a torrent of words. At times such activities reach dangerous proportions in terms of physical exhaustion. The smearing of urine and feces may be seen. Occasionally one finds open and almost constant masturbation occurring. These patients are unpredictable and may become impulsively belligerent at times.

Here again there is a wide variation in schizophrenic patients, ranging from the mute individual who will not answer questions at all to the hyperactive agitated patient who produces a constant but unintelligible tirade of words. This may be in the form of accusations for his fancied abuses, long conversations with hallucinated voices, or meaningless jargon or *word salad*. *Verbigeration*, which is a kind of stereotypy in which the patient repeats a word or phrase over and over again, is common with agitated schizophrenics. *Neologisms*, or newly coined words, are word condensations which have a special meaning for the patient. Whereas ordinary speech has to be submitted to the censorship of the ego and put in understandable form, this does not hold true for the speech of the schizophrenic. He displaces, condenses, reverses in a way that is seen in the formation of dreams. A previously puritanical patient may reveal a remarkable vocabulary of obscene words.

Occasionally one finds the phenomenon of *echolalia*, which is the repetition of statements or questions of the examiner by the patient. *Echopraxia* is another and somewhat more rare phenomenon in which the patient repeats the acts of the examiner.

Blocking, or the sudden cessation of word flow, is fairly characteristic of schizophrenics. They will suddenly stop in a conversation and, at least temporarily, be unable to go on. This can result from painful affects surging up from the unconscious. As one attempts to converse with the schizophrenic, one finds it a tedious and frustrating process, since the patient's thinking is dominated by the so-called *primary process*. It is dereistic thinking which shows a disregard for the laws of logic, reason and experience. It is characteristic of the unconscious, as compared to logical thinking dominated by the secondary process produced by a healthy ego. These patients show the phenomenon of *skidding* in which the answer to a question may begin properly but very soon "skid" off onto some irrelevant subject. A frequent change of theme without adequate reason is again characteristic of such patients and results from inadequate ego functioning. *Perseveration,* or the repetitious giving of one answer to several questions, is occasionally seen, although it is probably more characteristic of organic psychoses.

MOOD

It is considered characteristic of schizophrenic reaction that the *affect* becomes blunted early in the condition. It seems flat in that one does not get the feel of the usual fluctuation of emotions that we find in normal people. At times marked temper outbursts may occur with only minor provocations. It is more usual to feel a lack of warmth toward the schizophrenic and to feel vaguely perplexed by his speech or behavior. Many psychiatrists say that they can "smell" a schizophrenic, by which they indicate that their own emotions are stirred in the particular manner just described. Whereas the manic depressive patient who is in a manic phase has a sort of contagious humor to his productions, the agitated and hyperactive schizophrenic does not convey this type of humor. Eventually in some deteriorated schizophrenics the affect becomes almost completely flat and they respond only rarely with any show of emotion.

MISINTERPRETATIONS AND DELUSIONS

Perhaps the two most important findings in schizophrenic patients are those of delusions and hallucinations. *Hallucinations,* or false sensory perceptions without external stimulation, are most frequently of the auditory type, although occasionally visual hallucinations are seen and sometimes one finds the olfactory type. Typically the patient begins to hear voices, which are often of an accusatory nature. For instance, in the paranoid schizophrenic these voices are apt to tell the patient that he is a homosexual or that people are saying he is a homosexual. The patient is convinced of the reality of the voices and, under certain circumstances, is capable of acting on "command" of the voices. One occasionally finds visual hallucinations in schizophrenic patients, although this is ordinarily considered more characteristic of toxic psychoses. The content of the hallucinations depends upon the dynamics of the patient's personality.

Delusions, or false beliefs, are again seen commonly in schizo-phrenic reactions. The patient may think he is being laughed at, discriminated against, followed, or talked about by various people or groups. The paranoid person tends to spend a great deal of his time mentally involved in his delusional system. For instance, he may believe that the Masons are plotting against him and that they have assigned men to follow him and report his actions. He may believe they have installed a microphone in his room to listen to his conversations. They may be tampering with his food, perhaps to poison him. Or, he may believe he is Jesus Christ and conduct him-self accordingly even though confined to the hospital. Attempts to reason with such patients and to present to them proof of the false-ness of their beliefs is futile. At times the physician who tries to show the patient the falsity of his belief is then included by the pa-tient in the delusional system.

Ideas of reference are feelings on the part of the patient that var-ious events are related to him even though they are not. He inter-prets innocuous actions of others as having some special meaning toward him.

Somatic delusions are part of the hypochondriasis often seen early in the psychosis. Patients begin with complaints about various parts of their bodies and gradually these complaints assume a more bi-zarre nature. One patient feels his stomach is "dissolved and gone" while the next feels that his hands are becoming progressively smaller. Such patients often become preoccupied with some minor variation in their body structure or with a small scar. They then de-terminedly relate all their difficulties to this. For instance, a patient will decide his nose is not straight enough even though he has a very minimal variation. He will then find a physician willing to change the contour surgically. Following surgery he is content for only a short time and then feels that either not enough or too much has been done and the situation is just as bad as ever. Had the sur-geon questioned the patient more thoroughly before operating he would have seen the delusional content. He might have discovered that the patient felt everyone was watching him and laughing at him because of his "ridiculous nose which looked like a homosex-ual." At this point surgery could have been avoided. In an early stage of the psychosis the delusional material is not evident without some questioning. Suspicion should be aroused when a patient requests medication or surgery for a difficulty that seems of very minor consequence and which causes him undue concern.

Schizophrenic patients sometimes show the phenomenon of *depersonalization*, which is a loss of the feeling of being a real person. This results as the libido is gradually withdrawn from the environment and there is a loss of the ordinarily distinct boundaries of the ego. In small children with schizophrenic reactions we characteristically find a confusion of first- and second-person pronouns. The child is apt to say "you" when he means "I," again because his ego boundaries no longer are distinct and do not separate him as an entity from others. In adults this removal of libido from the world may lead to overinvestment of an organ, with consequent hypochondriacal complaints or somatic delusions. Needless to say, physical examinations and laboratory tests on such patients have little if any benefit as far as removing the delusions goes.

SENSORIUM

Measurement of the intellectual capacities of a schizophrenic by intelligence tests usually leads to an I.Q. below normal. However, if each section of the test is plotted we find that, while some are very low, others are above average. This is a phenomenon known as *scatter*. In mental defectives test sections are uniformly low, as compared to the wide variation seen in schizophrenics. The longer the schizophrenic psychosis has been present, and the more "deterioration" seen, the more the I.Q. results tend to approach true mental deficiency. Much of the difficulty the schizophrenic has with such tests is due to impairment of the use of his intellectual functioning by the severe ego disturbance. Orientation is often preserved in this psychosis but may not be if the patient becomes severely disturbed. Judgment is impaired, again usually because the patient has withdrawn his interest from the world and no longer evaluates adequately what goes on about him. Questions designed to test judgment are often answered with illogical or irrelevant answers because of the patient's associative difficulty. Insight is characteristically lacking, at least after the psychosis has become chronic. Early in the disease the patient is often aware of marked emotional changes within himself and may seek aid. More frequently, however, we have seen such patients show great concern with their mental state and yet be too suspicious or too wary to trust any physician with their problem. In such cases they are not seen medically until their symptoms become of sufficient gravity to cause the family to seek aid.

ETIOLOGY

The etiology of the schizophrenic phenomenon has thus far eluded investigators. It is entirely possible that when the whole story is eventually known it will be found that there is no single causative agent for this psychosis but rather, as has been proposed, several possible factors involved, which if operating simultaneously produce the psychosis. However, it is often not easy to determine whether these factors are the cause or the result of the psychosis itself. For instance, certain biochemical changes and endocrinological variations are seen in a schizophrenic reaction. However, at our present level of knowledge it is not always possible to understand all the intricacies of the relationship between the psyche and the hormonal balance. Certainly we have ample evidence to indicate that emotional factors are capable of influencing endocrine levels. For instance, it is well known that anger can be responsible for an increased output of adrenalin with all the resulting changes which are then produced by this hormone. If we consider the far-reaching psychic changes that accrue in a schizophrenic reaction it is reasonable to postulate that many of the biochemical changes and variations found in this condition are secondary to the psychic process itself.

At the present level of our attempts to understand this psychosis, the etiological investigations can generally be divided into the functional concepts and the organic concepts. Included in the latter, or possibly a third avenue of approach, is the constitutional theory. A great deal of data has been accumulated in each of these areas and while none has thus far proven the final answer, certainly each has added to our over-all understanding of this personality reaction.

Following are some of the present-day theories related to these concepts.

FUNCTIONAL CONCEPT

Perhaps the best way to summarize the functional approach to a schizophrenic reaction would be to say that we now know a great deal about the underlying psychopathology which is seen in this condition, but we cannot be certain of all the factors involved in the production of this particular type of personality disintegration. Modern dynamic psychiatry considers severe and conspicuous regression to be the important element in the schizophrenic psychosis. This regression is to a much earlier phase of development than is true in the neurotic patient. It reaches back to the time when ego formation was just beginning. The ego itself disintegrates and thus allows expression of the so-called primary thinking processes which always hold sway in the unconscious but are ordinarily elaborated into secondary thinking processes in normal individuals by the ego. When these unconscious processes break through they seem to be highly illogical and, from the standpoint of the normal ego, they are. It is to the lack of ego-synthesizing and reality-testing functions that we owe the odd and bizarre character of the schizophrenic pattern. Truly the unconscious has been exposed to the world.

In the early stage of the psychosis we notice a gradual giving up by the patient of his object relationships with people about him. He no longer invests his environment with the normal amount of interest. Put in another way, his libidinal ties begin to weaken. Very often the schizophrenic senses this gradual withdrawal and it may lead him to a feeling that the world is coming to an end. At times he may suffer from the feeling of depersonalization or the loss of the feeling of one's self. Another regressive symptom often seen relatively early in the disease process is that of hypochondriasis. This is the result of a change in ego stability and a difficulty with the body image. The latter is the intrapsychic representation of the body and all its parts. During the schizophrenic process the body image is disturbed so that various portions of the body have a heightened awareness. At times these hypochondriacal sensations reach the proportion of somatic delusions in which the patient becomes convinced of a marked change or even absence of an organ or part of the body. Rather typical is the impression occasionally found in patients that the brain is literally rotting away.

ORGANIC CONCEPT

Endocrinology is prominent among the organic approaches in a search for the etiology of schizophrenic reaction. The broad field of the interrelationships between endocrines, emotions, and autonomic function is too complex to be dealt with in any detail here. Certainly, however, many thought-provoking facts are coming to light through recent research in this direction. At the present time it is apparent that we are not yet close to any final understanding of this complicated problem. However, we do know that these three important "systems" are closely interrelated and the function of each influences the others. Our methods of measurement are far from adequate in any of the three and with so many variables and "unknowns" it is extremely difficult to standardize results. While it would be desirable to find some endocrine substance or combination that would "cure" psychiatric disorders there is little evidence at present that this will occur. Man, with his complicated psyche, tries hard to achieve an adjustment to the fast-moving, complicated world he has created. When he fails and his psyche begins to malfunction, his soma suffers. Treatment of the soma, at least with what we have now available, for psychiatric disorders is usually inefficient and nonproductive.

Some of the most thorough and scientific work done on the biological aspects of schizophrenic reactions has been going on since 1927 at the Worcester State Hospital in Massachusetts. Hoskins [3] calls attention to "the apparent paradox that although well-marked endocrinopathies and psychosis are seldom seen in the same patient, many schizophrenics show deviations from normality that are suggestive of less severe endocrine disorders." He suggests that the difficulty is not necessarily one of levels of hormone production but possibly one of "inadequate reactivity to hormones." In reporting on

[3] Hoskins, Roy G. *The Biology of Schizophrenia.* New York, W. W. Norton & Company, 1946.

thyroid in schizophrenic reactions he finds that about 10 per cent of hospitalized cases show evidences of thyroid deficiency and that in such cases the administration of adequate dosages of thyroid over a period of time results in improvement in such patients. However, he finds that this medication in other cases does not produce improvement.

Attempts have been made to correlate adrenal function with the psychosis. Hoskins says "the schizophrenic patient is handicapped in most cases by a failure of his adrenals to respond adaptively to the changing needs of the body. It is this characteristic, rather than any marked failure of secretion, that is impressive." His group also has attempted to use androgens in the treatment of schizophrenics. Again results were mildly encouraging but not conclusive. Another more recent study is that of Gerard [4] at the University of Michigan and Ypsilanti State Hospital. His findings in this area were inconclusive.

Sakel [5] and his group at the Creedmoor State Hospital have studied many of the biological aspects of schizophrenic reactions. They have been particularly interested in histamine and have shown that schizophrenics tolerate, as a group, at least 50 per cent more histamine than psychoneurotics. They also found that sex steroids and thyroid reduce the resistance of these patients to histamine. Sex steroids raise the resting eosinophile level and adrenal cortical hormones lower it, which, at least in this respect, poses these two groups as antagonists. It was postulated and now seems to begin to be proven correct that ACTH would perhaps contribute to rather than diminish emotional disturbances.

The oxygen metabolism and carbohydrate metabolism have also been studied extensively in this psychosis. Hoskins found that oxygen uptake was deficient in schizophrenic patients but presents fairly good evidence that the cause is to be found in the tissues of the body, probably in the enzyme systems. Gerard's results did not show any clear abnormality in this function. Many writers have

[4] Gerard, R. W., et al. "The Nosology of Schizophrenia" *American Journal of Psychiatry*, Vol. 120 1:16–29, July, 1963.
[5] Sakel, M. *Pharmacological Shock Treatment of Schizophrenia*. Washington, Nervous and Mental Disease Publishing Co., 1938.

shown that a high percentage of schizophrenic patients show a diabetic curve as determined by the Exton-Rose procedure.

It is easy to see that although much data is being accumulated, there is still a great deal of unexplored territory. Again the autonomic nervous system must be reckoned with in the triad of emotions–endocrine–autonomic nervous system.

CONSTITUTIONAL CONCEPT

Another interesting approach to the understanding of schizophrenic reaction is concerned with constitutional or body type. There is a higher incidence of the asthenic or leptosome type seen in schizophrenic patients. This more or less approaches Sheldon's ectomorph type,[6] which is predominately ectodermal, and the patient is nervous, high-strung, and sensitive. Kline and Tenney, using the methods of Sheldon, somatotyped 2,100 consecutive admissions to a Veterans Administration hospital and found that paranoid schizophrenics tended to be mesomorphs rather than ectomorphs but that this was reversed in hebephrenic schizophrenia.

The subject of heredity in schizophrenic reactions has been studied but the results are not conclusive. Monozygotic twins have proven to be the most valuable source of information, but investigators have not always been careful to give adequate weight to environmental factors. Heredity may play a role in a schizophrenic reaction but not as great as it apparently does in a manic depressive reaction.

Dr. Lauretta Bender [7] believes that an important factor in the production of schizophrenic reaction is a lag in prenatal neurological development. This lag, she believes, is such that even the best of environmental conditions (the best maternal care) cannot effect a healthy and normal environmental reaction in certain children. These children's concepts of spatial relations are faulty, giving rise to anxiety and symptoms of depersonalization.

[6] Sheldon, W. H. and Stevens, S. S. *The Varieties of Temperament*. New York. Harper and Brothers, 1942.

[7] Bender, Lauretta. "Childhood Schizophrenia: A Clinical Study of 100 Schizophrenic Children." *American Journal of Orthopsychiatry*, XVII. 1947.

SCHIZOPHRENIC REACTION TYPES

Ever since Kraepelin first gathered together under the name of "dementia praecox" several syndromes it has been the usual procedure to classify schizophrenic patients into four types. They will be discussed here under five headings, approximating the current APA nomenclature and thus including the schizo-affective type. The five subdivisions are:

1. simple type
2. hebephrenic type
3. catatonic type
4. paranoid type
5. schizo-affective type.

It must be recognized that whereas these are ordinarily defined as clear-cut types, one often sees a case which has elements of two or more of them. The main factors to be considered are those of the underlying dynamic mechanisms which are responsible for the personality disorganization. The original classification was made primarily upon the presence of certain overt symptoms rather than upon the more important underlying mechanisms. It is also not at all rare to see a case in which one finds a transition from one type to another of these various divisions.

SIMPLE TYPE

This particular type of schizophrenic psychosis is ordinarily a chronic and insidious form. It develops slowly over a period of years and leads to a gradual withdrawal from people and a slow deterioration of personal habits. Associated with it are the classical emotional changes resulting in a *blunting of the affect* with occasionally a more obvious dissociation of the affect from the ideational content. During the process of development of the psychosis these patients are not always easily recognized as schizophrenics, at least until the later stages. By the time the psychosis is full-blown, they present a clearer picture of a blunted affect with occasional silly, incongruous emotional reactions, lack of interest in the world about them, preoccupation with their fantasy world, and a general disinterest in leading any type of constructive life. Hallucinations and delusions are seen at times although they are not ordinarily thought of as characteristic of this particular type. In these cases the deterioration often proceeds steadily over a period of years until patients finally reach a vegetative state where they are inaccessible to any type of ordinary relationship with other individuals. Many of these people are to be found on the fringes of society where, before the full-blown psychosis develops, they drift from one job to another, often becoming involved in minor encounters with the law primarily because of their inability to conform to the ordinary social standards and their tendency to drift and wander from one occupation to another.

Case History: Schizophrenic Reaction, Simple Type

A twenty-four-year-old single girl was referred for psychiatric help because her family had been increasingly concerned about her behavior during the previous two weeks. She had begun repeatedly calling her boy friend on the telephone but then would be unable to carry on a reasonable conversation with him. She would often try to make an appointment to meet him someplace but immediately changed the date, the time, or the place. She had begun writing notes on bits of scratch paper, for instance, "I must not disgrace my parents," or "I will do it, I must do it." She had become increasingly bizarre in her conversation and activity. It was very difficult to have a logical discussion with her because she would frequently change the subject and not be able to follow one line of thought for any period of time. She had become increasingly indecisive, often deciding to do one thing but then immediately changing her mind and deciding to do something else. She had not wanted to see a psychiatrist but had been coerced into doing so by her family.

The first interview was typical of the patient's disorganized thinking in that it was difficult to get a clear, concise history from her. Initially she said that all of her trouble was caused by the fact that she had changed jobs many times. She said that she did not like the business world. Suddenly she said that she had had whooping cough at the age of seven and after that, asthma. She went on to say that she had seen two psychologists about her worries over the asthma. Her talk was not spontaneous and considerable urging was necessary. She would begin to talk about something in a few jerky phrases and suddenly change the subject and talk about something completely unrelated. She had had many jobs, never for any longer than eight or nine months at a time. She was extremely anxious to gain financial independence from her family and yet at the same time was vague as to the methods by which she would do this.

Much of her concern was in the sexual sphere. She said that she had had intercourse with a boy friend approximately two years previously and that ever since then she had been very worried about it. She had enjoyed it, she said, but felt thereafter that "sex has changed me. I am no longer a virgin, I shouldn't wear white." She also thought that she should use tampons rather than ordinary menstrual pads, again because she was no longer a virgin. She had the impression that her family also knew this. She felt that she and this man had the proper conditions for a good love affair because they both had suffered from asthma in the past. During one of her conversations about him she spoke of "having fallen in love with the image of myself."

Because of the obvious personality disorganization that was present in this patient she was hospitalized, and remained in the hospital for three months. During this time she received sixteen electroshock treatments and thirty-six treatments with insulin. In addition, she was seen frequently in psychotherapeutic interviews.

Her condition did not improve a great deal even with this treatment. She remained quite distractable. It was very difficult to get her to concentrate on anything for more than a very brief period of time. Occasionally she gave the examiner the impression of listening to something as if she were hallucinated in the auditory sphere but she always denied this. Her family provided more information about her background. She had been a rather shy individual with feelings of inferiority and had been rather asocial. She had voluntarily stopped school before graduation and had always been unpredictable, and unstable in her living habits and employment. She had never talked easily to anyone and tended to be rather secretive about her personal life. There was one paternal uncle who had been institutionalized, and who had eventually committed suicide. Other than this there was no history of mental disease in the family.

Discussion

This patient was diagnosed as a simple schizophrenic and she presented a rather typical history of the gradual transition from a schizoid, withdrawn, asocial personality into an overt psychotic. At the time of the development of her psychosis she focused most of her emotions on the sexual sphere. She became increasingly delusional to the point where she felt all of her family as well as other people were aware of her sexual indiscretion.

Her early childhood had not been happy. Her parents had never gotten along well and had often fought with each other. When she was smaller both parents had worked. The family had not been very social and few friends ever visited. Her school life had also been difficult because of the neighborhood in which she lived. Occasionally she stole from the cash register in her parents' store to bribe some of the children in school to leave her alone. She had withdrawn increasingly within herself and developed the schizoid type of personality which had persisted until she became involved in the sexual affair at about twenty-two. At this time, although she claimed to have had some enjoyment from the experience, her ego was unable to handle the subsequent guilt and then became delusional saying, "Everyone can see what has taken place."

The prognosis in this case was rather poor. At the end of her hospitalization the patient still talked in the same indecisive and disorganized way and was still preoccupied with the sexual experience. She had become somewhat more accessible but still had a very tenuous hold on reality, and considerable difficulty in establishing any sort of relationship with people. As is rather typical of many of these schizophrenic patients this girl showed little if any insight into her condition even after her therapy.

HEBEPHRENIC TYPE

This type of schizophrenic reaction is characterized by a more marked and obvious *dissociation* of affect and ideational content, with resulting silly laughter and grimaces. Delusions and hallucinations are more frequent. It may come on acutely or in a chronic manner. In hebephrenia the regression is usually more malignant than that seen in the other types of schizophrenia. The patient's ego seems literally to "give up."

Case History: Schizophrenic Reaction, Hebephrenic Type

A twenty-two-year-old single woman was brought to the hospital by her family because of bizarre behavior at home. She had over the previous three weeks gradually lost interest in people and in her work. She had kept more and more to herself. She was often to be found alone, laughing, grimacing, and posturing. She no longer was able to maintain an acceptable appearance and frequently wet and soiled her bed. Her remarks were often inappropriate and it was impossible to converse with her in a logical and coherent manner. Eventually she began to refuse to eat.

At the time of admission she appeared to be an unkempt and not particularly attractive woman who showed numerous facial grimaces and twitchings which were apparently meaningless. She often moved her hands and fingers as if performing some magical gesture. She rolled and unrolled her hair on her fingers. It was difficult to talk to her because every few minutes she would jump to her feet and laugh for no apparent reason. She was rather poorly oriented and, although she knew the month, was unable to give the proper day. She was obviously quite confused and was unable to give any coherent history of her past, remote or recent. She was very distractible and often interrupted the conversation by asking irrelevant questions. From time to time she would look at a corner of the room in an attentive and listening fashion and it was obvious that she was having hallucinations of some type, although she would not discuss them. She was often blocked and when asked a question would begin to give an answer only to stop for a long period in mid-sentence.

A history was very difficult to obtain because of the general lack of interest of the relatives. They rarely came to visit her and many attempts had to be made before anyone in the family would come to the hospital to give a history. When this was done the history was brief and vague. The patient was the youngest of six children, three of whom had died in their earliest years. As far as could be gathered she had done satisfactorily in school, or at least there had not been many complaints. Her father, who gave the history, was an uneducated and not particularly intelligent individual who had never paid much attention to his children and felt their care was the duty of his wife. The mother had been equally uninterested and had always been busy with a variety of activities outside the home. She was content to leave the children alone as long as no complaints about them came to her.

The patient had never been active socially, and had few friends. Her heterosexual experience had been minimal. Apparently she had begun a relationship with a service man some months prior to her breakdown. This had ended in her being rejected by the man and it was approximately two weeks afterward that her present psychotic episode had begun.

The patient was begun on tranquilizers. Initially she began to respond and for a brief period of time was in contact with reality. At that time her affect was much more appropriate and her answers more logical and coherent. However, in spite of a continuation of therapy, the patient soon regressed back to her original state. She was given a series of electroshock. She did not respond and continued to manifest the original signs of her psychosis.

Discussion

This patient represents a rather typical example of hebephrenic schizophrenic reaction. Characteristic were the silly grimaces and mannerisms which she revealed along with her markedly inappropriate affect and general personality disorganization. The prognosis with this patient is extremely guarded as it is in many such hebephrenic individuals. The possibility of improvement through the use of continued tranquilizers and active psychotherapy remains.

CATATONIC TYPE

There are two subtypes of catatonic schizophrenic reaction which may alternate with each other. They are the *agitated* or excited state and the *stuporous* state. In the catatonic excitement one sees marked hyperactivity of a disorganized and purposeless nature. These patients are most difficult to control because they may impulsively attack an innocent person without provocation or indulge in some type of destructiveness for no apparent reason. They tend to be generally negativistic and irritable. Speech production may or may not be increased but if so it tends to be constant, incoherent, and extremely difficult to comprehend. Such patients are apt to use obscene language and speak vituperatively to anyone who happens to be nearby. Hallucinations are frequent and although usually auditory may occasionally be visual.

The catatonic stuporous reaction is on the other end of the scale of motility from the excited state. The patient is extremely withdrawn and often totally unresponsive, at least from a verbal standpoint. His face is immobile and he seemingly pays little if any attention to things which are going on around him. Whereas in the excited state the patient is apt to smear urine and feces, in the stuporous state he is apt to retain his excreta. Mutism may be present. The previously described phenomenon of waxy flexibility is seen from time to time: if a patient's arm is raised he will keep it there for a long period. In this type of patient one may see edema developing in the dependent parts because of the long-maintained positions. These patients have reached such an utterly complete passive state that literally everything must be done for them. As mentioned above, there may be a rapid transition between the stuporous and excited states. Occasionally, however one may see a catatonic schizophrenic who remains in either the stuporous or the excited phase without ever reverting to the other type. While we have no clear or complete knowledge of the mechanisms of the catatonic schizophrenic reaction, certainly it is fairly obvious from many cases that regression is present to the point of infantile or even fetal characteristics.

Case History: Schizophrenic Reaction, Catatonic Type

A thirty-three-year-old unmarried woman was brought to the receiving ward of the hospital by the police. Early that morning she had been picked up wandering around the streets. She had been detained at the police station during the day and was brought to the hospital because of her disturbed and unusual behavior. She had not talked all day long, nor had she eaten anything. Attempts had been made to spoon-feed her, but they had been unsuccessful.

When brought to the hospital she presented a very disheveled, untidy, and obviously infantile picture. She sucked her thumb constantly, she crawled about on the floor like a baby and licked dirt from her fingers. She was attracted by various shiny objects in the room, but obviously feared touching them. She would often whimper and cry, but spoke no words.

She was placed on a psychiatric ward where this infantile, regressed behavior continued. A solution of sugar and water was placed in a nursing bottle with a nipple, and offered to the patient. She responded eagerly and drank the entire bottle voraciously. During the process she had an obvious orgasm manifested by thrashing of her legs, flushed cheeks, and clear signs of great emotional pleasure, followed by relaxation. She then curled up and went to sleep in a typical fetal position.

An anamnesis obtained from relatives revealed the following material. The patient was the third of four children. She had an older brother and sister and a younger brother. Her father and mother had been divorced when the patient was approximately four years old. The mother had been an alcoholic who had intermittently been engaged in active prostitution. The patient physically resembled her mother. Following the divorce, the father remarried. The stepmother made it plain to everyone concerned from the beginning that she wanted nothing to do with her stepchildren. She had two other children of her own whom she brought into the new marriage and was unwilling to accept the added burden of her new husband's previous children. Since the patient's father had been given custody of the children, he elected to place them in an orphanage. This was done, but within a short time all of the children except the patient were returned home. At the age of ten the patient ran away from the orphanage and subsequent to this, because she had proven difficult to manage, was sent to live with a distant relative. This particular woman was an extremely rigid, punitive person who had little interest in the youngster other than requiring complete and total obedience. Eventually the patient's other siblings were sent to live with this relative. Each of them grew up to manifest severe personality disturbances. One was a criminal, one an alcoholic, and another a psychotic.

When she was sixteen, the patient was punished severely for something for which she had not been responsible. Shortly following this, there was a history of what apparently was a psychotic episode. The patient had threatened suicide and was sent to a state hospital. A diagnosis of schizophrenic reaction was made, but the family would not give permission for either insulin therapy or electroshock. The patient remained in the state hospital with the exception of a few brief paroles for a period of sixteen years. Each time she was paroled, her behavior soon became so disorganized that she had to be returned to the hospital.

Later in the hospitalization under discussion, the patient's I.Q. was found to be 125. She was continued on the regimen of bottle feeding every four hours and treated in every way as if she were a very young child. She was given one of the phenothiazine tranquilizers. All of her various manifestations of regression were indulged by the doctors and nurses, and after approximately a month on this regimen she gradually began to talk and to assume a more mature adjustment. She remained in the hospital for a period of three months. Psychotherapeutic interviews provided her with some beginning insight, but generally were more supportive in nature. Following her discharge from the hospital, she obtained a position doing simple tasks and has been successful in maintaining this job for the past two years. She continued on smaller doses of tranquilizer, which undoubtedly helped maintain her improvement.

Discussion

This patient represents a fairly typical example of catatonic schizophrenic reaction. She showed the mutism, negativism, and other catatonic features that are so prominent. The rather dramatic way that she revealed her regressive tendencies is typical of this type of psychosis. She literally nursed from a bottle and assumed the fetal position. We find in her past history many evidences of severe psychological traumata. Her parents' separation and the fact that neither of them was mature contributed largely to her faulty personality development. Then there was added to this placement in an orphanage where little if any love or understanding came her way. Then, to make matters worse, she was transferred to an uninterested and unloving relative whose demands upon her were excessive. All of these factors helped to contribute to a very poor ego development which left her susceptible to ego disintegration such as was seen in her psychosis.

PARANOID TYPE

This particular type of schizophrenic reaction is characterized chiefly by the development of poorly systematized paranoid delusions. The patient is constantly concerned that various individuals are working against him. His system of delusions may involve anywhere from one individual to the entire human race. The important element is that of the involved individual or individuals plotting against the patient. Frequently one finds the presence of paranoid hallucinations in these patients. In these cases the hallucinated voices inform the patients of the evils that are being perpetrated against them by other individuals. Such a psychosis is generally manifested later than the other four types. It most frequently comes on in the thirties and forties and proceeds insidiously, but may occur more abruptly in a younger person.

The paranoid schizophrenic, at least early in his psychosis, tends to retain his grasp on reality more than any of the other schizophrenic types. While early in the development of the psychosis the delusions may be relatively limited, as the process spreads so also do the delusions until they finally occupy most of the patient's waking hours. These people are ordinarily resentful, suspicious, and irritable. They may go through a period of years during the development of their psychosis where their relationships with people gradually become tinged with a paranoid coloring. Legal actions are often resorted to by these patients for fancied wrongs done them by their neighbors. During the developmental stages of the psychosis, before they have completely lost contact with reality, it is not unusual for them to make a very good impression upon legal authorities.

It is very common for the delusions and hallucinations in this type of schizophrenic reaction to involve accusations of homosexuality directed toward the patient. Our modern dynamic understanding of the underlying mechanisms in this process makes it clear that latent homosexuality is responsible for many of the symptoms seen in this condition. The paranoid schizophrenic is one of the most difficult of all psychiatric patients with whom to deal. The prognosis is guarded and tranquilizers or even the shock therapies are often ineffectual.

Discussion of paranoid conditions would not be complete without mention of another rather uncommon condition. *Folie à deux* is a term indicating a sort of "communicable" psychosis, usually paranoid in nature. One member of a closely associated pair becomes psychotic and then the other, mainly through suggestibility, becomes similarly psychotic. This may occur for instance between mother and daughter or husband and wife. It is ordinarily found that there has existed between the two a very close and pathological relationship with one being more active and one more passive. The active one becomes psychotic first and then the passive one. The prognosis of the second patient varies with the degree of psychopathology. Some are more accurately diagnosed as dissociative-reaction, and others are essentially psychotic. Where the condition involves more than two persons it is called *folie à trois* (for three) and so on.

Case History (1): Schizophrenic Reaction, Paranoid Type

A thirty-one-year-old married woman was brought to the psychiatrist by her sister because of what the latter described as "confused periods" which the patient had been having. During these times the patient talked disconnectedly and related many bizarre ideas, particularly involving the numerous catastrophes for which she felt herself responsible. Most of these latter ideas had developed approximately two weeks prior to her referral.

This patient brought forth primarily during her first interview her concerns about her marriage of seven months. She said that she did not think that her husband had originally wanted to marry her. She went on to relate how both she and her husband had had hormonal injections prior to marriage. She complained that ever since marriage she had had sex on her mind especially when her husband was at work. However, she added that they had rarely had intercourse. She said that perhaps the marriage was a mistake and that she could never really grow away from her mother. Her husband was fifty years of age, nineteen years her senior.

Then she went on to relate a great deal of delusional material. She felt that she was causing all of the troubles in the world. For instance, she was responsible for all the recent fires about which she had read in the paper. She then said that if her husband did not love her and she refused to have sex relations with him four times and finally accepted him the fifth, things would eventually be all right. She then immediately changed the subject and said that a recent rise in food prices was her fault.

Because of the obviously psychotic material presented by this patient in the first interview she was referred for hospitalization where she remained for approximately three weeks.

At the time of her first interview in the hospital she appeared a rather nice-looking young woman, well dressed but obviously anxious and making a considerable effort to control herself and give a proper impression. She told the examiner that she had decided to come to the hospital for a rest for two or three days, at the end of which time she would go home. She made it very clear to him that she did not feel that she was at all ill but that she had been somewhat upset because of her recent marriage. She went on to say that she felt that she now had the marriage situation in hand and that she planned very soon to return to her husband.

Soon after her admission she became disturbed and irritated at the fact that she could not come and go freely or telephone any of her relatives when she desired. She became extremely agitated and approached an assaultive state when told that she would not be able to see her relatives during the first ten days of hospitalization. As soon as it became obvious to her that the rules of the hospital would have to be obeyed she changed her tactics completely and became submissive, docile, and superficially friendly. She spoke of her great desire to co-operate in any therapeutic endeavors and felt that the only thing that she wanted was "to get well." In spite of her seemingly co-operative demeanor the patient remained on a very anxious level and refused to discuss anything of great importance. She minimized all the difficulties that she had and seemed bent upon producing the best possible impression upon the examiner.

This patient's family history revealed that she had four sisters, three of whom were older than herself. The second sister was at the time a patient in a state hospital where she had been for the past ten years, diagnosed as a schizophrenic. The other three sisters were all working and none of them were married. The patient's father had died ten years previously. He had been a professional man who was described as easy-going and completely dominated by his wife. He had been a Protestant while his wife was a Catholic. The mother was still living and had made a marked effort to keep all of her children around her, having discouraged any marital ventures that any of them had considered. She was a very domineering, overly religious, and hard-working woman who had ruled the family with an iron hand. She had strenuously disapproved of the patient's marriage.

The patient's husband was fifty years of age. He was a Protestant while she had been raised in and still practiced Catholicism. She had gone with him for ten years prior to their marriage and he had constantly urged her to marry him. She had declined for a long time because of the difference in their ages, the difference in their religions, and her concern that she would not be able to carry on a satisfactory sexual relationship with any man. The patient's mother had been the source of a great deal of difficulty during the courtship, and things had finally culminated in the patient breaking relations with her mother and marrying her suitor. At this time her mother told her never to return home again.

Following her marriage the patient had been completely ignored by her family until the onset of her illness. The husband reported that during the brief marriage there had been considerable difficulty in their sex life and it had been unsatisfactory for both. Following the acute outbreak of the psychosis the husband became upset and took the patient back to her mother where she improved for about a week. She then wanted to come back to her husband and this was arranged. However, as soon as she returned to her apartment she again became confused, upset, and delusional.

After approximately three weeks of hospitalization and phenothiazine medication the patient's mother decided that she should return home and she was therefore discharged against advice. It was felt at that time that she needed longer hospitalization, and psychotherapy should be given. She had stopped talking about her delusional material but this presumably was because she recognized that such talk diminished her chances for release from the hospital. The patient evidenced almost no insight into her condition. She would frequently say that she knew that some of her delusions were ridiculous yet she steadfastly maintained the veracity of them.

Discussion

This patient was diagnosed as paranoid schizophrenic primarily because of her marked ideas of reference and her tendency always to find hidden bizarre meanings in things which were said to her. She never had had a good work history, frequently changing jobs because of difficulty in adjusting to those with whom she worked. She came from a family where the mother was a dominating and oppressive figure. The father, on the other hand, had been a passive, easy-going individual whose influence in the family was not strong. Following his death the mother kept all five daughters single and within the home until finally the patient had broken away and made a very unsatisfactory marriage. Her greatest concern prior to marriage was that she would not be able to have adequate sexual relationships with men. It is interesting to note that she picked a man nineteen years her senior, who himself had suffered from many neurotic complaints. Obviously she felt very insecure about her own sexuality and one can easily postulate the presence of a latent homosexual trend, particularly in view of the close attachment that she had always had to her mother as well as the extreme concern she had had regarding her ability to make a heterosexual adjustment.

Interestingly enough we see in this patient a phenomenon that is not infrequently seen in schizophrenic reactions, especially of the paranoid type. They seem to sense that they are suffering from a difficulty in thinking which may result in their institutionalization if they are persuaded to talk about it. Soon after their hospitalization they become aware of the importance to the physician of their delusional material and therefore begin to deny its presence even though they are still convinced of the truth of their delusions. They do this obviously in the hope of being released from the hospital. This patient's main conflict seemed to center around her ambivalent attachment to her mother who did not and never had met her daughter's needs. The conflict became intolerable and projection began to play an important role which resulted in her delusional material. It is difficult to ascertain the specific dynamics of her delusions regarding sins for which she felt herself responsible, but one can easily postulate that these again had their origin in the sexual sphere, particularly in view of her delusion that if she were to refuse her husband intercourse four times in a row, but accept him the fifth, then everything would be all right. But, in contrast, if she refused him three times, a fire would break out in the city—a displacement of his or her sexual "fire."

Case History (2): Schizophrenic Reaction, Paranoid Type

A forty-seven-year-old single male came for an outpatient consultation which he himself had arranged. He was an obese, untidy individual who obviously had been suspicious in his original telephone conversation regarding the appointment. When he presented himself for the interview he was extremely interested to know whether records would be kept. He was unwilling to give his address or his telephone number and, in fact, seemed hesitant as to whether he should have come at all. He did not present a picture of anxiety, but of marked suspiciousness. He said, "I have a tendency to make enemies. People take offense at me without any reason. Recently there have been some attempts to get into my room. These have been occurring over the past few years. On one occasion, somebody attempted to hold me up and on another occasion they attempted to wreck my car." The patient described in minute detail the date, time, and place of each of these occurrences with remarkable memory. He then went on to say that waiters at the hotel where he was currently living had been putting things in his food so that he had to be extremely careful what he ate. He had begun sending out for his food and was careful to pick a new restaurant each time so that no one would be aware of where he was getting his food.

The examiner's questions, if they concerned his personal life, were resented by the patient and were ignored or brushed aside. However, persistence on the part of the examiner brought out some facts. The patient did not make friends very easily. He was an attorney who had built up a small practice which was sufficient to maintain his own needs. He always worked alone and did not spend many hours in his office. He said he had accumulated enough money to marry and had proposed to several girls, but had never been accepted. He then went on to say, "Things happen to me that don't happen to other people. I get singled out in an unfavorable way." He claimed that such things had been happening to him since he was six or seven years of age, and felt "astrology is probably where the answer lies."

He had seen two or three psychiatrists before, but had only gone once to each physician because "they didn't give me enough." He pointed out that one of the psychiatrists had agreed that perhaps someone was following him. He felt that this was the best psychiatrist he had seen. He denied having any close friends now nor had he had any since he began high school. He said that he frequently invited girls to go places with him, but that they turned him down. He often went to dances alone, but never seemed able to make any friends. Once again he launched into his delusional system claiming that he "did not look right," and that people often told him so.

This patient after about forty minutes felt that once again the present psychiatrist was not offering him anything and decided to leave. He refused all invitations for another appointment, and still refused to give any address or telephone number.

Discussion

Here again is a typical example of a schizophrenic reaction, paranoid type. It brings up an important element which one sees from time to time with psychotic patients, namely the decision of disposition. Obviously this patient was psychotic and might even be considered potentially dangerous. Yet he had refused any further psychiatric help and had refused to allow the psychiatrist to contact anyone else in his family. If such patients are considered by the physician to be seriously dangerous to the community, measures must be taken to see that they are given a thorough psychiatric checkup. Obviously this individual had never made a good adjustment. He had been relatively asocial all his life and was now, for the most part, estranged even from his own family. He was thoroughly involved in his own delusional system although still capable of carrying on a limited work schedule.

SCHIZO-AFFECTIVE TYPE

This type refers to those patients who show a mixture of schizophrenic and affective reactions. At times the elation or depression are quite marked yet there is a bizarre, obviously schizophrenic process present also. Usually such patients, when they have been observed over a period of time, reveal themselves to be basically schizophrenic.

Case History: Schizophrenic Reaction, Schizo-affective Type

This thirty-four-year-old married male was admitted to the psychopathic hospital at the direction of the municipal court. His wife had taken him there because of his behavior and he had been seen by the court psychiatrist, who recommended hospitalization. This psychiatrist reported that the patient had unrealistic ideas about making a great deal of money and had on one occasion purchased an automobile with a worthless check. He had shown a personality change from being thrifty, exceedingly industrious and serious, to using obscene language, and being irresponsible, quarrelsome, and constantly complaining that his family had tried to "frame" him. This patient, when seen upon admission, was an attractive, well-built, physically adequate individual who seemed to be in contact with his environment. He began the interview by making numerous demands upon the psychiatrist, stating that he must be released from the hospital at once. He said that it was really his wife who was insane and not he. He said that he had only come into the hospital in order to "receive clearance" and that he would arrange for the hospitalization of his wife as soon as he was able to bring it to the attention of the authorities. He said that the court physician who had examined him had made a "terrible mistake" in hospitalizing him and he felt that this particular physician had "blown his lid," was insane, and needed an examination in order to "protect the public." He said that this doctor was suffering from a psychosis because he never looked anyone in the face and this was a certain sign of his severe mental illness. The patient suggested that this particular court physician had hypnotized a patient and "he lost his subconscious to that patient." He went on to say that he was planning to sue this physician as soon as he was released and to force the physician to subject himself to a mental examination. These delusional ideas formed the primary basis of the patient's initial interview. He was in good contact with his environment otherwise. He was oriented, his memory was excellent, and he gave the impression of being of better than average intelligence. He completely lacked insight into his own mental illness.

Following admission this patient became a chronic troublemaker on the ward. He constantly requested permission to leave the hospital, and frequently threatened to sue everyone connected with the hospital. He often incited other patients, for instance, telling Negro patients that they were being discriminated against in order to stir them up to create a disturbance on the ward. On one occasion he attacked an attendant and subsequently explained, "I antagonized him to see his reaction and to see if he was well trained to handle such situations." He mentioned the name of a book dealing with psychological subjects which he felt that all nurses and attendants in the hospital should be required to read. He was particularly bitter against one intern who, he said, was a Southerner and should be removed from the hospital because he was prejudiced against Negroes. When this physician was absent from his duties for a couple of days because of illness, the patient proclaimed, "I had him removed." He stated that fifteen people had already been arrested as a result of his incarceration and the investigation that he had begun. He frequently prescribed for fellow patients, not only suggesting to them what they should request in the way of medication, but talking with them about their emotional problems. Whenever a new patient was admitted, this patient would go to the nurse and remark, "Take a history and see that he gets penicillin." On one occasion he was overheard instructing several patients to scream and to create trouble so that the nurses would pay some attention to them "for a change." He refused to go to bed at night, removed most of the bedsprings from his bed, and tried to remove the lock from the door. On one occasion he broke into the nurses' office and called the telephone operator of the hospital to get his lawyer for him. He was constantly hyperactive about the ward, talking to other patients and to every physician or visitor who entered the ward. He talked to every nurse, always pointing out the faults and shortcomings of the ward routine. He soon became one of the best-known patients on the ward. He arose early in the morning, began his hyperactivity, and continued it unabated until long after bed time.

The history obtained from the patient's wife revealed that he had been married ten years. He was described by his wife as a "quiet, thoughtful, kind, sympathetic person who was a good provider and who didn't drink, smoke, or use profanity." His family, his wife said, was not close and she felt that they had never had sufficient regard for their own children. The father was described as having made one suicide attempt several years previously. The patient had never gotten along well with his mother, who was described as high-strung and irritable. The patient's wife said that when she and the patient adopted a child two years previously the patient's family had opposed the idea. She said that approximately three years prior to admission the patient had had a job during the day, and had spent his evenings on a second job in order to accumulate enough money to buy a house. It was during this period of hard work that he gradually became depressed and was unable to sleep. He changed jobs, and within six weeks was fired because he was belligerent and unable to get along with the other employees. After that, according to his wife, he regressed, sat around the house, would not work, had crying spells, could not sleep, and did not eat well.

He had been sent to a private sanitarium where he received twelve electroshock treatments with considerable improvement. He returned to his job, but when his wife was hospitalized for a surgical procedure, he became involved in an argument with his mother-in-law. Actually, he and his wife had lived with her ever since they had been married. At the time of the argument, he left his mother-in-law's home and rented an apartment. A few months later he again became depressed because of difficulty in obtaining a new job. He began to worry excessively about financial matters and yet at the same time expressed a great desire to buy a car. Once more he developed crying spells and had periods where he would sit around dejectedly and be unable to do anything for hours at a time.

The situation proceeded to a point where the wife was unable to go out and leave him with their child, since he paid absolutely no attention to the needs of the youngster. It then became necessary for them to move back with the mother-in-law. Arrangements were made for them to pay half the phone bill because of the patient's tendency to make numerous calls. Despite this arrangement and despite his continuing to make many phone calls, he never paid the bill and this resulted in another argument with his mother-in-law. At this point he became quite overactive. He left the house frequently and was often not seen nor heard from for an entire day at a time. He borrowed a considerable sum of money from a bank without informing his wife. He wrote a worthless check to purchase an automobile. He later said that he planned to sell this car and split the proceeds with the company from whom he had bought it.

When his mother-in-law asked him to leave, the patient rented a truck and moved all his belongings, along with his wife's, to a friend's home. When his wife objected that the friends might not be willing to have them live there he continued with the move. It was at this point that she went to court and requested his hospitalization.

The father gave a history that the patient was born in the Middle West, the oldest of seven children. His childhood was described as "normal." He had been a good student, had graduated from high school, and had taken some college work in the evenings. His family had always been relatively poor and it was a constant hardship to obtain enough money to make ends meet. The patient's family had asked him to cut short his education and contribute to the support of the family. The wife's family were Catholic and the patient's family Protestant. The two families did not get along with each other either before or after the marriage. The patient's family were extremely frugal and always resented any of the wife's expenditures even for necessary things. The father felt that visits to the pediatrician when the child was sick were not called for, since he had raised his own seven children by having them seen in a clinic.

Psychological tests revealed an I.Q. of 115 with considerable "scatter." The diagnosis at the time of admission was schizophrenic reaction, schizo-affective type. This was subsequently confirmed as the patient's manic-like behavior became increasingly bizarre and tinged with paranoid elements. His basic schizophrenic process became increasingly obvious. He was put on a tranquilizer and showed considerable improvement.

This patient, at the time of admission, presented many of the symptoms ordinarily associated with an affective disorder of the manic depressive type. He was hyperactive, continually on the move, showed a rapid change of ideas, and seemed under great pressure. However, even at the time of his admission there was a certain bizarreness or oddness about his behavior which lacked the normal "infectiousness" of the manic's behavior. This patient had, in his prepsychotic state, shown a more or less compulsive type of personality. He had been exceedingly industrious, hard-working, perfectionistic, sober, thrifty, and fussy. When his psychosis began there was a large element of depression present, and yet the schizophrenic delusional type of material eventually predominated and made the diagnosis of schizo-affective schizophrenic reaction the correct one.

PROGNOSIS

The prognosis in schizophrenic reactions runs the gamut from poor to fairly good. In the main, prognosis is rather grave and many thousands of patients who show the signs described as schizophrenic reaction move out of the main stream of human productiveness and live useless lives at home or have to spend much, if not all, of their lives in mental hospitals. The integration of the personality in these people has been inadequate and when disorganization and retreat from reality begins to take place, it is not easy to reintegrate the personality and produce a robust, well-functioning individual. Nevertheless, it can be done and has been done and there are some people who show the symptoms of schizophrenic reaction who can, with no more treatment than is given to the average psychoneurotic, take their place in life again and live perfectly normally. Neither the family nor the family physician should despair if a patient is showing schizophrenic signs. For even though the majority of patients to date have had a bad prognosis, more and more work is being done to change this. What we can honestly term "cure" takes place relatively rarely, but a satisfactory social adjustment can be brought about in many. With an increasing number of psychiatrists to do psychotherapeutic work with the schizophrenic, we can produce better results, even though we are dealing with a very serious condition in which many do not get well permanently. The tranquilizing drugs have been of great value in many of these patients but do not necessarily improve the prognosis in terms of increased maturity.

TREATMENT

Treatment in schizophrenic reaction should be oriented toward helping the individual achieve a more adequate level of personality organization and adjustment. Since the psychosis itself represents a process of total personality disorganization, it naturally follows that the treatment will be concerned with all the facets of adjustment. The most important thing that a schizophrenic has to do is improve his relationships with people. In our scientific search for newer and more dramatic ways of treating these patients, we must not forget that the element of human interest, kindness, and thoughtfulness on the part of those responsible for the treatment is of utmost importance. Inherent in the schizophrenic process is a gradual withdrawal from people and from reality. As the psychosis progresses these patients become less and less able to build relationships with those about them. In order to help them re-establish this ability, considerable time and effort are necessary on the part of those concerned with the therapy.

One of the greatest difficulties stemming from the understaffed mental institutions of today is that these schizophrenic patients are of necessity given little time or attention. Their own mental disease forces them further and further from relationships with people until finally they reach a so-called "vegetative" state. Therefore it can well be repeated that at whatever stage we are considering the treatment of the schizophrenic, one of the most important, if not the most important, points to bear in mind is the necessity for helping the patient to re-establish contact with those about him. This means presenting to him every encouragement possible in terms of friendliness, warmth, and understanding.

It should be remembered when dealing with the schizophrenic that his relationship with us will be tenuous at best. Frequently one must spend a great deal of time and effort before the results of therapy begin to be noticeable. Disappointments are frequent, particularly in the form of negative reactions from the patient. Ordinarily, as physicians, we derive a good deal of satisfaction from our work through sensing and being told by patients of the gratitude they hold toward us for our help. With the schizophrenic one is apt to be unrewarded from this standpoint, at least for a long period of time. However, if the therapist reacts with discouragement or hostility, it tends only to further the processes which weaken and finally dissolve the relationship completely.

One of the first decisions which must be made in the plan of treatment for a schizophrenic is whether hospitalization is necessary. Generally speaking, one should institutionalize such patients whenever their psychosis has reached proportions that make it impossible for them to be responsible for their own well-being outside an institution. Since ordinarily the patients who have reached this stage of disorganization are not capable of utilizing their own judgment, family consent and commitment forms must be resorted to.

In addition to overtly psychotic individuals, there are many so-called ambulatory schizophrenics whose disorder has not progressed to the point where they are incapable of caring for themselves or getting along at least to a limited degree in their environment. With such individuals the decision of hospitalization rests primarily upon how amenable they are to therapeutic efforts on an outpatient basis. They may possibly be so disturbed in their relationships with other individuals that it is literally impossible to produce any therapeutic effect as long as they remain in their usual environment.

Hospitalization, in order to be of maximum effectiveness in the schizophrenic reactions, should include certain definite procedures. Obviously, complete physical study is essential. The schizophrenic, with his poor attention to living habits, is prone to develop tuberculosis as well as other physical diseases. To be of the most benefit the entire hospital staff, from superintendent to orderlies, should be oriented toward a kind, friendly therapeutic approach. During his hospitalization the patient needs a good deal of encouragement and help to counteract his tendency to withdraw. At least in the early part of his hospital stay most of his daily schedule will need to be planned for him and he will require considerable encouragement to undertake activities, even of minor types. Occupational therapy plays an important role in the redevelopment of the schizophrenic's interest in the world about him. Social and athletic activities help him to feel an integral part of his environment. In addition, there are the all-important periods spent with him by the staff psychiatrist. It is truly rewarding to see how many seemingly inaccessible patients will gradually respond to consistent friendly and understanding treatment on the part of those about them. The "total push" method of Myerson [8] and Tillotson [9] has had its greatest use in so-called deteriorated schizophrenics.

At the present time the various tranquilizing drugs, particularly of the phenothiazine group, play a large role in the treatment of schizophrenic reactions. It cannot be overstressed that such medications do not constitute the entire treatment approach, but must be supplemented and complemented by psychotherapeutic interviews and a healthy daily routine.

Insulin shock therapy introduced by Sakel [10] in 1928 was used

[8] Myerson, A. "Theory and Principles of the 'Total Push' Method in the Treatment of Chronic Schizophrenia." *Am. J. of Psychiatry*, XCV, 1939.

[9] Tillotson, Kenneth J. "Practice of the 'Total Push' Method in the Treatment of Chronic Schizophrenia." *Am. J. of Psychiatry*, XCV, 1939.

[10] Op. cit., p. 354.

extensively for twenty years in public and private mental hospitals all over the world. While great results were expected from its use, it gradually became evident that this type of treatment did not produce any lasting beneficial results and its use has been almost entirely discontinued.

The giving of insulin to the point of shock led to the application of an electrically induced convulsive shock three or more times weekly in the hope that it too would have a beneficial effect upon this illness, but EST proved only partially and sporadically effective and today is used much less than previously. It can at times be helpful in improving rapport in the depressed or markedly withdrawn or overly active schizophrenic.

Generally speaking at the present time tranquilization is more widely used in schizophrenia than any other treatment. This stems not from the fact that it produces a basic and permanent improvement, but rather from the fact that it is easier to write a prescription than it is to deal, over a long period of time, with a difficult schizophrenic patient. As is discussed in Chapter 22 (Other Treatment Procedures), the whole field of psychopharmacology is developing rapidly and new drugs, or varying combinations of drugs, continue to appear frequently on the market. It is reasonable to assume that with continued research the efficiency of the tranquilizing drugs will improve, but it is still doubtful that this approach will ever lead to a medication which will eradicate the basic problems of the schizophrenic patient.

Because of the average schizophrenic's difficulty in relating to anyone, including a therapist, it is no easy task to treat this type of patient. Ordinarily one must be unusually sensitive to the make-up of schizophrenics in order to establish and maintain rapport with them. The training for this type of treatment and the techniques that go with it reach beyond what is required in the daily treatment of psychoneurotic individuals. The frankly psychotic schizophrenic person has lost many of his ego functions and openly reveals many of the so-called "primary processes" of the id. Whereas these processes are present in everyone, the average person keeps them unconscious by virtue of his ego strength. Therefore, in dealing with the schizophrenic, the therapist is liable to be either completely mystified by the patient's productions, or else have anxiety created in himself by these productions because of the threat to his own ego structure.

The raw material produced by the schizophrenic patient stemming directly from the unconscious without the usual censorship activity of the ego is difficult to evaluate, understand, and even tolerate as far as the therapist is concerned. Interpreting the meaning of the symptoms and productions of these patients requires skill as well as special training. The efforts of the patient and physician to synthesize the various emotions and ideas into a new way of thinking goes on at a different pace than is true of the ordinary psychoneurotic. This puts a much greater strain upon the therapist and it is generally agreed that working with these patients is quite difficult. It would be impossible for the average therapist to spend his entire day, every day of the week, working with schizophrenics. The therapist gains little in the way of narcissistic satisfaction from such patients, and at the same time is bombarded with a constant stream of uncensored, unconscious productions which threaten his own ego.

This brings us back to a reconsideration of the various tranquilizing drugs in the over-all treatment of the schizophrenic. These medications often produce sufficient improvement in the patient so that both he and his family, and possibly even the physician, are content to leave well enough alone. Further arduous psychotherapeutic efforts may not only be time-consuming and inconvenient, but to a degree involve a burdensome expense. It is important that the entire family of such a patient must be made to realize that a serious mental disease exists and that prolonged and skilled therapeutic efforts will have to be made in order to bring about reasonable rehabilitation. During this time the family themselves will often require psychiatric counsel and advice in order to assist in helping the sick individual in his adjustment both during and after the therapy.

As to the actual procedure of psychotherapy itself, both Dr. Frieda Fromm-Reichmann [11] and Dr. John N. Rosen [12] have accentuated

[11] Fromm-Reichmann, Frieda. *Principles of Intensive Psychotherapy*. Chicago. University of Chicago Press, 1950.

[12] Rosen, John N. "The Treatment of Schizophrenic Psychosis by Direct Analytic Therapy." *Psychiatric Quarterly*, XXI, 1947.

certain aspects. Dr. Fromm-Reichmann, because of her long experience with these individuals, felt that a constant, unwavering, almost maternal loving approach, with gentle interpretations, served the best purpose. She accepted all that the patient had to say both positively and negatively, and reacted with an understanding, albeit interpretive approach. Each individual patient was helped to see, and gradually accept as well, the enormous need for love that he had.

Dr. Rosen has found a considerable measure of success through his approach. Generally speaking, he attempts to understand and interpret to the patient, often dramatically and forcefully the true meaning of the conflicts which are so distortedly and bizarrely expressed. In a certain sense he joins the patient in his psychosis, helps him understand what he is trying to express, and gradually leads him out of his psychotic picture by demonstrating to him that psychotic thinking and behavior is less rewarding than the use of normal values and behavior. This particular approach obviously demands a great deal of intuitive understanding on the part of the therapist as well as special training in this particular technique. Only the most thoroughly skilled therapists can be expected to have success with Dr. Rosen's methods.

There are several institutions around the country treating schizophrenia by psychotherapeutic methods, and it is quite possible that this will eventually prove to be the most effective and lasting therapeutic procedure even though it is expensive and time consuming. These latter factors will probably limit its broad usefulness for a number of years until such time as we become more sophisticated in learning some of the earlier emotional roots of this disorder.

The senior author [13] has outlined some of the philosophy in this type of psychotherapeutic approach to these patients. They do require much more activity on the part of the physician than is true in the accepted patterns of psychoanalytic technique. In some ways they have to be reared again as if they were children, but in new kinds of human experience. They must be given certain experiences

[13] English, O. S. "Seven Years' Experience in an Effort to Define and Treat Schizophrenia." Presented at annual meeting of American Psychiatric Association, St. Louis, May, 1963 (unpublished).

which they could never have undertaken or initiated by themselves. They need more approval, encouragement, support and clarification of various facts of life from the therapist. They require protection against self-destruction and from criticism or ridicule of others. Active explanation by the therapist to other family members is frequently required. Transference does not develop easily in these patients, but often must be fostered and encouraged by the therapist. In general, the physician must make social adaptation more gratifying to the schizophrenic than his previous mode of adjustment. These patients do not have the desire to participate in life in the usual sense that even the neurotic patient has. Instead, they tend toward inaction and a retreat from real living. This means that the therapist must be more flexible and more basically involved in the treatment process itself.

Such an approach to the treatment of the schizophrenic patient is time consuming, demanding of the therapist, and yet oriented toward the basic difficulties of the psychotic individual. The schizophrenic must be helped to understand that his distorted value system is useless and that life can be lived under more realistic conditions.

It is probably important at this point to re-emphasize that the basic etiology of schizophrenia, or perhaps better that group of syndromes we subsume under the label of schizophrenia, is not understood. The roots of the disorder obviously lie early in life and when the pressures and tensions become sufficient, the individual gives up his hold on reality. Undoubtedly there are potent emotional forces contributing to this eventual personality disintegration. There may also be certain biological forces. At the present time it is important that every available technique be utilized in order to assist these patients in regaining their hold on the real world, and we must continue to explore every avenue of improved therapeutic techniques.

CHAPTER 15

Affective Reactions

THE affective reactions are characterized by a severe disturbance of affect with concomitant disorders of thought and behavior corresponding to the mood changes. Patients either show a depressive affect far beyond normal mood variation or a euphoric affect, again far exceeding the bounds of normality. At times patients show a cyclic alternation of these moods. The term manic depressive psychosis was originally given to this syndrome by Kraepelin, who described both the depressed phase and the manic phase.

MANIC DEPRESSIVE REACTIONS

These groups comprise the psychotic reactions which are severe affective disturbances in which the patient has phases of hyperactivity with elated moods, or hypoactivity with depressed moods, or both. In the typical manic depressive patient, one finds a cyclic type of disturbance in which the affective swings are from euphoria to depression to euphoria. There are often periods between these extremes of affect during which the patient appears comparatively normal—or at least he does not suffer from either mania or depression. The average normal person has periods when he feels quite good, even exuberant, and other periods when he is less full of drive and energy and when his problems seem of somewhat greater magnitude to him. Such phases in the normal individual are to a great degree dependent upon what happens to him in the environment. In the manic depressive, however, one finds an extreme exaggeration of these mood swings to the point where the patient is unable to carry on his life activities realistically.

In practice one does not often see the typical cyclic manic-to-depressive swing repeated endlessly. One is more likely to see an individual who periodically sinks into a depressive state, from which he eventually emerges some weeks, months, or even years later, depending upon his treatment. One may less frequently see an individual who occasionally goes into a mild or severe manic phase which is not followed by a depression. It is possible to see any combination of these two opposite poles represented over a period of time in a single patient. While we no longer adhere to Kraepelin's original limitations placed upon this reaction, it is nevertheless true that the manic and depressive phases are closely related to each other and stem from similar underlying psychopathology.

Although the number of patients admitted to mental hospitals with this reaction is less than the number of schizophrenic patients, it still remains a formidable figure. About 3.5 per cent of all patients admitted to mental institutions are suffering from this particular type of disturbance. Manic depressive reaction is the fifth most common psychosis, following schizophrenia, psychosis with cerebral sclerosis, senile psychosis, and involutional psychosis. As is true in schizophrenia, there are many patients in the incipient stages of this psychosis who never reach mental hospitals, but who remain burdens and problems to their families for many years. Milder evidences of manic behavior or depressive behavior ordinarily do not lead to hospitalization, but are certainly capable of disrupting family life for months and even years.

SYMPTOMATOLOGY

DEPRESSIVE PHASE

In the depressive phase of an affective reaction there is a progressive slowing up of all psychic and physiological activities. This process may reach any degree from mild to severe. The onset of a depressive phase is often insidious. At times it develops so slowly that neither the patient nor his family are aware later of exactly when it began. There is a gradual development of difficulty in performing ordinary tasks that the individual has long been used to doing. The patient seems to find them much more arduous than he had previously. Each duty becomes a painful labor rather than a pleasant task and is performed slowly and often inaccurately. There is a heightened awareness of physical sensations, along with a feeling of lassitude. The entire outlook toward life becomes increasingly pessimistic and a sense of guilt begins to make an appearance. The individual feels guilty that he cannot complete easily the tasks which he has set for himself. He also feels guilty that he seems to have lost his drive. Gradually he begins to develop self-recriminations that he is useless, worthless, or lazy. Finally, as his guilt increases, he begins to feel responsible in some unknown way for many of the difficulties in the world. He exaggerates his past misdemeanors and feels that they are serious sins and that by having committed them he has subsequently brought on much of the world's misery. Concurrently with the developing depression comes an increasing degree of insomnia.

Ordinarily one thinks of the depressive patient as being very critical of himself, yet he often shows outbursts of obstinacy, irritability, and selfishness. As these various psychic manifestations increase, there is also a slowing up of physiological processes. Constipation becomes a problem. The appetite is diminished and voluntary movements are slowed. Eventually the patient reaches a severely depressed state in which he has lost contact with reality, feeling himself responsible for innumerable sins as well as for great social difficulties elsewhere in the world. He relates poorly to everyone and takes little heed of what is said to him. He may or may not begin to talk about suicide. It is a common fallacy to think that a patient who mentions suicidal intentions will not go through with them. Many of these patients feel themselves so guilty and worthless that ending their own lives appears to be the only solution. Since these patients suffer under such great guilt, their suicidal attempts are ordinarily not histrionic, but are quite determined and end fatally. In any depressed patient it is wise to keep in mind the possibility of suicide and attempt to find out what ideas the patient has along this line. In many instances families and even physicians fail to recognize the degree to which the depression has progressed, and therefore fail to take adequate precautions to prevent suicide.

Several types of depressive reaction have been described. It would seem to us that the most useful way to classify these is in terms of the degree of the depression and the presence or absence of complicating factors. For instance, there may be a pure depression, mild or severe in degree, characterized by the same slowed-up psychologic and physiologic activities, as well as an increase in self-recriminations and guilt feelings. Or there may be a so-called agitated depression in which there is an increase in psychic and physical activity, thus giving the appearance of agitation. The patient seems to suffer more acutely and walks about wringing his hands and talking a great deal about his anguish and feeling of worthlessness. He is generally more irritable than the pure depressive patient, and does not sit and stare morosely with a suffering countenance as does the latter. There is another possible subtype called "stuporous depression" in which the patient seems literally to progress into a stupor because of the pressure of depressive forces. One common ingredient of all of these types of depression is the severe affective disturbance. The individual is far below the normal line of feeling of well-being.

Case History: Manic Depressive Reaction, Depressed Type (Pure)

This single woman, thirty-two, office worker, began to lose her appetite and suffer from indigestion. She lost interest in meeting people and slowed up in her work. As her work piled up she began to worry but could not work faster. She became irritable with her family and self-critical and felt that there was no future and that she might as well give up. She asked for a leave of absence, sat at home, and would not seek out former friends or permit them to share their social life with her. She said, "I used to think that life was good but I've lost that and it doesn't seem I shall ever find it again." She was seen three times in psychotherapy without any evidence of change through either proffered ego building or efforts at insight.

She was given one of the psychic energizing drugs and gradually regained her sense of well-being and felt well enough to return to work and her former social life.

In follow-up psychotherapy the history showed a girl who had an older brother, a father who was a mediocre insurance salesman and a mother who was an unimaginative housewife, concentrating on keeping her daughter (the patient) a good girl, i.e., an unobtrusive nonentity who would give her teachers no trouble, also little pleasure. The patient was brought up without feeling that wifehood and motherhood were pleasurable goals; instead they were the unpleasant lot of the girl who was not clever enough to do something else. So the patient sought to do that something else, but without pleasure. She had had three opportunities to marry, but she could never be sure that any was the right man. She had petted a little and found it "a little thrilling" but said she would have thought less of her suitors had they sought sex relations with her. She thought marriage might be a happy way of life in spite of her mother's low opinion of it, but still was unable to commit herself to it.

Here, then, was a girl with limited libidinal investments of such low intensity that she was destined to come to a point where life did not have either zest or meaning.

She came, through psychotherapy, to free her emotions somewhat for a more courageous and generous investment in her work and social life. But it was felt that she might become a victim of depression again. It is not yet certain in her case whether through psychotherapy the libido was freed from its narcissistic investment and anchored in reality with sufficient satisfactions being gained to preclude future depressions. A followup study of analyzed manic depressives would be valuable to determine statistically how many such patients remain permanently free of depression. If enough personality change is effected an individual should be free from future depressions.

Case History: Manic Depressive Reaction, Depressed Type (Stuporous)

An elderly-looking woman of sixty-two was admitted to the mental hospital because of having gone to the cellar and thrust herself into the door of a burning furnace. The fire had burned her hands, forearms, and face and scorched most of her hair. She sat mute, would not eat, took no interest in her surroundings, and had to be dressed, undressed, bathed, and fed a liquid diet through a nasal tube.

Her history revealed that as a young girl she had been brought up in eastern Europe under conditions of poverty and privation and had lived a frustrated, joyless existence during most of her developmental period. She came to the United States at the age of fifteen, worked long hours, and lived a lonely existence until she married at twenty-three. She and her husband worked hard to establish a business and to care for and educate three children. She denied herself pleasures—in fact, had little interest in social life of any kind. The result of this deprived existence, against which she rebelled inwardly, brought her to a point of giving up all interest in life. For six weeks before entering the hospital she had sat at home, speechless and uninterested in her surroundings. Her family was reluctant to hospitalize her until her suicidal attempt by self-cremation occurred. She did not respond to a psychic energizing drug, but eight electroshock treatments restored her to activity and a few of her former interests. A few psychotherapeutic interviews in which her past life was reviewed made her less vulnerable to another attack.

The psychotherapeutic interviews revealed that this woman had a rigid type of personality with a severe superego. She had always made great demands upon herself, never learned to truly enjoy people or activities, and generally had led a constricted type of life. As is true with many people who are severely deprived in early years, she retained within her unconscious much orality, ambivalence, and instability. She had erected a severe conscience which forbade expression of inner emotion and she felt a constant pressing need to be more hard-working and conscientious. She had allowed herself few of the ordinary pleasures of life. She derived only a minimum of pleasure from her few friends and from her family. She had never been sufficiently flexible to thoroughly adopt the atmosphere of her "new" country though she had been here for many years. During the interviews she was helped to see how many excessive demands she had always made upon herself. She was encouraged to re-establish and improve her previous friendships. She had resented her children achieving independence and had come to feel useless without their continued dependence. She was helped to understand the need to add more interests and activities to her life to compensate for her diminished maternal duties. At the same time she was helped to realize the changed but still important relationship she had with her children. As she verbalized her resentments about her difficult life and her many vicissitudes and found not only an understanding listener but a helpful counselor in her physician, she assumed sufficient flexibility to prevent another depression of suicidal proportions. She was by no means cured, but became a more pleasant, relaxed, and comfortable person.

Case History: Manic Depressive Reaction, Depressed Type (Agitated)

A fifty-one-year-old female was brought to the psychopathic hospital after having made a scene in church where she threatened dramatically to kill herself. She could not be physically examined at the time of admission because of extreme modesty. She had to be held, and screamed as if she were being sexually attacked whenever she was touched by the physician. She refused to answer many of the questions which were presented to her, claiming that she would only give the answers to a priest in confession. She complained that the police had no right to bring her to the hospital without the presence of another woman on the trip. She went on to say that she was extremely ashamed of herself for having made this trip without another woman present and worried, "What will Father C. think of me?"

History revealed that this patient had been in the hospital on two previous occasions, both for depressions. She had been given ten electroshock treatments on her first admission and discharged as improved. The second admission had been for a similar agitated state with suicidal intention and marked depression and she had been given nine electroshocks and discharged as improved. On both occasions she had failed to follow up a recommendation for outpatient psychotherapy.

A hastily written and barely legible note was sent to a physician at the hospital shortly after this patient's admission. It was from a woman who was apparently the patient's only close acquaintance and it was remarkably clear in its description of this patient's depressive episodes. It read, "Spells of depression have overcome Annie during the twelve years she has been living here with me. Lately she may turn, in a period of twelve hours, from a quiet and industrious person to one who is depressed and brooding, and continue in this state of mental lapse for ten weeks. Then she is silent in her work, easily angered at the least disturbance, and after hours goes to her room, will not speak to me and locks the door. Then the spells gradually wear off and eventually leave her for about one month. Then the sickness resumes in the same pattern. The attack may at first leave her speechless so that she cannot complete a sentence. Sometimes she will begin a sentence with one thought and in a fit of irritation, finish with a foreign thought. She gets to be uncommunicative, brooding, angry, lazy, and loses her appetite. She grows careless of her personal hygiene. She regards everyone as if there were some personal insult involved. She has been getting sick now for some nine or ten days as usual and then this great dip occurred this afternoon in church."

History revealed that this patient had lived with the writer of the note for the past twelve years. She had a job in the local Catholic rectory, was extremely religious, led a very constricted life, and had no masculine acquaintances as far as anyone knew. She had never married and had lived with her parents until they died. She was extremely attached to her mother and very much upset by the latter's death.

Following her admission, the patient continued to show an agitated, restless, self-depreciatory attitude. She felt at times that she was a very unworthy person who could never possibly be forgiven by the priest. She said suicide was the only solution. At other times she was extremely irritable and resentful of the physician's attempts to examine her or even to talk to her in a room alone. She accused him of being indecent in wanting to talk to her without the presence of a nurse. Her sensorium was relatively clear. She was oriented and able to answer questions about general information with reasonable accuracy. On one occasion a physician accidentally bumped into her and she screamed at him as if she was being raped, "How could you do that? Stay away from me. Don't touch me. Nurse, nurse." The patient was given a phenothiazine tranquilizer and a course of fifteen electroshock treatments, by which time she had regained her composure, lost most of her depression, and become much calmer. She was feeling physically quite well and looking forward to her previous job in the church. She became a helpful patient on the ward and got along quite well with most of the patients, revealing little of her previous hostility.

This patient was discharged in a markedly improved condition, but once again refused to follow up with the recommendations for outpatient treatment.

MANIC PHASE

Hypomania

The manic phase of manic depressive reaction is characterized by hyperactivity from the physiological and psychological standpoints. The individual increases his tempo of life. He moves rapidly, thinks rapidly, and gives the impression of being quite happy, often far too happy. Just as there are variations in the severity in the depressive reaction, there are also degrees of mania. The one closest to normality is called "hypomania." It is characterized by hyperactivity from the physiological and psychological standpoint. There is a more or less exuberant, hyperactive type of behavior which does not completely leave the realm of reality. The individual is constantly on the move, but if watched closely is found to be superficial in his activities. He changes from one pursuit to another and rarely does a complete or thorough job on any of them. While his exuberance is somewhat contagious, this contagiousness soon wears off when one discovers that the hypomanic's interest in others does not go very deep. Thinking processes are speeded up and to the uninitiated may seem quite acute, but to the more discerning person the hypomanic's thinking is not well founded on reality principles. The degree of psychopathology may escape many persons in the hypomanic's environment, especially those not in his immediate family. Milder degrees in hypomania often lead to an increased output of work and give an excellent impression, at least temporarily.

Case History: Manic Depressive Reaction, Hypomania

A woman of thirty-five, a secretary, began to be unduly cheerful and overactive. She became boringly expansive about her past life and the status of her family. She made many phone calls, including expensive long-distance calls, to friends she had not been in touch with in some time. She spoke of the fact that she had a good voice which had never been cultivated and she was going to study singing. She was also going to study dancing, do dressmaking, learn French and Spanish, and travel extensively. She thought it not necessary to explain where she would find either the time or the money for these activities. She slept poorly and her efficiency dropped off and it became evident that she was emotionally unwell. However, she did not want any interference with her way of life and it took a great deal of strong persuasion from her family and friends to get her into the hospital. Tranquilization lessened her exuberance, and she was able to understand that she had been unduly active, planful, and unrealistic.

Subsequent psychotherapeutic interviews with this woman produced additional insight into her personality structure. She was the overprotected, overindulged only child in her family. Her parents had not only provided her with too many material things but had never required any efforts from her in return. She had been praised constantly and unrealistically even though her real accomplishments had been few. The parents boasted of her talents even in areas where she obviously had none.

As the patient grew up and had to assume increasing responsibilities in her own life, she became unable to tolerate what she felt to be the harshness of reality. She found competition at work difficult and losing very painful. She related poorly to men and considered them unappreciative of her even though she really did little for which she could be appreciated.

Finally, as her severe conscience began to punish her increasingly for not measuring up to its unrealistic standards, she took refuge in a flight into hypomanic activity. This, of course, involved at least a partial denial of reality. She became, to herself, the possessor of many attributes, talents, plans, and activities.

Mania

The more obvious manic phase is an exaggeration of the hypomanic phase. Motor activity increases, as does superficiality. The individual becomes more grandiose in his ideas and jumps rapidly from one thought to another. He may become involved in large but unrealistic schemes. If not confined in an institution, he is prone to invest money in obviously ill-founded ventures. He may make great plans for travel, business, or investment which initially have a grain of reality in them, but which are obviously unsubstantiated in the main. The manic individual is very forward in his contacts with others and readily tells his life history to anyone who will listen. In doing so, he reveals what usually are regarded as close personal secrets. Sexual drive becomes enhanced and the patient may be bold and lewd in advances to the opposite sex. Sexual excesses often occur. Sleep is generally diminished because of the hyperactivity and the patient gets by on amazingly little rest. As the manic phase increases, the patient finds little time for either sleep or food and is involved in a constant torrent of words and activity which shift rapidly from one subject to another.

While the manic patient may appear pleasant or even humorous, it is evident after a short period of time with him that frustrations lead to irritability, stubbornness, and even violent temper outbursts. The manic is essentially a selfish, narcissistic individual with many self-centered fantasies. The world literally revolves about him. At times manic hyperactivity reaches proportions that endanger physical health and require strong sedation, lest complete physical exhaustion result.

Hallucinations are extremely rare in manic patients, but delusions, while not common, are occasionally seen. The delusions are ordinarily of a grandiose nature. The manic patient on the closed ward of a mental hospital may be found casually writing out a million-dollar check to a person who has just befriended him. He may be found boasting about the great plans he has for buying yachts or mansions. He may give a lengthy discourse on his recent conversation with the President of the United States. Frequently manics become involved in planning various types of inventions which they are certain will make them very wealthy. While these inventions may appear to have a superficially correct orientation, they are obviously founded on nothing but fantasy. Manic behavior has often been described as a flight from reality and truly it is so: the patient is unable to slow up and meet reality as it is about him. The manic patient also presents a *flight of ideas,* which is the extremely rapid production of various thoughts without true regard for maintaining logical processes. In this flight of ideas, the patient rapidly states a thought, then follows it quickly with another, more or less irrelevantly based upon the first, but connected to it at some minor point. In other words, there is a connection between the two thoughts, but it is far too tenuous.

Case History: Manic Depressive Reaction, Manic Type

A man of thirty-seven, married and father of two children, began to stay up late nights writing letters to all and sundry, describing his ideas for the use of atomic energy. He was irritable and demanding of his wife. He was impudent to his employer, curt to his fellow employees. He laughed loudly and made rather pointless jokes at everyone's expense. He kept the lights burning in the house all night, rearranged his belongings, and thought it best to keep a loaded gun in his room in case anyone wanted to "make trouble." He would barely touch food, so feverishly was he occupied in rummaging through old belongings, writing letters, and making phone calls. When it was thought best for safety's sake to take the key of his car, he became enraged and threatened to do violence to his wife. After twenty-four hours of this behavior, he was hospitalized. In the hospital he took the bed apart and sat naked upon the mattress, singing songs, making ribald jokes, and making a poor attempt to write poetry. He would shout out of the windows, make requests for cigarettes and water, and make improper proposals to the nurses when they came near his room. He needed large doses of sedation and was only partially improved with a series of electroshock treatments. He remained in a fairly marked overactive state for five months and required coaxing to eat, but finally became more quiet, even shy and withdrawn, and remained so for several weeks after leaving the hospital. In fact, after leaving the hospital, he felt so chastened and sensitive about his having "behaved so badly" that it was several weeks before he could return to work. We see in this manic attack the breakthrough of selfishness, self-centeredness, lack of consideration, and expressions of hostility toward those above him in authority as well as those dependent upon him. He threw off responsibility and regressed to the wild, untamed megalomania of the most untrained, irresponsible delinquent. The id impulses threw off the restraining forces of the superego and the ego ideal, and took possession of the ego.

Following his return home this patient was encouraged to return periodically for further outpatient psychotherapy. He continued to be extremely sensitive about his psychotic episode, however, and refused to accept treatment. His history, obtained primarily from his wife during his hospitalization, revealed he had always been a very moody, sensitive, and irritable person. He was overly conscientious in some things and sloppy in others. The apparent precipitating event of the psychotic episode had been the promotion of a rival of his in his business. He had hoped for the promotion himself and had felt his superior did not adequately appreciate him when his rival was promoted. Follow-up history was obtained one year later when the patient was readmitted in a depression. He had maintained his marginal adjustment for about six months after discharge and then had begun to show increasing signs of depression. This had culminated in a serious but unsuccessful suicidal attempt which led to hospitalization.

This patient, during both his manic and depressive phases, related very poorly to others. Thus, as is true with the majority of these patients, psychotherapy was impossible. He was, during the psychotic episodes, so wrapped up in himself that forming a therapeutic relationship was out of the question. Many manic depressive patients, however, unlike this man, are willing and able to benefit by psychotherapy when the acute episode has been surmounted with tranquilizers or electroshock treatment.

ETIOLOGY

The etiology of manic depressive reaction would not seem to have surrounding it the same confusion and multiplicity of theories as does that of schizophrenia. Generally speaking, there have been three main concepts put forward to explain manic depressive reaction. The most useful and probably the closest to the eventual answer is the psychological approach. The second is that of heredity and the third has to do with body type. We will discuss these briefly in reverse order.

Various statistical studies have been accumulated which tend to show that there is a high incidence of the pyknic type of body habitus among manic depressive psychotics. This would correspond rather closely to the endomorph type of Sheldon.[1] It is characterized by a tendency toward obesity rather than slenderness or muscularity. However, this particular theory would seem open to many arguments, not the least of which is the large number of individuals one sees with this particular type of mental disorder who by no means fit into this morphological classification. Many patients with this disorder are found to be of an entirely different type of body structure.

The second, or hereditary, theory is again based upon several statistical surveys which have shown a higher incidence of manic depressive reaction where others in the family have suffered from this same syndrome. Here again there seem to be certain difficulties. One questions the broadness of various surveys and whether they have included a sufficient variety of patients. Also, there is the fact that if a child is raised by a mother suffering from this psychotic reaction, the child's chances for a mature adjustment are much less than if he had been raised by a mature mother. The old saying that "neurotics beget neurotics" can be applied here. Certainly it is true that psychotic parents are not capable of providing an emotional atmosphere conducive to normal healthy development in their children. Therefore, it would stand to reason that statistically we might

[1] Sheldon, W. H. and Stevens, S. S. *The Varieties of Temperament*. New York, Harper and Brothers, 1942.

find a higher percentage of psychotics in families in which psychosis had existed previously, and yet would not have to assume that this incidence was based upon a hereditary factor. However, it must be stressed that these studies do show a higher incidence of manic depressive reactions in certain families than they do of, for instance, schizophrenic reactions.

The psychological approach to an explanation for this psychosis rests chiefly upon modern psychodynamic understanding. Once the apparently meaningless self-accusations and the depressive mood of a patient have been understood in terms of his unconscious, it becomes easier to discover why such an end condition has resulted. Similarly, if the excessive thought productions and elated moods of a manic patient are subjected to intensive study based upon modern dynamic principles, definite comprehensible reasons are found to lie behind them as well as factors which have precipitated and led to this particular condition. Freud[2] laid the foundation of our present understanding of the psychodynamics of manic depressive reaction in his paper, "Mourning and Melancholia." Abraham,[3] one of Freud's original pupils, went on to further elucidate the relationship of both mania and depression to fixations in the early psychosexual development. When the various symptoms and behavior patterns of these patients are explained in the psychoanalytic manner the psychological etiology becomes much more acceptable. This etiology becomes even more valid when it is realized that many manic depressive patients have been relieved of their symptoms through psychoanalytic procedures.

Freud, in his paper, "Mourning and Melancholia," compared the mourning and melancholic states of mind and found similarities between them. The individual in mourning is going through a temporarily painful period following the loss of a loved one. During this process, he is literally working at detaching his libido from that loved person and reinvesting it in other individuals in his environment. When this process of reinvestment is completed, the indi-

---

[2] Freud, Sigmund: "Mourning and Melancholia," in *Collected Papers,* Vol. IV. London. Hogarth Press and the Institute of Psychoanalysis, 1949.

[3] Abraham, Karl: "Notes on the Psychoanalytical Investigation and Treatment of Manic Depressive Insanity and Allied Conditions," in *Selected Papers on Psychoanalysis* (Abraham). London. Hogarth Press, 1948, Basic Books, 1953.

vidual resumes his more normal state of mind and is no longer depressed. In the case of the psychotically depressed patient, we find a similar sort of unhappiness, but without the obvious external loss of a loved object.

In proceeding further with the research into this subject, both Freud and Abraham found that the answer lies essentially in the manic depressive's original type of relationship with the so-called love object. It was found that much of the manic depressive's psychosexual development had been arrested in a very early phase, namely that of the late oral and early anal periods, making for a defect in all subsequent human relationships. At such an early phase in life, the individual's relationship with those about him is markedly ambivalent and he is unable to love without hating or hate without loving. As this person grows older chronologically, the love tends to be retained in consciousness, while the hate is relegated to an unconscious position. With such a state of affairs existing, even minor rejections or frustrations by the so-called love object are interpreted, at least unconsciously, by the patient as complete and total rejection. He is then in the position of having been deserted by a love object in somewhat the same way as a normal person is when the love object dies.

However, he is also left struggling with much unconscious hostility, which then is turned upon the patient himself. It is literally taken over by his conscience and turned upon him in the form of self-recriminations. Close observation has shown that the innumerable accusations directed by the depressed patient seemingly toward himself are really unconsciously directed toward the presumed lost love object. In other words, when the depressed patient says, "I am no good, I cheat, I lie, and I have sinned," he really is, without realizing it, directing such accusations toward the other person whom he feels he has loved but who has now deserted him.

When subjected to the microscopic searchings of psychoanalysis, such patients are found to be very narcissistic, egocentric individuals, with many early infantile drives still present within them. However, they are struggling with an extremely severe and rigid superego. It is this punitive superego which takes over and turns against them the unconscious hostility which they have held toward others. They are extremely sensitive people, prone to be obstinate and selfish. They are apt to show many childish characteristics if observed for any length of time. Ordinarily they cannot show or even consciously become aware of the extreme degree of unconscious hostility which they possess because their rigid superego prevents it. It is perhaps easiest to think of these individuals as essentially very small children with strong and punitive consciences.

The early life experiences are of great importance in the etiology of manic depressive reaction. The very early mother-child relationship determines whether a child will successfully pass through the first two levels of psychosexual development. Probably there is also a certain constitutional factor present which predisposes an individual toward this type of illness. However, it behooves us as physicians to recognize and work with any factors which are recognizable and amenable to change rather than to adopt the more pessimistic attitude that the condition is largely constitutional and therefore not changeable.

The psychodynamics of the hypomanic phase have not been discussed as thoroughly as those of the depressed phase. However, it may be said that in the hypomanic phase the presumably weak but childish ego achieves a victorious overthrow of the cruel and punitive superego. As it escapes from this previously ever-present watchdog, it literally runs wild with exaggerated self-esteem. Since it is no longer controlled by its rigid governor, the ego is able to show more clearly its narcissistic, megalomanic qualities. It must continue to run rapidly lest it be captured and again subjugated by its rigid master.

As the typical manic depressive passes from one to the other extreme of his psychosis, he may go through a temporary period of so-called normality. It is interesting to note that in this particular period there is no true normality, since these patients by and large at this time are typically obsessive-compulsive. Their main personality characteristics are of a rigid, perfectionistic, meticulous, parsimonious, compulsive kind. Such a situation lends credence to the psychoanalytic theory, since it is in the anal phase of development that the obsessive-compulsive person is stagnated. However, in these psychotic individuals, the balance is precarious and the instincts as well as the environment can easily upset the balance and send the individuals off into one or the other of the phases of the manic depressive psychosis.

DIFFERENTIAL DIAGNOSIS

State hospitals differ markedly in their statistical estimates of the percentage of manic depressive patients admitted to their institutions. Much of this variation probably lies in the different criteria for making the diagnosis. In all probability the biggest area of confusion in differential diagnosis is between schizophrenic reactions and manic depressive reactions. The agitated schizophrenic may show many of the symptoms of the manic patient. He is hyperactive; his thoughts seem rapid and his activity purposeless. This, of course, is true also of the manic patient. However, the latter does not possess the bizarreness of the schizophrenic. The manic comes closer to making sense. In addition there is the all-important factor that the hyperactivity and seeming euphoria of the manic patient is much more contagious than is that of the schizophrenic. After spending fifteen minutes with the agitated schizophrenic, one tends to be perplexed and at a loss to understand the patient's productions. However, after such a time with a manic patient, one is apt to see at least some humor in the situation. The schizophrenic's rapid thought processes come more clearly from the unconscious in a completely illogical and seemingly not understandable way. The manic's rapid thought processes, on the other hand, do bear links to each other, even if somewhat tenuously. The agitated schizophrenic is essentially unhappy and therefore cannot convey a sense of pleasure to the examiner, while the manic patient seems more euphoric and does convey a certain elevation in mood to the examiner.

Another area of possible difficulty in the realm of differential diagnosis is with the paretic patient. As the process of general paresis progresses, the patient is apt to reach a pseudo-euphoric state wherein he may claim to own a million dollars or exhibit some other such megalomanic fantasy. However, a thorough physical and neurological examination will show evidence of organic central nervous system damage in the paretic, while it will not in the manic. In addition there is the history to be relied on—particularly of the primary and secondary stages of lues. Such things as Argyll-Robertson pupils, changes in reflexes, and other organic signs are not found in manic patients and are in paretics. The final evidence may also be gained through laboratory tests for syphilis on the blood and spinal fluid.

PROGNOSIS

The prognosis of the individual psychotic episode in manic depressive reaction is comparatively good, especially if it is the first such attack. The vast majority of patients recover with treatment from the initial attacks, but about three-quarters of them will suffer future episodes. The prognosis of manic depressive reaction from a general standpoint depends upon a variety of factors. Attacks early in life, during the teens, indicate a poorer prognosis. As years pass future episodes tend to become more severe, prolonged, and difficult to treat. All of these factors are also dependent upon the amount and type of treatment which the patient receives. While electroshock treatment produces improvement in many of these cases, the ultimate prognosis rests upon adequate dynamic psychotherapy being given during the ensuing "quiescent" period. Family or patient resistance to this measure only makes the ultimate prognosis poorer.

The individual episode of manic depressive reaction does not seem to leave a "psychic scar" on the personality which would impair function and predispose to further attacks in the way which is seen in schizophrenia. A patient with a manic or depressive episode can return to his prepsychotic state following his attack while the "recovered" schizophrenic usually appears to have suffered some permanent psychic damage.

TREATMENT

Fortunately, the treatment of manic depressive reactions is much more efficacious than that of the schizophrenic reactions. It would seem that there is one major contributing factor to this. Schizophrenic reaction may be thought of as a more malignant type of personality disorganization than manic depressive reaction. A manic depressive who, by one means or another, has recovered from an attack does not appear to have suffered any particular residual damage. It is true that he may, in the future, have further attacks, but his recovery from each would seem to leave him essentially the same. In the schizophrenic patient, however, there is a tendency for each attack of the psychosis to leave its mark upon the personality and permanently hamper its future adjustment, at least to some degree. This does not mean that we have an unalterably pessimistic view toward a "recovered" schizophrenic. Such individuals need and deserve psychotherapy as well as other measures to insure their future mental health. However, the ego resiliency is lessened by a schizophrenic attack more than by a manic depressive attack.

Generally speaking, there are two large questions to be answered in the treatment of manic depressive psychosis. First, when is treatment essential, and second, what treatment is most advisable?

In some ways the manic depressive problem is not unlike that of the schizophrenic. When the psychosis is not of great proportion and the individual seems not to have lost complete contact with reality, there is often a reluctance on the part of the family or the patient to seek psychiatric care. In regard to the depressed patient, if the depression is mild, the individual is more than apt to seek general medical help for some lassitude and weakness which he considers organic in nature. Undoubtedly most general practitioners have been consulted by such individuals. Physical examination is more than apt to show, in almost anyone, certain minor abnormalities. In the mildly depressed patients, such findings as hypotension of a minor degree or chronic constipation may side-track the physician into treating these ailments as the primary difficulty. It is quite obvious that a laxative will have little or no effect upon the depressed patient. As the depression becomes more pronounced and the deviation from normality more obvious, even the family, and often the patient himself, are able to recognize the psychogenic nature of the difficulty.

However, in spite of their apparent severe suffering, such depressed patients may resist a psychological approach to their problems. Generally speaking, however, they are more amenable to this type of referral than are incipient schizophrenics. They seem to be more prone to recognize the psychological nature of their problems and therefore are more willing, at least if some pressure is applied, to seek aid in this direction.

The physician who is careful in his history-taking will usually be able to elucidate factors dating far back in the patient's life which would lead him to believe that the case is one of psychological depression rather than organic disturbance.

The mildly hypomanic patient again is somewhat of a problem from the standpoint of treatability. His sense of well-being usually precludes his acceptance of any offer of medical advice. If his hyper-activity does not reach great proportions, even his family is apt not to become disturbed. However, if, as is the usual case, it reaches the point where the individual begins to enter into unwise schemes or to spend his money foolishly and excessively, the family then becomes more concerned about his condition. Hypomanic patients, generally speaking, are more difficult to convince of the need for medical help than are depressed patients. Both, however, are fairly refractory to ordinary superficial psychotherapeutic talks. Their ability to relate to the physician, or as a matter of fact to anyone, is so limited that anything that is said to them makes little impression.

Once either the manic phase or the depressive phase reaches formidable proportions, the family of the patient is apt to seek medical advice. Hospitalization is ordinarily an advisable procedure. Occasionally one sees either mildly manic or mildly depressed patients who may be treated on an outpatient basis. However, the physician who does so must accurately evaluate and calculate the risks involved. Certainly the risk of suicide is never absent in the depressed patient, although he may not appear to have contemplated it. The risks in the manic patient are of another kind, for he is perfectly capable of getting himself into all sorts of difficulties, financial, sexual, and personal. Where there is doubt, it is wise to refer such patients for expert psychiatric opinion, or to seek hospitalization so that the actions of the patient can be adequately controlled.

Suicide, as we have mentioned previously, is a common problem with depressed patients. They may or may not discuss it, but the threat must always be borne in mind. Perhaps it is greatest when the patient begins to suffer from insomnia. The continued periods of self-recriminatory torture and guilt suffered by these patients during the long lonely night hours are apt to stimulate a suicidal attempt. Well-meaning friends and family who attempt to "talk him out of it" are often only contributing to the seriousness of the difficulty. Even the physician who understands psychopathology and attempts to help the patient out of his depression may postpone hospitalization until it is too late, because suicide has intervened.

Once hospitalization has been accomplished, one of the most useful and efficient ways of treating the manic-depressive psychotic is with the psychoactive drugs. Tranquilizers are helpful in diminishing excitement and agitation while psychic energizers are useful in alleviating depression. Not all patients respond successfully to these drugs, however, and the use of electroshock may be necessary. When the latter is required it is often given in conjunction with medication of the above types.

The advent of the psychoactive drugs has markedly diminished the amount of electroshock being used throughout the country. The administration of these drugs is not without risk, however, and signs of toxicity should be watched for carefully. When EST is necessary, the total number of such treatments is usually less than it would have been in the past, prior to the availability of the drugs. The use of insulin coma or psychosurgery in these patients has all but disappeared from the scene.

While in the hospital, the manic or the depressive patient often requires considerable nursing attention. Precautions against suicide should always be undertaken with the depressed patient. Any means by which he might accomplish this act are removed. In addition to the ordinary hospital routine, the depressed patient is encouraged wherever possible toward all types of activity. While the "total push" method was originally designated for schizophrenic patients, it is not inadvisable to use such a method upon certain depressed patients. Occasionally one sees a depressive who literally goes on a hunger strike and refuses to eat for the stated purpose of starving himself to death. In such cases, of course, tube feeding is essential.

A careful watch must be kept upon the individual's physical condition lest he develop some type of concurrent illness. These patients often seem to welcome the onset of an organic illness as a form of martyrdom and do not call it to anyone's attention or complain about any pain that may result. In the manic, the problems chiefly evolve from hyperactivity. These individuals are capable literally of running themselves to death. At times it becomes necessary to resort to considerable tranquilization to calm them down. The use of electroshock may also be required. These patients also have little regard for their physical health. At times they refuse to eat, primarily because they will not take time out to do so. They often shout, yell, and scream until they develop a chronic laryngitis. They are also careless about incipient signs of organic illness such as pain, and will not report them to the physician. Therefore, again, their physical condition must be watched closely either for signs of developing illness or for signs of exhaustion.

Perhaps one of the most important measures in the treatment of this particular psychosis is psychotherapy. It is ordinarily not possible to utilize this method on depressed or manic patients during the severe phases because their ability to relate is remarkably limited. However, following the successful use of drugs and EST, these patients usually return to a reasonable degree of normality, even though it be of the compulsive type; and they can benefit by follow-up psychotherapeutic interviews.

If manic depressive patients can be led into a better understanding and insight into their inner processes, it is possible to prevent or minimize the recurrence of manic or depressive episodes. They must be helped to recognize some of the sources of their inner problems, particularly in terms of their severe consciences as well as some of their more infantile drives. Even a beginning in this direction is apt to ameliorate future psychotic breaks. Unfortunately the dramatic and seemingly permanent improvement that follows a short course of medication is apt to discourage the patient and his family from seeking further help. It is wise to warn the family prior to the beginning of such treatment that improvement, while it may be very quick and seem quite satisfactory, must be followed by more extensive interview-type therapy, or else it is very likely to prove unsuccessful in the long run.

When one works psychotherapeutically with a manic depressive patient who is between psychotic breaks, one finds certain more or less characteristic problems. These patients have suffered very early-life traumata to their developing egos. The phenomena of "relatedness," empathy, and capacity for identification are greatly impaired. Their feelings of being loved, of being lovable, of wishing or caring to love someone else, are greatly impaired at the height of the illness and remain impaired during the "quiescent" phase. Such difficulties in the personality of the patient make therapy quite difficult because of the patient's problem in relating to the therapist and using the relationship to get better. He seems to have great difficulty in putting value on the friendship that is given to him either in therapy or out. He cannot seem to feel that people are sincere when they indicate that they like or appreciate him. The result of this is unfortunate, because just as he belittles himself, he belittles the efforts of those who would make him feel better.

One such patient said, "I don't see how anything that I would have to say would be important or would be of interest to you." Such individuals have great difficulty in allowing themselves to love comfortably or to feel that they are loved. A characteristic attitude was expressed by the patient who said, "To fail to come up to the expectations of people makes me want to die. If what I do or say has not been accepted unconditionally, I feel that it has been absolutely worthless. Either I am wonderfully right or I am dead wrong and ostracized." Later this patient said, "I never let myself love completely. I feel ridiculed, criticized, rebuked, and rebuffed. I constantly fear exploitation. I fear that I may become putty in someone else's hands, that I can no longer shape my own destiny. To love someone is an invitation for that person to hurt me."

Such feelings obviously stem from the early-life relationships between parent and child which were pathological. The parent did not meet the needs of the infantile ego as it began to grow, and left in the child a basic difficulty in the all-important area of loving and being loved.

Obviously it is of great importance that the patient learn, among other things, how to relate on a more satisfactory level to the therapist. If he can accomplish this task, it will improve his ability to relate to others outside. By improving and learning about his relationship with the therapist, he will understand more clearly what some of his hitherto unknown difficulties have been in the realm of interpersonal relationship. He will begin to see how, on the one hand, his unconscious demands for love and attention have been excessive, while, on the other, he has constantly punished himself for making such demands, or at least for having been resentful that they were not met. The manic depressive patient has characteristically a severe superego which is harsh and intolerant of the extremely immature drives and urges and needs which lie within him. Much of his life is a constant battle between himself and this severe superego. Psychotherapy has as its goal helping the patient to understand and modify his rigid superego as well as understanding and bringing closer to maturity his unconscious infantile needs, which have been of such an excessive degree.

CHAPTER 16

Involutional Psychotic Reaction

"INVOLUTIONAL psychotic reaction" is a term used to indicate certain mental reactions, primarily depressive and paranoid in type, characteristically appearing during the fourth and fifth decades of life and associated fairly closely with the change of life. There is a widely held belief among psychoanalysts that most cases of this condition are not remarkably different in dynamics from the depression seen in the depressive phase of manic depressive psychosis or in the psychoneurotic depressive reactions. Clinical psychiatry has been much more active in separating this syndrome from other types of depression than has psychoanalysis. The analyst, concerned primarily with unconscious dynamics, has tended to look upon these individuals as examples of depression, rather than separating them into a category of their own. This syndrome has attained its own diagnostic label primarily because of its association with the endocrine changes occurring at the menopause and absence of previous clinical depressions during the life history.

Involutional psychosis is of importance because of its frequency and its potential severity. It accounts for almost 5 per cent of first admissions to mental hospitals in the United States. A far larger number of cases are not represented in such statistics, either because many patients were treated on an outpatient basis without hospital admission or because an improper and often organic diagnosis was made as a result of the concomitant physical complaints which are so frequent. The strong possibility of suicide in unrecognized and untreated involutional reactions makes proper understanding, evaluation, and treatment extremely essential. Prior to the advent of electroshock treatment, twenty-five per cent of these cases committed suicide.

This syndrome is most frequently associated with the female sex, but is by no means rare among men. Generally speaking, the syndrome in men tends to occur somewhat later than in women, perhaps toward the late fifties, and may be somewhat more difficult to diagnose because of the lack of such an obvious physical involutional change as the menopause in women.

ETIOLOGY AND PSYCHOPATHOLOGY

The final word as to the etiology of involutional psychotic reaction has yet, undoubtedly, to be said. Its occurrence at that time in life when the reproductive period ends obviously has led to the assumption that gonadal changes are responsible. However, extensive experimentation with the administration of endocrine substances has not produced particularly encouraging results. There has been evidence presented which would seem to indicate that in these patients the previous balance between pituitary and ovaries is upset by the change in ovarian hormonal excretion at the time of the menopause. The resulting imbalance has been blamed for certain emotional symptoms. However, the administration of ovarian hormones is, more often than not, unsuccessful in diminishing the symptoms.

It is true that the hormonal changes occurring during the menopause may at times be capable of producing certain physiological symptoms. The so-called "hot flushes" are the most outstanding example. These consist of temporary episodic generalized feelings of flushing and then chilling on the part of the patient. It is also true that in the fourth and fifth decades of life, physiological reactions and adaptive reactions are not as rapid and efficient as they have been earlier in life. Such changes may lead to mild constipation, autonomic imbalance, or slower circulatory adjustments. Some of these symptoms, particularly the hot flushes, may be improved by the administration of endocrine substances. Such an improvement may even lead to a temporary remission in the depressive picture. However, it is unwise to expect endocrines to completely eradicate a condition which contains many emotional elements.

From a psychological standpoint, patients with involutional reaction frequently present a picture that is indistinguishable from the depressions seen in the manic depressive psychoses. They do, however, lack the previous history of repeated manic or depressed phases. Typically, the involutional patient has a past history which more closely resembles that of an obsessive-compulsive personality. Such patients are usually rigid, perfectionistic people who have led constricted and inhibited lives. Instinctual drives have been denied expression and innumerable psychic defense mechanisms are present in the personality functioning. The patients often give a history of having been ambitious and hard-working, as well as demanding. Many of them have been considered excellent mothers who literally gave their all in the raising of their children. They sacrificed their own pleasures in order to insure their children more luxuries. They lived to do their duty and were intent upon doing the right thing rather than the pleasurable thing. They appear to have lived only to fulfill their chosen task, whether it was motherhood or a career. Unfortunately, however, their lives have been limited in the main to this one particular area and they lack the flexibility, warmth, and spontaneity which is found in the more mature individual. Praise as it comes is rejected as nonessential to them or insincere on the part of those who give it.

It is at the time of the menopause that such patients begin to be overwhelmed by the relative emptiness of their past lives. They begin to realize that now they have reached the end of their procreative existence and face a generally downward course. Past unfulfilled wishes, unrealized ambitions, and goals which they have somehow felt they would attain now seem beyond their reach. Children are grown and married and are no longer dependent. Often these patients have hoped for greater achievements from husband or children than have occurred. Retirement from motherhood means a great decrease in their sense of usefulness. Such patients have managed to achieve a limited type of adjustment by channeling all of their energy into one very limited field. Now this area is gone and the entire personality structure begins to suffer. Such patients can no longer be given the previous degree of recognition for their arduous labors and begin to feel less essential. With this comes a feeling of worthlessness and concomitant anger at those responsible. Men are prone to feel discriminated against by associates or circumstances.

Exactly why the entire defense system of the personality begins to break down at this age is not always completely clear, but it seems to be a cumulative matter arising from repeated frustrations and disappointments. The general distribution of libido is possibly affected by the endocrine imbalance and change which occurs at the menopause. Yet if this were the sole contributing factor, the administration of endocrine substances should result in amelioration of all symptoms and, as we have said, this does not occur. Moreover there is no evidence that the male suffers from any such rapid decline in gonadal activity as does the female. Undoubtedly, the changes in the external environment of the patient which result from his reaching this age, the slowing up of his body processes, the changes in his reproductive activities, and many other factors, are contributors to the over-all factors seen in involutional reaction.

The personality structure of the involutional reaction patient is, as has been mentioned, similar in many ways to that of the obsessive-compulsive person. The involutional patient may be said to represent a sort of "decompensated obsessive" whose psychological structure has finally broken down under the strain of advancing age. A severe conscience similar to that seen in the obsessive patient makes open expression of inner frustration and anger impossible. All types of instinctual expression have always been guarded closely by the involutional patient. Such an individual has for years worked arduously and perfectionistically in an attempt to mollify his severe conscience. Such a patient's adjustment to life has perhaps appeared laudable to the casual observer, but it has been based on unhealthy psychological principles, primarily including an excessive use of pathological mechanisms of defense. Such an adjustment has required the expenditure of considerable mental effort in rigidly confining instinctual forces into a narrow type of living which includes very little in the way of flexibility, warmth, or pleasure. Such a delicate balance is shattered at the time of menopause. As these individuals reach a change in life, they begin to feel less important to their employer or to their children. This stirs up within them resentment of which their consciences forbid open expression. This resentment is then turned back on themselves and they belabor themselves with criticisms. At the same time there is a turning inward of much libido which was previously invested in occupation or family, so that these patients become increasingly aware of and involved with their own body functions. Such turning inward of the libido may reach the point of a hypochondriacal state where the patient is constantly preoccupied with the functions of his own body. This, of course, is made easier for the patient by the fact that his own physiological functions are not as efficient as they have been earlier in his life. It is not at all unusual for an involutional reaction to be ushered in by a hypochondriacal phase. All the mental energy which was previously invested in a child may now become focused upon the lower bowel and its sluggish action, or on some other portion of the body. A vicious circle develops in which the patient begins self-medication along with his preoccupation. This often results in further malfunction of the organ and thus increases the preoccupation.

In summary, then, it may be said that the involutional reaction patient often presents a history which ten or fifteen years previously would have been diagnosed as an obsessive-compulsive reaction. A severe superego, punitive in nature, combined with inner unconscious immaturities, ambivalence, and anality are characteristic. At the same time, there is an elaborate system of defenses typical of the compulsive patient, which includes overcompensation, intellectualization, and isolation. The entire personality structure may function sufficiently well to carry the individual along without overt symptoms until the menopause, at which time the entire structure breaks down, precipitating a depression. Internalization of the conflicts has been of psychotic proportions. There is ordinarily a history of difficulty in expression of all instincts, both sexual and aggressive. Frigidity and impotence are common finding in the past history of involutional patients.

SYMPTOMATOLOGY

The symptomatology of the clinical picture seen in involutional psychotic reaction varies considerably as to its severity and content. Typically, the onset of this condition is gradual. It is difficult for the family, or even the patient, to tell exactly when it started. At times, however, it is found to date back to some physical illness, often transitory in nature. The initial phases are frequently ushered in by a hypochondriacal stage during which the patient becomes excessively preoccupied with his own bodily functions. The sparsity, irregularity, or cessation of menses may lead the patient to focus on the lower abdominal region. Constipation is a common concern. During this early phase of the illness the patient may make many visits to physicians complaining of varied and vague physical discomforts, apathy, loss of pep, headaches, general abdominal discomfort, insomnia, and poor appetite. Physical examinations in individuals of this age will usually reveal minor abnormalities of one type or another. Such finding as mild hypotension, hypertension, constipation, and anemia are not unusual. Treatment of these conditions may give transitory improvement, but this is usually followed, even though the treatment is continued, by a relapse or by the development of new symptoms.

Gradually the physical complaints become more and more important to these patients. They feel themselves failing and then begin to criticize themselves for not keeping up with their previously active modes of living. Insomnia becomes more marked, as do the self-recriminations for present as well as past demeanors. The patients begin to assume a demanding, bitter, self-critical, self-condemnatory attitude which not only makes life difficult for them but also for those around them. As close relatives begin to sense the importance of the emotional factors rather than the somatic elements, and suggest more activity and co-operation, these patients are prone to become bitter against such relatives, who, they feel, fail to recognize the severity of the condition.

Some involutional reactions have a marked paranoid coloring to them. If suspiciousness played a prominent role in the patient's prior life, it becomes exaggerated to the degree of paranoid feeling at this time. Such patients may reach the point where they have ideas of reference, feel people are talking about them, looking at them, and intending to do them harm. The best intentions and efforts of family and friends are often regarded by the patient as having an ulterior motive. In some of these individuals, the differential diagnosis from paranoid schizophrenic reaction is rather difficult, although the personality disorganization common to the latter is not seen. This attitude often delays the early and appropriate treatment and impedes its progress when once begun.

As the depressive picture increases, the patient gradually withdraws his libido from the outer world and invests an increasing amount of it in himself. He becomes more demanding, more difficult to live with, and increasingly self-depreciatory. There develops a general slowing of speech and motor activity, as well as thought. Such patients present a picture of sadness and dejection. They respond little to efforts which are made to interest them in things going on in the world. Agitation with increased motor activity, increased self-recriminations, and self-accusations may be more prominent. The patient may pace the floor, wring his hands for hours each day. There is a tendency to ruminate about past mild wrongdoings. These patients feel that they have made failures of their role in life and consider themselves useless and unloved. Insomnia becomes increasingly noticeable and is a good barometer in many cases as to the severity of the depression. The patient awakes early—around 3 or 4 A.M.—ruminates about his deficiencies, and complains bitterly about the harm he feels his insomnia is producing in him. Chronic severe insomnia is a deeply disturbing symptom and the wise physician is on the alert to recognize the serious suicidal possibilities in a patient who suffers from it.

PROGNOSIS

The symptoms of involutional reaction vary greatly in their severity and in their duration. Some patients may undergo a few months of mild depression and emerge, with very little treatment, to reassume the personality picture which was present earlier. In other individuals the depression is much more prolonged and severe and may remain for months or years if not treated. From the prognostic standpoint, pure depressive elements are easier to treat than those which are colored with paranoid element.

TREATMENT

Numerous factors must be taken into account before the proper therapeutic approach to a case of involutional reaction can be decided upon. These patients vary not only in the degree of severity of their illness, but also in symptomatology. The foundation upon which any useful treatment of this syndrome is based is an adequate and thorough evaluation of (1) the physical condition of the patient. This evaluation, however, by no means excludes the necessity of (2) an adequate survey of the patient's personality structure and (3) his present living conditions. It is of extreme importance that the physician neither exaggerate nor minimize any of these three factors. They must all be weighed carefully and each given its due consideration. There are many cases where major therapeutic concentration on one of the factors along with some attention to the other two factors will be of sufficient value to re-establish the patient's psychic equilibrium. For instance, attention should be paid to the fact that iatrogenic illnesses of a depressive type are particularly common in this age group. Hastily given, ill-advised statements by a physician to a patient with a psychological predisposition to a depression may be the precipitating factor even in an involutional reaction. A hard-working, overly conscientious, worrisome, forty-nine-year-old man who is carelessly told by his physician that his cardiac action is not all that it might be, may brood, worry, and ruminate about this statement until he begins the whole chain of events toward a real depression. Similarly, a single, inhibited, constricted forty-five-year-old woman who has never faced her advancing age may be thrown into depression by a sudden, callous, and thoughtless recommendation by her physician that a hysterectomy may very soon be required. It is in such situations as these that the physician must, first, truly know his patient; second, make an accurate evaluation of the physical condition; and, third, impart his recommendations to the patient in such a way that the latter will not be unduly upset.

From a therapeutic standpoint two important elements require special mention. First, patients with involutional reaction are often wrongly diagnosed because of the vague and numerous physical complaints which they present. While it is true that such complaints may require some type of medication, it is essential that the physician not feel that the whole symptom picture results from the particular complaint. Mild anemia or mild constipation are not basic causes of true depression and should not be treated as such. Second, to continue to treat such patients on an organic basis invites the serious possibility of suicide. Such patients may or may not verbalize their suicidal thoughts occasionally, but it suffices to say that when they do attempt suicide the attempt is usually successful. After making a proper diagnosis and recognizing the need for psychiatric care, there often follows the difficult problem of convincing both the patient and his family of the need for such treatment. When these patients have become so depressed themselves as to be extremely uncomfortable they are usually amenable to the suggestion of psychiatric assistance. However, prior to this stage of depression both they and their families are apt to be resistant to any form of psychiatric approach. It is wise at this point for the physician to advise a responsible member of the family as to the degree of seriousness of the illness and the possibility of suicide.

From the psychiatric standpoint an early and accurate decision must be made as to whether an involutional reaction patient may be treated on an outpatient basis or whether the patient is sufficiently ill as to require hospitalization. This decision, of course, is based primarily upon the possibility of suicide, but also, to some degree, on the environmental situation of the patient and the family dynamics. It is at times wise to hospitalize an involutional patient in order to remove him from an environment which is contributing to and exaggerating his depressive picture. Another decision which must be arrived at by the therapist is whether the patient is still capable of relating sufficiently to the physician to make use of psychotherapeutic interviews. In severe depressions, where the withdrawal of interest in the outer world is great, psychotherapy is difficult if not impossible. The patient relates no better to his therapist than he does to the rest of his environment, and therefore the treatment interviews are of little benefit. If the patient retains sufficient ability to relate to the therapist so that he can use the advice, suggestions, and interpretations of the physician, then psychotherapy is the treatment of choice.

For those patients who are severely depressed and cannot be reached by ordinary psychotherapeutic methods, electroshock is indicated. This illness is the one most successfully treated by electroshock treatment. In more than three-quarters of such cases considerable, and often dramatic, improvement follows the administration of perhaps from eight to twelve shock treatments. However, as many as twenty-four treatments may be necessary to gain the desired result. The improvement rate in these depressed patients may be higher if the depression does not have a paranoid coloring to it. Electroshock therapy, while certainly a boon to depressive patients, is not without its drawbacks. Perhaps the greatest practical difficulty is that the physician, the patient, and the family are so pleased by the rapid improvement produced by electroshock that further therapeutic interviews are not considered necessary. It is a cardinal rule that electroshock should only be considered a means by which the patient can be temporarily lifted from his depression to the point where he can relate to other individuals. To cease therapy at this point is only to invite future depressions. Once the patient's depression has been temporarily removed by electroshock therapy it is essential that psychotherapeutic interviews be utilized in order to effect some changes in the personality structure and thus minimize the possibility of future depressions.

The psychotherapeutic approach to the patient with involutional reaction, whether he has had shock or not, is concerned primarily with the particular dynamics of the patient. Such individuals, as mentioned previously, tend to be of a rigid, compulsive type and as such do not differ markedly from other rigid, compulsive people or other depressed patients. They have a severe, punitive superego which requires some modification therapeutically in order to allow them to live in peace with their instinctual demands. They suffer from having had too little love, tenderness, and acceptance during the pregenital period of development. Their critical conscience is the internalization of cold, strict parents. They are limited in the interests and recreational activities which are desirable for emotional health. Wherever possible—as with other patients—it is wise to help these individuals to understand, not only intellectually but also emotionally, some of the origins of their individual psychopathology. Discussions with patients of family background, childhood, and other early life attitudes are helpful in bringing about insight and establishing a more comfortable acceptance of themselves and others. Therapy should be pointed toward constructive activities and all successes should be stressed in order to strengthen the ego and ameliorate the rigid, sadistic superego.

Another extremely important aspect in the psychotherapeutic approach to involutional patients is concerned with the age period in life at which this syndrome occurs. Most of these patients are in their late forties or early fifties. They have a feeling, particularly because of their rigidity, that they have passed the useful, efficient, and worth-while part of life and are on the brink of old age. Their somewhat distorted relationships with their children lead them to surmise that they (the patients) are of no further use to them. The same thing holds true of their estimation of their marital situation. The general tendency of these individuals is to isolate themselves from their friends and from outside activities and to become increasingly dependent upon immediate members of their families in a pathological, ambivalent manner. They find themselves no longer willing, or apparently able, to seek companionship, interests, and pleasures from circles outside their own families.

Such a situation rapidly becomes a vicious cycle, where contact with previous interests is lost and friends no longer are of concern. Such patients obviously need a great deal of reassurance and encouragement to resume whatever activities they have had in the past, and to form new activities. They need help and understanding that life can and does hold many pleasures for those who are beyond fifty years of age. Practical advice must often be given as to where and how they may seek out companionship and activities which will stimulate their interest. The physician will not become discouraged at slow progress if he remembers that the patient has lived with his personality for some fifty years and it cannot be altered overnight. It is rigid and unbending and will not become flexible, warm, and resourceful in a short span of time. A great deal of effort, understanding, and patience is required to help these patients to establish a living situation which meets normal emotional needs. Wherever possible, as we have said, this should be done without electroshock, but if necessary the latter is useful in the early stages. Since the re-educational process is lengthy, there are some cases in which the benefit of electroshock is all that can be provided. The value of this treatment alone is considerable.

A word also should be mentioned about the transference which occurs in these patients. Those who are severely depressed relate poorly, if at all, to the therapist and therefore the transference is at a minimum. As for those who begin to relate, the physician soon finds them to be demanding, irritable, easily stirred to resentment, and at the same time frequently unable to express it. Such expressions of resentment as they make are subtle and usually unconscious and serve to alienate family and physician and thereby sabotage treatment efforts. These patients, in the early stages of treatment, attribute the severity of their own consciences to the therapist and expect rejection or criticism from him. Only gradually do they learn that he is different from their conscience and their family. As this point is learned they become more accepting of their instinctual needs and demands. At this point, however, they are often noticeably childish and demanding. Throughout the therapeutic program it is essential for the physician to remain friendly, understanding, and yet encouragingly firm in his approach. He must not allow these patients to "vegetate" or thwart the co-operative efforts being made by those around them for their recovery. He must praise each effort that the patient makes toward establishing new relationships. He must accept resentment, childishness, or coldness without resentment on his own part and must keep in mind the general goal of helping the patient understand more about himself.

Case History: Involutional Psychotic Reaction

This forty-nine-year-old married woman was referred to the psychiatrist by her own local physician. He had attempted for several weeks to deal with her complaints but had found that his therapy was not producing any improvement. The patient complained of a general loss of interest in her family and her friends. She said that she was becoming increasingly irritable and frequently suffered from crying spells. In addition to this she had a number of vague physical complaints for which no organic basis had been found by her local physician. She often suffered from headaches, constipation, and a general feeling of lassitude and weakness.

Upon questioning it developed that the patient's inability to sleep was a particularly bothersome symptom, and that much of her depression occurred during the early morning hours after a sleepless night. She had, on many occasions, entertained thoughts of suicide but, at least at the time she was referred, had not acted upon any of them. She felt that she was of no further use to her husband or to her two grown children, who had married and moved away. She was concerned about her general physical condition and also about her attractiveness, feeling that both were below par. She was no longer interested in pursuing the many social duties and obligations with which she had in the past occupied herself. She had resigned from most of the organizations to which she had previously belonged. She found herself no longer interested in her husband nor in his work. She could not even talk to him for any length of time without becoming irritable and critical of him. She was bitter about the fact that her married children visited her with decreasing frequency and yet, when pressed, made it evident that she treated them in an uncordial manner whenever they did come to see her.

This patient's past history revealed that she had always been a rigid person with perfectionistic, meticulous standards. She had led a life which appeared on the surface to have been full, yet which contained no deep emotional values. She had had many friends, but none of them had been close nor warm to her. She had always been an ambitious person striving for higher goals, many of which she now felt she had never attained. She had spent a great deal of time and interest in her home and yet had chronically been displeased with the results. Although she initially attempted to paint her earlier life as having been satisfactory, happy, and contented, it soon became evident that she had never achieved any measure of pleasurable living. She had been a chronically worrisome person concerned about everything in the life of her husband, her children, and herself. She watched over her family and had carried this tendency to the point of domination.

When this woman found herself in the menopause and realized that she was beginning to grow older, she became increasingly bitter about not having attained many of her goals. She resented the fact that her children no longer paid her the attention which they had previously. She resented the fact that her husband no longer found her as important as she thought he should. She began complaining of her physical symptoms, initially, and then made increased demands upon her husband and her children. She bitterly resented the fact that they did not respond as she wished to these excessive demands. As the situation continued she became increasingly depressed.

Three interviews, using a psychotherapeutic technique, did not result in any improvement and it was impossible to establish a useful relationship with this patient. Therefore, electroshock was recommended and the patient received a total of eight treatments. After approximately five she began to improve and by the end of eight her improvement had reached a more healthy pattern so that she was able to continue her psychotherapeutic interviews. Attempts were then made to help her re-establish her social activities and her interest in her children and grandchildren. She was also helped to understand how her previous life had been constricted, rigid, and lacking in joy. She was encouraged to make a more flexible adjustment and to appreciate the meaning and value of family and of friends. She gradually began to accept herself more thoroughly and to seek the companionship of others. She was seen in fifteen interviews over a period of several months. Her improvement was marked after electroshock and remained stabilized. After a follow-up of approximately four years, she suffered no relapse, as might well have occurred if she had not had the electroshock or had she received this treatment alone without any follow-up psychotherapy.

CHAPTER 17

Paranoid Reactions

PARANOID reactions are psychoses characterized by the presence of persecutory or grandiose delusions, but with the preservation of intelligence and with emotional responses appropriate to the ideas. Hallucinations are rarely seen and the patient does not show the personality disintegration so commonly seen in the paranoid schizophrenic. The present classification includes two subgroups within this category: *paranoia,* which comprises paranoid delusions that form an isolated, well-systematized, and almost encapsulated structure within the patient's personality; and *paranoid state,* which is characterized by less systematized, less isolated paranoid delusions which color the majority of the patient's thinking.

The term *paranoid* as applied to a person varies in meaning from a mild unrealistic feeling of being discriminated against to a delusion of persecution. Unfortunately, throughout the history of psychiatry and psychoanalysis, this term has been used in a variety of ways by different workers. There are numerous syndromes in which excessive suspiciousness, delusions of persecution, exaggerated jealousy, or grandiose delusions play a role. Much of the confusion surrounding the classification of various paranoid conditions is a result of a prolonged continuation of the Kraepelinian system of classification primarily based upon symptomatology. The newer, more dynamic psychiatry is far more interested in the underlying dynamics of patients than in the minute classification of their overt symptoms. Most present-day psychiatrists look upon paranoid symptoms, whether they occur in personality disorders, in paranoid reactions, or in paranoid schizophrenics, as having a common underlying origin. The current official nomenclature does separate these syndromes. The paranoid personality, as discussed in Chapter 12, is not psychotic, but is extremely sensitive and suspicious. The paranoid schizophrenic shows autistic and unrealistic thinking with paranoid delusions, ideas of reference, sometimes hallucinations, and a tendency toward total personality deterioration. The paranoid reactions, while psychotic, do not show the bizarre affect and behavior of the schizophrenic. The question of whether patients can be separated accurately into these categories has been answered differently by different authors, many feeling that all patients with paranoid reactions are really basically schizophrenic. While it is certainly important to recognize clearly how the patient outwardly deals with his unconscious conflicts, it nevertheless is also of marked importance to understand the unconscious origins of certain tendencies, such as paranoid feelings or delusions. For this reason it is valuable when dealing with the individual paranoid patient, no matter what his eventual diagnosis, to understand the basic roots of his tendency toward this form of mental aberration.

The definitely paranoid patient is one who attributes hostile motives to most of those who surround him. For instance, if he sees a group of people talking, and if one of this group looks casually in his direction, he becomes convinced immediately that they are discussing him and perhaps making fun of him. The paranoid husband is extremely suspicious of his wife's every move. If she is even a few minutes late meeting him for an appointment, he accuses her of lack of interest in him and assumes that she is interested in some other man instead. At work such a person feels discriminated against and is certain that his boss favors others and dislikes him. He is convinced that his co-workers discuss him behind his back and make uncomplimentary remarks about him. He reads into many chance and innocuous occurrences evidence that others are out to get his job or to have him fired. He tends to be meticulous, precise, uncompromising, and aggressive.

Paranoid thinking appears in varying degrees. The milder variety, as exemplified by the paranoid personality, is characterized by excessive suspiciousness, jealousy, and a constant tendency to feel disliked and unappreciated. As paranoid thinking increases in severity, it becomes more unrealistic and reaches a delusional stage, as is seen in paranoid reactions.

It is impossible to assess accurately the number of persons with paranoid reactions in the population. Many of these individuals go untreated for their entire lives. Personality disintegration, as is present in schizophrenic reactions, does not tend to occur in these persons and many of them are capable of maintaining their place in society, although at a marginal level of adjustment. Because of their heightened suspiciousness, it is not uncommon for them to resist any efforts others may make to have them seek psychiatric assistance. They are apt to take such suggestions as further evidence that no one around them is truly friendly and everyone has hostile motives toward them. They are particularly prone to lean heavily upon legal procedures to insure that no one will take unfair advantage of them. They may even seek legal redress for trifling or imagined transgression against their "rights" ("litigious paranoia"). Certainly it is true that paranoid thinking is an extremely important and common type of psychopathology in our society today. It is a type of thinking which is capable of producing great unhappiness both for the individuals involved and for those who surround them. At the same time, unfortunately, it often presents an insurmountable barrier preventing patients from taking advantage of any therapeutic efforts made toward improving their adjustment. In paranoid reactions it is not uncommon to find patients who have superior intelligence, great potential, and promising careers. Yet, unfortunately, they become enmeshed in distorted, suspicious, resentful thinking which destroys their relationships with others and markedly impedes or even ruins their future.

ETIOLOGY AND PSYCHOPATHOLOGY

One of the pillars on which paranoid thinking is built is the excessive use of the mechanism of defense known as "projection." The paranoid patient projects much of his own unconscious onto those in his environment and then reacts to this projection. This particular mechanism is used to some degree by many people, but fortunately it does not ordinarily reach the proportions that classify it as paranoid thinking. An example of the more common, and less pathological, type of projection is the Sunday golfer who shoots a very poor score. As his number of strokes increases, he becomes more critical of the condition of the golf course. The grass is too long or too short, or it's too wet or too dry. Each hole is too narrow or the rough is too thick. The general idea which he is trying to convey to himself and to his fellow players is that he is basically a good golfer, but the golf course itself is inadequate. Projection, like any other mechanism of defense, is an attempt to deal with an inner painful and unacceptable feeling. If, for instance, the golfer can project his inner feeling of inadequacy onto the golf course, he feels more comfortable than if he has to accept the painful fact that he is not a good player.

It is known that paranoid conditions have their roots early in life, most probably as a result, basically, of a disturbed and unhealthy mother-child relationship. The mother, or whoever is to take care of the infant, has the task of putting him at ease, making him feel important, accepted, loved. This is done in a variety of ways such as fondling, holding the infant tenderly, speaking softly and soothingly to him, keeping him warm and dry, feeding him regularly when he indicates his hunger, and, most importantly, giving him an hour-by-hour example of a buoyant, happy spirit. This buoyant happiness is introjected by the child. He literally "swallows and becomes like" the mother. Another way to depict what seems to happen is to imagine that a human being emanates an aura of happiness which other minds can tune in on. It is important that the mind of the infant be able to draw on this emanation which is coming primarily from the mother. In the paranoid individual early harmonious vibrations do not seem to get started. Instead distress, unhappiness, loneliness, resentment, and hostility are formed. When such a child leaves his mother's knee and begins to play with other children he is awkward, stilted, inept, lacking in friendliness and skill at play. As he is rebuffed, more resentment piles up along with the conviction that people are "against" him.

As adolescence is reached, reproaches against family and friends are more frequent and trifling occurrences assume an important personal significance. For example, the young girl who receives an invitation to a social affair and is unable to be happy about it concludes it came about because the hosts were sorry for her. Or the shy teen-age girl who is included in the conversation when guests arrive, instead of reacting positively and warmly thinks that her parents included her to show up her stupidity and thus embarrass her. Obviously such people do not add to their own happiness nor endear themselves to others. Those in the environment may try their best to be tactful and kind but to some degree they are likely to resent the special effort required to keep these people in a state approaching emotional well-being. In short, they make mountains out of molehills, have a constant chip on their shoulders, lack a sense of humor, and are usually incapable of seeing the other fellow's point of view. Some of these people retain this suspicious, hostile, truculent personality through a lifetime, while others gradually increase their rigidity until they lose all regard for the opinion and attitudes of others and are completely in the grip of their own distorted point of view. No amount of logic, evidence, or persuasion will influence them; a psychotic state of mind has developed.

The mechanism of projection appears very early in paranoid conditions, perhaps even within the first few months of life, and represents a deep psychological disturbance within the personality. The excessive use of projection involves a literal denial of reality, particularly the reality of a friendly environment. One such patient said, "I'll never accept the reality of what people think of me." This we see in paranoid reactions and, as a result, such a condition is truly a psychotic picture.

It may be said that there is a grain of truth in the paranoid patient's accusations of others. In a sense his unconscious is attuned with exquisite delicateness to the unconscious of others. He senses the ubiquitous unconscious that exists within everyone and magnifies it to a great degree. The term *empathy* serves well to illustrate this particular situation. All infants are adept at sensing the total feeling of the adults around them. This particular ability or situation we call empathy. The six-month-old infant who is fretful and disturbed when held by his own insecure, immature, and anxious mother may quiet down quickly when held by his grandmother, who has successfully raised many children and feels comfortable with him. He does not understand the words that are said to him, nor clearly perceive the actions that the adult goes through. However, he is acutely aware of whether there is anxiety, resentment, ambivalence, or other disturbed emotions in the atmosphere surrounding him. This property of empathy is unfortunately present to a heightened degree in a paranoid patient. One might compare the paranoid patient to an albino individual who is exquisitely sensitive to the sun. Most individuals are capable of achieving a healthy tan if they go about it slowly and gradually. Everyone is capable of getting a sunburn if exposed to massive doses of sunlight. The albino, however, is perpetually sensitive to even small doses of sun and must be extremely careful lest he injure himself through exposure. So it is with the paranoid patient, who is acutely attuned to many unconscious reverberations that the ordinary individual does not sense. He quickly senses minor hostilities in others. He cannot accept his counterreactions to these but must impute his attitudes to their alleged malicious thinking. "They" are out to harm him.

Another pillar on which a paranoid reaction rests has been shown by psychoanalysis to be a homesexual tendency present in the unconscious of the patient. This homosexual impulse is denied access to consciousness by the superego and is literally projected into the environment. It is at this point that the patient becomes delusional, often with the belief that others are accusing him of homosexual practices. It is unlikely that the latent homosexuality in the paranoid patient is any greater than in other psychoneurotics or psychotics, but it is inordinately unacceptable to the paranoid patient and he must project it in his delusional pattern. At the same time he is extremely uneasy about his own heterosexual relationships. He attempts to ward off his own feelings of inadequate heterosexuality. He unconsciously identifies himself with his female partner and subsequently accuses her of desires toward other men. His jealousy rises to extreme proportions and he is unable to believe that she truly loves him.

SYMPTOMATOLOGY

The essential feature of the paranoid reaction is the development of delusions of persecution or grandiosity. This delusional formation occurs without a concomitant interference with intellectual functions. The patient reacts to his delusions with appropriate emotions and reactions and, as has been mentioned, does not show the progressive personality disintegration so commonly seen in the paranoid schizophrenic. It is an extremely important point for the physician and student to remember that the paranoid patient cannot be "talked out of" or "reasoned out of" his delusions. This, of course, is what makes him psychotic. The average individual who utilizes projection from time to time will, if presented with the realistic facts of the situation, give up his projection and accept the facts. The paranoid psychotic patient, however, will not do so but will tend to include the individual who is presenting the facts in his paranoid system, and thus continue to ignore reality. Not only the families of these patients but many physicians harbor the idea that if they continue to present the patient with sufficient facts and reality, he will finally accept them. This, of course, will not occur as these patients are psychotic and cannot accept reality.

The difference between true paranoia and paranoid state is probably a matter of degree more than of type of pathology. The underlying dynamics of excessive sensitivity, a sense of inferiority, and a latent homosexual tendency, with an excessive use of the mechanism of projection, are present in both these conditions. The ego of the patient with true paranoia is somewhat more successful in that it manages to keep the paranoid delusional system systematized and localized in one particular portion of the patient's life. In this sense it is healthier than the ego of the patient with paranoid state, in which there is a spread of this pathological thinking that involves the majority of the patient's living experiences. As mentioned previously, there are many cases which on initial interview would appear to be true paranoia, but which, over a period of time, gradually show a spread of pathological thinking to the point where the diagnosis must be changed either to paranoid state or, in many instances, to schizophrenic reaction, paranoid type.

PROGNOSIS

The prognosis of paranoid reactions is generally guarded. Many paranoid individuals, as mentioned, never seek treatment and remain chronically ill. Others are referred by family, court, or physicians and present an extremely defensive attitude toward the therapist. The factor which most hampers a good prognosis is the suspicious, distrustful attitude of the patient and his frequent tendency to include the physician in his paranoid system. The patient's sensitivity is so great that he easily misunderstands remarks of the therapist and may stop treatment, feeling he is misunderstood and mistreated.

In order to effect a lasting improvement, the patient must gain some insight into his inner feelings. His narcissism is threatened as this insight approaches during treatment and he increases his defenses, particularly projection. Thus, unless he is in an institution, he may stop treatment then.

The ultimate prognosis is also influenced by the skill of the therapist. Treatment of the paranoid patient requires great skill and tact, and even small mistakes which would not seriously impede treatment of other types of patients will prove very deleterious in the treatment of the paranoid.

TREATMENT

The patient with paranoid reaction is psychotic. His delusions lead him to be suspicious of everyone and to falsely attribute hostile motives to many of those with whom he comes in contact. The patient reacts to his delusions as if they were true and in so doing is apt to show a variety of patterns of behavior. He may, primarily, withdraw from most of his contacts, feeling that it is useless to combat the hostility that he senses in everyone about him. Or he may aggressively attack what he considers to be the injustice to which he is being subjected. The essential point which the prospective therapist must bear in mind, however, is the marked impairment from which the patient suffers in his attempt to form good, useful interpersonal relationships. This impairment will make itself evident in the therapeutic relationship. The patient's delusional structure, as we have mentioned, is not subject to logical, rational disproof as would be true of the ordinary false belief of an average individual. After all, if this particular approach were of benefit it would already have cured the patient, since it is utilized extensively by the family and friends of every such patient long before psychiatric or medical help is sought. The mere possession of a medical degree does not lend sufficient additional weight to the therapist's words to have them thoroughly accepted by the patient.

An initial decision which must be made about the patient with paranoid reaction, as about any other psychotic patient, is whether or not hospitalization is required. This will depend upon two general questions: (1) whether the patient is so far removed from reality as to be potentially dangerous to himself or others, and so mentally disturbed as to be unable to conduct his own life without serious detriment to himself or others, and (2) whether such a patient can be helped therapeutically on an outpatient basis, or whether more intensive treatment with a regulated environment is needed to achieve improvement. The answers to these questions are difficult at times to determine. Whenever a part or all of a patient's life is being markedly influenced by delusional material arising from irrational, distorted unconscious factors, there is always a serious question as to how wise it is to allow him to continue to live outside an institution. On the other hand, there are paranoid individuals, particularly those with true paranoia, whose thinking and living is comparatively well regulated and who may be treated on an outpatient basis. Doing harm to others is foreign to their thinking. They may scold, complain, write letters, and accuse others over and over again of lack of consideration or unfairness but they do not plan anything destructive.

Too often, however, the decision whether to hospitalize or not is not made by the physician. Many patients enlist the support of their families to the point where it becomes impossible to hospitalize them even though the physician feels this would be advisable for security reasons. In such cases it is desirable to have at least one responsible member of the family realize the possible difficulties and dangers involved of harm to others and understand clearly the advisability of hospitalization. Generally the physician will be wise to lean in the direction of conservatism and hospitalize the paranoid psychotic during treatment. To do otherwise is to risk the possibility of innumerable complications and difficulties brought on by the patient's reaction to his own paranoid system. He may squander large sums of money on his grandiose schemes or travel great distances to convey his important messages to the world. Such actions are not necessarily serious in all cases but can reach alarming proportions, as for instance when homicidal tendencies occur. Unfortunately not every patient with such dangerous impulses can be recognized and apprehended before he does harm, but greater vigilance and insistence upon treatment may prevent many such incidents.

Perhaps the greatest difficulty encountered by the physician in the typical paranoid reaction case is getting the patient to undertake psychotherapy and enlisting the family's co-operation toward this end. Most of these patients, since they preserve their intellectual capacities as well as their seemingly appropriate emotional responses, can be extremely persuasive to their families in arguing against psychiatric treatment. As we have mentioned, these patients are in many instances prone to view relatives' suggestions concerning their need for psychotherapy as further evidence of the truth of their own paranoid systems. The delusion that someone or some group would like to put the patient in a mental hospital in order to punish him or remove him from his environment is not uncommon. In such a case, a suggestion that psychotherapy is needed usually brings a negative response from the patient. In many instances it requires a considerable period of time for relatives to decide finally that their "logical" approach will not benefit the patient and that he suffers from a difficulty which requires expert attention.

No matter how early or under what circumstances the patient comes or is brought for psychiatric help, he usually approaches the initial interview with considerable suspiciousness. This is, after all, only an exaggeration of the way he approaches all new relationships. If the treatment is planned on an outpatient basis, the initial interview may be unsuccessful in allaying the patient's suspiciousness and enticing him to return for more help. In such a case hospitalization may be the only remaining method. In a patient who is institutionalized this particular factor is not nearly so important, since the therapist exercises control over the patient's day-to-day living.

Once psychotherapy is instituted on a regular schedule the initial goal is to bring about a sufficiently good relationship between patient and therapist to enable the sessions to be meaningful to the patient in a beneficial way. Tranquilizers are somewhat less effective with paranoid psychotics than non-paranoid schizophrenics. This is often complicated further by the paranoid person's unwillingness to accept medication or his tendency to attribute harmful properties to pills. Nevertheless, tranquilizers may be useful in selected cases. There are many paranoid patients whose ability to relate to others is so disturbed by their delusions, or is so limited by the paucity of good will in the ego, that more drastic measures are required in the initial phases of treatment. For such patients electroshock, or at times even insulin shock, is necessary in order to initiate their ability to relate to a therapist. Neither of these forms of treatment should be thought of as "cures" for paranoid reactions. They may reduce the severity of the delusional system, and help any associated depression. As with depressive reactions, the purpose is only to enhance the patient's ability to relate to the therapist and then to use psychotherapeutic techniques. The percentage of patients with paranoid reaction who improve with either electroshock or insulin shock is not as large as it is with depressive patients, but is sufficiently good to indicate the use of one of these methods where initial psychotherapeutic approaches fail. Electroshock may at times be utilized on an outpatient basis if performed by a person well trained in this procedure, but the more formidable insulin shock method is always an inpatient procedure.

Once the patient has begun to relate more comfortably and less distrustfully to the physician the ordinary rules of psychotherapy apply. The general aim is to help the patient understand some of his unconscious motivations and to work them through in such a way as to remove the necessity of distorted symptom formation. For instance, the average paranoid patient must be helped to understand that he is attributing to other people a great deal of his own inner resentment and bitterness. He must be encouraged to understand how as a result of his suspicion, jealousy, and distrust he has brought on negative reactions from other people and how more friendliness awaits him when he himself is more capable of showing it to others. The homosexual problem must be worked through very slowly, delicately, and carefully. These patients have already become psychotic in an attempt to "disown" their homosexual impulses, or to deny or compensate for their feeling of inferiority. Therefore, they can only be brought into conscious contact with these impulses slowly, without criticism, and with understanding assistance toward a more mature adjustment.

Even if little or no insight is obtained the paranoid patient is helped to keep down the degree of his aggression and truculence against his imagined aggressors when he has a regular opportunity to vent his hurt feelings and his resentment. There is a "letting off of steam," a discharge of aggression; and after a session in which he has been "given a hearing" he is contented to hold some of his complaints in abeyance for a few days. Some paranoid patients will not have anything to do with a psychiatrist, even to use him as a listener. But if a patient does come the psychiatrist may do as the physician has often had to do in disease, i.e., alleviate suffering even when he cannot cure the disease.

One of the great difficulties, once a therapeutic relationship has been established, is an unconscious fear on the part of the patient himself of a homosexual attachment to the therapist if the latter is of the same sex. This requires judicious handling and often taxes the skill of even the best psychotherapist. The patient's reaction to such an attachment may be, for instance, to stop therapy without explanation or to become aggressive toward the therapist.

It should be re-emphasized at this point that the patient who utilizes excessively the mechanism of projection is an extremely difficult person with whom to deal. He is suspicious of everything and everyone. He is defensively guarded against finding difficulties within himself and instead finds them in those surrounding him. He is excessively sensitive to any deficiency within himself, and if such an inadequacy is even gently pointed out to him it is apt to hamper his relationship with the therapist severely. When the mechanism of projection reaches such proportions as to result in delusional formation it has truly assumed formidable proportions from a therapeutic standpoint. Therefore, as has been mentioned, the physician should never be misled into assuming that logical, coherent, argumentative proof will remove the delusions or even the suspicious character qualities. Patients with paranoid reactions are extremely sick individuals reacting in an unrealistic manner, and they are difficult people with whom to deal therapeutically. In short, the therapist should bring optimism to each case undertaken but at the same time know the nature of the disease well enough so that he is not personally traumatized should insight not be gained through his efforts.

Case History: Paranoid State

The wife of this forty-two-year-old male originally consulted the psychiatrist seeking advice as to the care and management of the obvious psychiatric illness from which her husband suffered. The latter had been in psychiatric treatment with another psychiatrist for about two months, at which time he had emphatically stated that he would not return for any further visits and that he was going "to put it all out of my mind." This patient had originally sought psychiatric help only because his wife had coerced him into it. This had followed an occurrence where the wife had awakened in the middle of the night to find her husband's hands around her throat. She had managed to dissuade him from choking her and had enticed him into a conversation about his motives. He complained that he had seen her masturbating and that he had known for a long time that she was "oversexed." He told her that he was going to leave her because of this difficulty. The wife managed to pacify him temporarily and later the matter was discussed more thoroughly. It required pressure from his wife, as well as several other relatives, to induce him to consult a psychiatrist.

However, even during the time that the patient was seeing the first psychiatrist, he had continued to observe his wife's every move closely, even to the extent of using a mirror. He continued to harbor the impression that she was masturbating. Such an accusation had no basis in fact. It was during this time that the husband became increasingly concerned about his own physical appearance. He was preoccupied with his inability to attain a full erection and his impotence became more noticeable.

The patient's wife stated that her husband had always been, even during courtship and marriage, an extremely jealous individual who could be described as a rigid, overly conscientious person. He had become progressively more religious following his marriage and this had been even more noticeable after the death of his father one year previously. He had begun to pray in a ritualistic and almost meaningless fashion about his deceased father. During the weeks prior to the consultation with the second psychiatrist he had shown more paranoid delusions. He believed that the telephone wires of his home had been tapped. He complained that he had been followed home on several occasions. He said that people did not understand him and were hostile toward him. Meantime, however, he had maintained his work capacity, as well as his limited social life, to the point where neither his employer nor his friends were aware of the seriousness of his difficulty.

This patient had, by the time his wife consulted the second psychiatrist, refused to return to his original psychiatrist. He also refused to consult the second psychiatrist in spite of attempts by his wife and other relatives to induce him to do so. His condition remained more or less static for a period of about three months. During this time he continued to work, and as far as could be discerned, showed none of the personality disintegration that might be expected in the schizophrenic. His wife reached the conclusion that she would not be able to live with him. She reached this decision only after many scenes during which she pleaded with him to seek psychiatric help. She steadfastly refused to instigate procedures to have him seen psychiatrically in order that commitment to a mental hospital might be arranged. Following their separation, the patient continued to visit his wife periodically and alternately accuse her of infidelity and hypersexuality, as well as to plead with her to return to him again. He was not regarded as homicidal, and these occasional scenes were less of a strain for his wife than when living with him. The separation made her freer to maintain her own emotional equilibrium and peace of mind and the patient seemed no worse for the move.

Case History: Paranoia

This twenty-eight-year-old male was admitted to the hospital, having been sent from prison where he had been incarcerated after his wife swore out a warrant charging him with beating her. The patient admitted that the charge was true but stated that he felt he had good reason to beat her inasmuch as she was repeatedly unfaithful to him and regularly mistreated the children. He said that he was quite certain of her infidelities although he had not actually caught her in the act. He knew the identity of her paramour, he said, but was unwilling to disclose his name, inasmuch as this was a personal matter.

On examination the patient was well-oriented, his reasoning was clear and logical, his memory excellent; he exhibited no hallucinations; and the only evidence of pathological thinking was the questionable issue of his wife's actions. He did not feel that he was mentally ill and did not feel that he should be held in the hospital. However, he was willing to stay for a short period of observation in order to prove that he was perfectly all right and that this was not just some strange idea of his.

Little was known of the patient's background, partly because he refused to discuss it, stating that this was irrelevant to the issue in question. However, according to his statement, he was the fourth of five children who came from a poor family abroad. He had had approximately ten years of schooling and had then enlisted, according to his statement, in the French Navy. His ship was one of those which was not lost during World War II and he spent a good deal of time in the ensuing years in the United States. It was during one of these periods that he met and courted his present wife, marrying her when she became pregnant. Four children were born of the marriage. After leaving the Navy he came to the United States and worked at various unskilled occupations after the war and had a fairly steady employment record.

The patient's wife, when seen by the social worker and the intern, denied all her husband's accusations and stated that he had always been very jealous and suspicious. She added that since they had little money, her time was so taken up with watching the children, who were fairly close in age, that she did not have time to cheat even if she wanted to. She stated that he varied considerably in his behavior to the children, sometimes being exceedingly indulgent and on other occasions either paying little attention to them or abusing them. Other relatives and one neighbor were seen by the social worker and these reports tended to verify all the wife stated.

The patient reacted well to hospital routine although he offered a number of complaints about the various inconveniences and the lack of freedom. He very quickly learned that ten days was the legal period for holding patients for observation and when the time was up managed to smuggle a note to a lawyer making demands for release. At about the same time the immigration authorities became interested in the case, as apparently there was some doubt as to the legality of the patient's entry into the country, and a move was made to begin deportation proceedings. The foreign Consul saw the man and apparently was convinced not only that he should remain in the United States but that he was being unjustly held in the hospital. A deportation hearing was held at the hospital. All witnesses were present, but just as the hearing got under way the patient demanded a lawyer, which necessitated postponing the hearing.

As time passed, the patient became more and more hostile toward everyone connected with the hospital and on one occasion accused one of the staff physicians of being in league with his wife to get him out of the way so that she could continue her extramarital adventures. Psychological studies were done which confirmed the clinical diagnosis of paranoia, the patient exhibiting rather strong latent homosexual trends, heightened ambivalence toward male figures, and a marked degree of suspicion and evasiveness. The patient was eventually placed on electroshock treatment, made a good recovery, and was discharged. He improved at least to the point of no longer being as suspicious toward his wife. Follow-up treatment could not be arranged due to lack of co-operation on the patient's part. The prognosis was guarded since a return of the systematized delusions seemed probable. The case was diagnosed as paranoia because of the delusions centered around his wife's infidelity. The remainder of his thinking, except as it related to this area, remained comparatively good and uninfluenced by the paranoid process.

Organic Brain Disorders

PART VII

Organic Brain Disorders

CHAPTER 18

Acute Brain Disorders

PERSONALITY function may be distorted by organic factors in syndromes that are both temporary and reversible. It is with this group of syndromes that the present chapter is concerned. The central nervous system, like any other system of the body, may have its proper function disturbed by disease, injury, or physiological malfunction. Organic changes within the parenchymatous, vascular, or interstitial areas of the brain are capable of producing varying degrees of personality change. The symptomatology resulting from such change is due primarily to the degree and location of the organic changes; it may be relatively mild or may reach psychotic proportions. Symptoms may be acute or chronic in type, again depending upon the pathological process.

The etiology of such processes varies from endogenous to exogenous. It includes such factors as infections, intoxications, trauma, physiological disturbances, tumors, and metabolic disturbances. The essential factor necessary for qualification under this category is the reversibility and temporary nature of the condition. Those which persist and produce irreversible changes are classified under chronic brain syndromes (Chapter 19).

In the past, the tendency has been to make a general subdivision of these organic syndromes into toxic psychoses and organic psychoses. Such a classification did not take into account, primarily, the temporal element, as is now done. It also had the disadvantage of implying that all psychological disturbances which were caused by organic and toxic agents were psychotic in nature, whereas this is obviously not true, since many are of a lesser kind. It is of great

439

importance, as is stressed in the present classification, to know whether the condition is acute or chronic. It is also important to know, as is to be specified in the present classification, what the particular etiological agent is.

ACUTE BRAIN SYNDROME ASSOCIATED WITH INTRACRANIAL INFECTION

This category includes those conditions occurring as a result of intracranial infection. Among the most common etiological agents are encephalitis, meningitis, and brain abscess. It should be remembered, however, that in order to qualify under this category these conditions must produce a temporary and reversible type of brain syndrome. Infection within the cranial cavity itself in many instances produces a chronic brain syndrome. However, there are a certain number of such infections which subside after an acute episode and leave personality function relatively unimpaired.

Case History: Acute Brain Syndrome Associated with Intracranial Infection

This forty-eight-year-old woman was admitted to the hospital with a history of a sore throat and increasingly severe headache developing over the previous three days. At the time of admission she was having difficulty swallowing anything other than liquids. She was rather lethargic but could be roused and at such times complained of severe headache.

Physical examination revealed an acutely ill woman, temperature 103.5°, rapid pulse and respirations. Her neck was stiff. Spinal fluid examination revealed an increased pressure, high cell count, predominately polys. Meningococci were demonstrated in the spinal fluid and a diagnosis of meningococcus meningitis was made. Antibiotic therapy was begun immediately. On the first evening of her admission to the hospital this patient became agitated. She complained of nausea. She attempted to get out of bed, claiming that she saw a woman walking toward her who was apparently going to hurt her. She was reassured by the nurses and quieted down. However, several hours later she became noisy, agitated, and quite anxious. She said she knew there was someone else in the room who would harm her. She mistook a small stand in the corner for a person crouching ready to spring at her. At this time she was disoriented, confused, and extremely fearful. Once again, however, she was reassured by the physician and nurse. She went back to sleep and by the next morning had shown considerable improvement in both her mental and physical state. She continued to improve and was subsequently diagnosed as cured. There was no recurrence of her acute mental syndrome. She remained lucid, co-operative, and in good contact.

A brief review of her history revealed some marital difficulties between her and her husband. She felt he was showing undue interest in another woman and she bitterly resented his attentions to this woman. The description she gave of the hallucinatory woman and her husband's friend were remarkably similar. There undoubtedly had been a good deal of resentment between the two women. In acute toxic situations the patient's delusions or hallucinations are influenced by his own personality and conflicts with which he is struggling. After the acute toxic condition subsides, the patient loses the psychotic evidences and returns to the premorbid personality adjustment.

ACUTE BRAIN SYNDROME ASSOCIATED WITH SYSTEMIC INFECTION

This category includes the disturbances in personality function, of a varying degree of severity, temporary in nature, which are produced by relatively severe general systemic infections. In such conditions the entire body physiology is mobilized to combat the infection. Frequent concomitants are a hyperpyrexia, difficulties in fluid balance, and other similar physiological distortions. The central nervous system is particularly vulnerable to such changes and may react with a distortion in personality function. Typical conditions which may result in this acute brain syndrome are pneumonia, typhoid fever, acute rheumatic fever, and other similar general systemic infections which involve relatively severe illness. It is especially important to realize that in children and infants the occurrence of an acute delirious reaction as a concomitant of hyperpyrexia in one of the childhood diseases is not uncommon. The immature central nervous system apparently is more sensitive to such physiological changes as are prone to occur in systemic infection; therefore, the acute brain syndrome is to be distinguished from severe latent emotional or mental disturbances brought to the overt level as a result of a relatively minor infection. For instance, an individual who has a schizoid personality may be precipitated into an overt schizophrenic psychosis by a minor temporary infectious disease which in and of itself is not capable of producing an acute brain syndrome. The proper diagnosis in this case would be schizophrenia.

Case History: Acute Brain Syndrome Associated with Systemic Infection

This forty-nine-year-old male was seen by the psychiatrist on consultation while he was a patient in the medical ward. The patient had been admitted with a history of a sudden onset of a sharp pain in his left lower chest and left shoulder, which pain was accompanied by hiccough. The pain was also exaggerated by respiratory movements. It had begun some twenty-four hours prior to the patient's admission. Physical findings were essentially negative, except for a temperature of 102° and moderate dullness to percussion in the left base, posteriorly. X-ray of the chest revealed pneumonitis of the left lower lobe. Serology was negative. The patient had been placed on 50,000 units of penicillin every three hours, and was seen by the psychiatrist on the evening of his first day in the hospital.

During that evening the patient had become confused and disoriented and had had visual and auditory hallucinations. He declared that his granddaughter was calling to him. He became quite restless and anxious to leave the hospital. He put his bathrobe on over his pajamas and started to leave the hospital in an attempt to go home to see her.

When he was reassured that his granddaughter was perfectly all right and that he should remain in the hospital, he was fairly tractable to suggestion and returned to bed.

The following day, the patient's wife was interviewed. She said that he had not been in particularly good health for the past two years. He had frequently suffered from rather severe colds. She also said that he had been quite nervous during the past two years. He often suffered from insomnia and would, at times, arise at three or four o'clock in the morning, being unable to return to sleep. There were one or two instances described by the wife, particularly when he had had a severe cold and was quite febrile, when he had apparently become hallucinated, claiming that his mother was calling him. It was difficult to ascertain from the wife's history whether he was talking in his sleep or was actually awake.

The patient was seen in the hospital the following morning and was completely oriented. His sensorium was clear. He talked about the episode the previous night as if it were a joke. He was somewhat apprehensive and childish during the interview, but there were no other symptoms of psychosis. The patient, by this time, had begun to respond to the therapy for his pneumonitis and his temperature was down. He continued to improve, and when seen one week following his admission, was found to be mentally clear, with memory intact, and no evidences of visual or auditory hallucinations.

It was felt that this patient, although certainly suffering from some emotional problems, primarily of a psychoneurotic type, had had on several occasions, including his hospitalization, acute psychotic episodes brought on by systemic infection.

ACUTE BRAIN SYNDROME, DRUG OR POISON INTOXICATION

Intoxications due to drugs and poisons are capable of disturbing and distorting personality function. The type and degree of this disturbance and distortion varies with the particular type of toxic agent, the amount of it which is present, and the time over which it acts. We are here concerned primarily with those intoxication syndromes which are acute in nature and are reversible. It is of great practical importance, obviously, to know the particular etiological agent.

Generally speaking, most toxic brain syndromes are reversible, although some are capable of resulting in chronic brain syndromes if the toxic agent acts to a sufficient degree or is continued over a long enough period of time. It has been estimated that up to 10 per cent of psychiatric hospital admissions are due to various types of toxic conditions. It is difficult, if not impossible, however, to estimate the total number of such toxic brain syndromes. Many of them are temporary in nature and do not result in hospitalization, since they do not reach psychotic proportions. In addition, many of them are secondary features of more life-endangering conditions which take the primary role in the medical treatment. The effect of toxic brain syndrome on our national life in terms of absenteeism from work, disrupted family life and impairment of physical health would be difficult to overestimate.

There are certain general personality changes which are ordinarily associated with the toxic syndrome: a broad outline of these will be presented here. The changes obviously vary to some degree, depending upon the particular toxic agent, the quantity in which it is present, and the time during which it operates. Also it is necessary to take into account the previous personality characteristics of the individual. However, the following are some of the features which are often seen.

Of primary importance is the appearance of an impairment in the patient's degree of consciousness. This may come on temporarily only to disappear and subsequently recur. The impairment varies from mild to severe and may at times reach complete unconsciousness. There is a clouding of the sensorium which impairs the patient's thinking as well as his reaction to his environment. Another prominent difficulty is the misinterpretation by the patient of his surroundings, particularly in the form of illusions. At times such patients may become acutely delusional and even hallucinated. Especially in the early phases of the toxic condition there is a tendency to misinterpret various sights and sounds, often attributing to them a frightening quality. It is fairly characteristic of many toxic conditions for the patient to become acutely agitated and fearful because of the misinterpretations he makes concerning his surroundings. He finds danger everywhere and is apt to become terrified and remarkably frantic in his attempts to escape his supposed dangers. As mentioned, these toxic conditions often wax and wane so that when a patient is seen at one time he may be fairly clear and coherent in his answers, while at another time he may be absolutely terror-stricken and extremely difficult to manage. It is a general rule that many of these patients can be quieted merely by the reassuring, friendly, and understanding presence of another individual who talks quietly with them, thereby assisting them to maintain a better contact with reality. At times a patient in an acute toxic episode may become so agitated that he is extremely difficult to control, will not eat or sleep, and proceeds with this type of behavior to the point of exhaustion and even death.

The general therapeutic regimen for toxic conditions is initially directed toward the toxic agent itself. However, such patients have often reached a state of general physical ill health that makes many supportive measures essential. Any therapeutic measure which conserves the patient's strength is of value.

The various etiological agents involved in the toxic syndrome are such drugs as bromides, barbiturates, and opiates, and such poisons as lead, other metals, and some gases. It has been suggested that alcohol be listed in a separate category because of its frequency of use, and it is given a special statistical category of its own. Barbiturates and opiates represent such widespread and important problems in the psychiatric field that they are covered in Chapter 12, which deals with personality disorders.

The most important etiological agent, therefore, remaining within the category for discussion here is bromides.

It has been repeatedly shown how prolonged administration of even relatively small doses of preparations containing bromides results in accumulation of this substance within the body and in the production of a psychotic picture. Undoubtedly psychoses resulting from bromides were more frequent in the past before the medical profession was adequately alerted to the dangers which accrue to its prolonged administration. However it is still by no means a rare event to find a patient who has, either through prescriptions or otherwise, been taking some type of sedation containing bromides over a sufficient period of time to cause a bromide psychosis. Ordinarily the onset of this condition is rather gradual. One expects to find psychotic symptoms appearing whenever the blood bromide exceeds about 75 to 150 mg. per 100 cc. of serum. It is impossible to give any definite level, since bromide tolerance and excretion vary markedly from one patient to another.

Initially in the development of this psychosis there are periodic spells of confusion, disorientation, and illusions. Often hallucinations subsequently develop. Such patients are prone to suffer a noticeable personality change over a period of time. Many of them are in middle or later life and have been taking sedation to combat their insomnia. As the bromides accumulate within the body there is a tendency for the sleep pattern to change, and particularly there is wakefulness during the night when the illusions and hallucinations play a more noticeable role. Visual hallucinations in the form of brightly flashing lights are often said to occur. There is associated with this some difficulty in thinking and in concentrating. There is a clouding of the sensorium with some agitation and an indistinct type of speech. As mentioned, the psychotic difficulty comes on periodically in the beginning, but if the patient continues to take bromides the episodes gradually merge with each other until there is a constant loss of contact with reality.

The treatment for bromide psychosis consists of the administration of from thirty to sixty grains of sodium chloride three to four times a day. The chloride gradually replaces the bromide in the body and the latter is excreted. Obviously some attention must be paid at the same time to the general physical condition of the patient and an inquiry must be made into the underlying psychogenic reasons for which the individual became a chronic user of bromide sedatives in the first place. Attempts must be made toward substituting other sedatives or, preferably, instituting psychotherapeutic measures in order to negate the need for further sedation.

Case History: Acute Brain Syndrome, Drug Intoxication (Bromidism)

This fifty-five-year-old woman was admitted to the medical service of the hospital, having been referred by her physician in a small outlying town. The history revealed that the patient had been having difficulty for approximately two years. The most prominent symptom was severe headache, which became increasingly incapacitating. Such headaches were related to exercise and excitement and were occasionally accompanied by dizzy spells. Approximately one month prior to admission the patient had begun to develop new symptoms. These included confusion, loss of memory, periods of irrational speech, depression, crying, anorexia, constipation, and vomiting. There was also a history of hematemesis and melena.

Physical examination revealed a dehydrated, bedridden, malnourished woman. There was evidence of avitaminosis. She showed considerable mental confusion and had difficulty in speaking. There was a slight nystagmus on lateral gaze. There was also a slight bilateral ptosis. Complete blood count and urinalysis were not remarkable. Further inquiry revealed that this patient had been taking rather large daily doses of a proprietary drug containing bromide. This had been going on for several years. A blood bromide test revealed a level of 95 mg. per 100 cc. of blood serum.

During her first two nights in the hospital this patient was actively hallucinated in the visual sphere. On one occasion she claimed that she saw a red fire engine drive up in front of the hospital in the middle of the night and spray water on the first-floor windows. Several times during the second night she became quite frightened when she suffered from illusions. She misinterpreted several inanimate objects in her room, feeling that they were dangerous animals. This patient was given intravenous fluid and electrolytes, together with tube feedings to restore her nutritional state. Particular attention insured the fact that the patient received an adequate amount of sodium chloride in her daily intake. Her condition rapidly improved and within a few days all evidences of the psychosis had disappeared.

ACUTE BRAIN SYNDROME, ALCOHOL INTOXICATION

Where, when, and how primitive man first discovered the effects of alcohol are unknown. However, since that day thousands of years ago this drug has played a prominent role in every society and certainly ours today is no exception. Alcohol owes its tremendous popularity to the particular effect which it produces upon the psyche. In moderate doses it results in a diminution of tension, a feeling of well-being and even exhilaration, a false sense of ability, and lessening of inhibitions. In a topographical sense, alcohol begins its action by diminishing superego functions. The normal or often exaggerated demands of this particular mental division are "anesthetized" first, thus allowing the release and expression of underlying impulses which are often of a more immature, childish nature. There results a feeling of being free of terrors and worries and also a heightened sense of importance. The exact reaction of an individual to moderate doses of alcohol depends to a large degree upon his underlying psychological structure. There are certain people who have a large amount of underlying aggression which is held in check by a fairly severe superego. If such an individual imbibes a sufficient amount of alcohol to immobilize his superego, there may occur a sudden release of aggression. Generally speaking, the mores, rules, and regulations of the conscience become progressively diminished under the influence of alcohol until the imbiber shows a previously invisible type of immaturity. Obviously, if there is little superego structure to start with, the person is already quite immature in general and the alcohol is more than apt to accentuate this condition.

It is impossible to estimate the importance of alcohol, since it affects so many areas of living. It has been estimated that about nine and a half billion dollars is spent annually in the United States on beer, wine, and other liquors. At the same time it has been estimated that approximately seven hundred and fifty million dollars represents the annual cost in disease, crime, and property damage directly attributable to alcohol. The moral and legal implications of alcohol are not within the scope of this book. We are concerned here primarily with the psychological factors in the use and abuse of alcohol.

The term *social drinking* is used to indicate a "normal" use of alcohol. It refers essentially to that type of drinking which a person does at social gatherings in an atmosphere of congeniality. To qualify as social drinking the alcoholic intake must not be excessive and must not assume pathological importance to the individual. In other words, alcohol must not become essential to the person. It must not become a crutch upon which he constantly leans. It is always difficult to find the dividing line between social and pathological drinking. Most frequently it is easier for others to see when a person has passed this imaginary line than it is for the individual himself to see it.

Drinking may be said to have become pathological when it is excessive in amount, interferes with the individual's working and social adjustment, or produces a pathological emotional reaction. Generally speaking, a person may imbibe excessive amounts of alcohol either because of outside environmental pressures which are chronically tension-producing but inescapable or because of various types of internal psychopathology. The so-called reactive alcoholism, which results from excessive environmental pressures, should theoretically cease when these environmental pressures are removed. The various internal psychological factors because of which an individual drinks excessively are numerous. At times chronic alcoholism may result from an underlying and possibly latent psychosis of a functional or even organic nature. At other times such drinking results from a structuralized psychoneurosis or personality disorder and at still other times mental deficiency may be one of the basic contributing factors. However, there are a large number of chronic alcoholics in whom psychosis, psychoneurosis, and even mental deficiency are not clearly demonstrable. These individuals have been referred to as belonging to the "chronic alcoholic" group. It has been shown that they are characterized by deep oral needs. They have a poor ability to tolerate frustration and tension and easily seek refuge in alcohol. In the ordinary chronic alcoholic one finds an underlying depressive trend which may, if the patient is forbidden to drink, reach overt proportions and become clearly manifest. Essentially these individuals seek a reduction in tension and guilt. They feel inadequate, bitter, frustrated, and depressed and find solace in escaping through drinking. Life literally has become too difficult for them and they yearn for the protected dependent position of infancy. Responsibilities, duties, and obligations are resented. Through drinking the alcoholic achieves a false sense of well-being, potency, ability, and relaxation.

There are several types of difficulties associated with pathological drinking which are of an acute type and therefore essentially reversible: pathological intoxication, acute hallucinosis, and delirium tremens.

PATHOLOGICAL INTOXICATION

This syndrome, described many years ago by Krafft-Ebing, indicates the sudden onset of a relatively severe behavior reaction which is brought on by a mild to moderate intake of alcohol. Actually there is some question as to the advisability of the term *pathological intoxication,* since it indicates that the alcohol itself is of major importance, while in reality the underlying psychological problems are merely brought to the fore by the alcohol. Certain individuals suffering from latent psychosis or from various types of dissociative reaction or personality disorders may react violently to relatively small doses of alcohol. Such people literally become transformed and may reveal an excessive degree of aggression, combativeness, at times illusions, or even delusions, depending upon the particular type of underlying psychopathology brought to the fore by the alcohol. The removal by alcohol of the more or less superficial inhibitory effects within the personality gives the deeper problems free access to expression and this may result in behavior and characteristics not otherwise seen in these persons. Such individuals may attain and even maintain a reasonably satisfactory adjustment in the absence of alcohol but may, while under its influence, become belligerent, disoriented, delusional, aggressive, confused, or even at times hallucinated. Ordinarily this condition has a relatively rapid recovery period when the alcohol is withdrawn. The recovery takes place in twenty-four to forty-eight hours: this fact is of importance diagnostically, since several of the other syndromes associated with alcohol are much more chronic in nature.

ACUTE HALLUCINOSIS

This particular syndrome refers to those individuals who with varying intakes of alcohol begin to suffer from hallucinatory experiences, often of a paranoid nature. They react to these hallucinations as if they were real and consequently become extremely frightened, anxious, and at times even belligerent and destructive. They ordinarily do not reveal the complete personality change seen in pathological intoxication, and the sensorium, except as influenced by the hallucinations, often remains relatively clear. The hallucinations are apt to be of an auditory rather than visual type, but occasionally are olfactory. Most often they are persecutory in nature and represent a projection of the patient's unconscious homosexual drives. Again, as with pathological intoxication, the exact content of the delusions or illusions is determined by the underlying psychopathology. There is considerable evidence to indicate that a latent type of schizophrenic reaction may be brought to the fore by the use of moderate doses of alcohol and may result in the syndrome which we call "acute hallucinosis." This condition does not usually last over a long period of time—possibly only a few days to a week—although occasionally one finds a case in which the hallucinations persist and the pattern eventually becomes indistinguishable from schizophrenia.

In these cases, even though alcohol seems to be the precipitating factor, the proper diagnosis is schizophrenic reaction.

Case History: Acute Hallucinosis

This thirty-eight-year-old man was brought to the hospital by the police, who had found him in a stuporous, disoriented state. Approximately twelve hours elapsed after his admission to the hospital before it was possible to locate someone who could give at least some of his history. This patient was a mechanic who lived alone and had been divorced for about ten years. According to his history he had been on a week-long drinking party prior to his admission, during which time he had consumed an estimated two quarts of whisky a day. He had become progressively weaker, unable to remember things or to recognize his surroundings. He had complained a couple of times of a "buzzing noise" in his head and had heard the voice of a friend named James. This voice said over and over, "Do you want another drink? How about one more?"

At the time of admission to the hospital the patient was greatly agitated and disturbed. He talked about "James," who was "after me with a shotgun for messing around with his girl." At one time during the examination the patient emitted a loud scream and crawled under the table in great fright, saying that he was getting away from "James." Physical examination was done under sodium amytal sedation, but even so the patient continued to be so frightened that a complete examination was impossible. The main factors revealed were the patient's dehydration and a temperature of 102°.

This patient was sedated for two days following his admission, after which he became essentially clear but still amnesic for much that had occurred to him during his disoriented, disturbed period. He admitted that he did drink frequently but claimed that he had not been intoxicated for two years. He said that approximately two years previously he had had an illness similar to the present one and he described it with some show of anxiety as "in the bats." After approximately one week's time this patient had improved sufficiently to be discharged. It became evident that he had a long history of excessive alcoholism and had had at least one, if not more, acute episodes of hallucinosis characterized by the appearance of delusional material as well as vivid auditory and at times even visual hallucinations. The patient was unwilling or unable to follow through with further psychiatric help and, at the time of recovery from his psychotic episode, demanded his own discharge and was subsequently released. He failed to follow up with the further treatment which had been recommended for him.

DELIRIUM TREMENS

This syndrome refers to an acute psychotic toxic episode coming on in a chronic alcoholic who has imbibed an excessive amount of alcohol over a long period of time, usually for a number of years. This has been combined, as a rule, with a chronic state of malnutrition secondary to the excessive alcoholic intake. Delirium tremens ordinarily begins rather rapidly with the patient becoming exceedingly anxious, tense, and fearful, and then proceeds on to a typical psychotic reaction. The latter is characterized especially by illusions and hallucinations, particularly of a visual type. There is confusion, disorientation, and a general clouding of the sensorium. The patient often becomes quite hyperactive. There are marked tremors of the mouth, tongue, and outstretched fingers. The individual is fearful of everything about him and constantly misinterprets his surroundings, feeling that he is in great danger. He becomes so anxious and terrified that he may seriously injure himself trying to escape from his (hallucinated) tormentors. The hallucinations seen by an individual with delirium tremens are often of animals which are distorted in size, shape, and color. In many instances they are multiple, minute, and motile. Perhaps it is from this that the traditional pink-elephant stories have arisen. At times the patient with delirium tremens suffers hallucinations which are not particularly frightening and do not assume the fearful proportions that are more characteristic. We remember one such patient who saw small green men who apparently seemed to him quite comical in their behavior. He was not in the least afraid of them.

The reaction of delirium tremens goes on from perhaps three to ten days or longer and is an exhausting experience to the patient. This is particularly true if, as is usual, he is in a state of chronic malnutrition, and it is not at all rare that a patient dies literally from exhaustion during this syndrome. Such individuals may be unwilling to sleep or to accept food. Forcible restraint only makes matters worse and leads the patient to exhaust himself more completely. Frequently one finds that the most severe exacerbations of delirium tremens come at night, which is the time when the patient is most prone to misinterpret his surroundings, particularly with illusions.

During the period of recovery the patient may be reasonably clear during the day, only to become again overtly psychotic during the night.

Case History: Delirium Tremens

This thirty-seven-year-old male was admitted to the psychiatric ward after a four-day drinking spree which had terminated when he slashed his left wrist with a knife. The patient was obviously very agitated at the time of admission and still suffering from the effects of his alcoholic intake. He was unkempt and unshaven and appeared somewhat undernourished. It was impossible to get an adequate history from him on the night of his admission. General physical examination showed no obvious pathology except for the slashed wrist, which had not resulted in any great blood loss. He fell asleep shortly after the wrist was sutured and slept until the next morning. At that time he was somewhat more coherent and able to give a history. He stated that he had always made a fairly good adjustment in his work and in his general living pattern until approximately seven years prior to admission. At that time his wife divorced him in their seventh year of marriage. The patient stated that his wife had begun to run around with other men a year or two prior to their divorce. She had seriously neglected their two children and finally she had been arrested for drunkenness. Following this she was sent to a sanitarium where she remained for eight months. When she was released the patient, "like a fool," took her back with him after her promises that she would improve her behavior. Soon, however, she began to be unfaithful to him and at this time he divorced her. He said that he had always been an easy-going type of person and that he no longer felt upset about his divorce or the loss of his wife. After the divorce he began drinking heavily himself. Prior to this time he said that his drinking had been negligible. He enlisted in the Army shortly after the termination of hostilities and was overseas for approximately six months. During this time he drank quite heavily and gave a history of having had delirium tremens with auditory and visual hallucinations. These hallucinations concerned his children and his mother dying. He was returned to the United States because of this and was hospitalized for six months and finally given a medical discharge.

Since that time he had held innumerable jobs, usually working for three or four days and then spending his accumulated money on alcohol. He had delirium tremens twice after his Army discharge and prior to his admission to the hospital. Each episode ended in his slashing his left wrist. He stated during the history that he chose this wrist because he was a right-handed person.

During the ensuing days of his hospitalization, the patient appeared anxious, harassed, and restless in the daytime. At night he became more panicky and frequently complained of seeing snakes and bugs crawling around on the floor. At such times he would become extremely disturbed, yelling loudly for someone to help him. He would complain that he was tired of living and on several occasions threatened to commit suicide at the first opportunity. During the day, when the patient was more rational and tractable, he freely admitted the fact that he used alcohol as what he called an "escape." It served him as a means of forgetting his present and past unhappiness. He said that he did not like the taste of alcohol and very much wanted to stop drinking. He had heard of Alcoholics Anonymous but had never sought their help. He had found himself, on the other hand, totally unable to leave liquor alone as long as it was available to him. He said that he was the only member of his family who abused alcohol and could not visit his family because "all the other members lecture to me about this."

His family history revealed that his mother and father had separated when he was fifteen years old. They had never gotten along well. His father had been generally disinterested in his children and had been irritable with and unkind to the patient's mother. She, on the other hand, had been overworked, having had six children and little support from her husband. She had grown gradually more careless and uninterested in the children so that at the time of and after the patient's birth very little care had been lavished on him. He quit school at the time of his parents' separation and went to work in order to help support his mother and ease her burden. He had never been a particularly happy person but felt that he had made a satisfactory adjustment until his unhappy marriage, which had finally culminated in divorce.

This patient was put on a high-vitamin diet supplemented with additional doses of vitamins. His general physical condition slowly improved and evidences of delirium tremens diminished. He was finally discharged approximately three weeks after his admission and was encouraged to seek the help of Alcoholics Anonymous. It was felt at that time that this organization would be of the most use to him because of his difficulty in profiting adequately from individual psychotherapeutic sessions. It was suggested to him that he could continue his psychotherapy as long as he wished but that this should be supplemented by his joining Alcoholics Anonymous.

TREATMENT OF DISORDERS DUE TO ALCOHOL

The abuse of alcohol signifies the presence of psychological problems. Any treatment, if it is to be successful and efficient, must be directed toward this underlying problem. Therapeutic measures directed solely toward the removal of superficial symptoms are of questionable value. The situation can be compared to the one existing when the patient presents a chief complaint of abdominal pain. To merely use measures toward removing this superficial symptom with no regard for its underlying etiology would be considered poor medicine. The underlying difficulty might possibly prove to be a temporary and relatively innocuous type of gastroenteritis, but it might possibly be a tumor. The physician who pays little heed to the underlying pathology is certainly not practicing good medicine.

The individual who abuses alcohol is psychologically sick. This is true whether he is the ordinary chronic alcoholic or whether he is suffering from acute hallucinosis or even delirium tremens. Unfortunately, in the usual case, only extraordinary abuse of alcohol leads to medical consultation being obtained. Prior to this the ordinary individual is resentful of any reference to his excessive intake or pathological use of alcohol and is more than apt to resist attempts to help him. His own narcissism prevents him from recognizing that he is rapidly becoming a victim of the abuse of alcohol.

As with any other psychiatric condition, the will and consent of the patient to seek help are extremely important ingredients in successful therapy. Until such time as the patient can be convinced of the fact that he has difficulties with alcohol, it is often impossible to be of much assistance to him. The inept approach utilized by many close relatives and friends of alcoholics is unfortunately unsuccessful in most cases. For instance, the woman who is married to a chronic alcoholic probably married him with a full knowledge of his immature characteristics and his tendency to abuse alcohol. She fancied herself in the role of a reforming mother, even though intellectually she was aware that the cure of alcoholism is not possible by this means. Investigations have frequently revealed the presence in such women of a large masochistic element which leads them, in spite of their conscious objections, to an inner acceptance of the disgrace, punishment, and sadism heaped upon them by such husbands.

We may therefore say that the initial and probably essential foundation upon which the successful treatment of the patient who abuses alcohol is based is his recognition that alcohol is a problem for him. Such a recognition may come slowly or perhaps rapidly, as, for instance, after an acute attack of pathological intoxication or acute hallucinosis. It is unfortunately true that such patients utilize repeated alcoholic orgies to soften the painfulness of the difficulties into which they get themselves. It tends to be a progressively frequent retreat into the hazy unrealistic world of an alcoholic stupor. Such patients prefer not to face what they consider to be a harsh, cruel, unloving world. Actually, the world is not as harsh and unloving as they would seem to feel: they are really looking for a nirvana-like existence in which all of their wants and needs will be satisfied immediately and in which they will suffer no frustration at all.

Perhaps it can be seen by now that the cure of the average abuser of alcohol is an exceedingly difficult process. Such patients have been given a pathological start in life which has left them unable to tolerate the ordinary tensions and frustrations of living. They have found in alcohol a retreat to a more "pleasant" type of existence which is without cares or worries. Gradually, as their use of this retreat increases, they become less and less able to attain an adequate outer adjustment. The "morning after" is extremely painful with its return of reality and punishment from the superego and therefore these alcoholics are apt to resort to a further use of their drug. With many alcoholics, there is literally no point at which the therapist can begin. Any attempts to make the patient face again some of the realities of living are apt to cause him only to retreat once more to alcohol. As he begins to form an attachment to the therapist, even a minor frustration or unintended slight may result in another alcoholic debauch.

The most hopeful treatment of the alcoholic occurs when the patient himself recognizes the problem as one of some magnitude and comes of his own free will, seeking help. One of the prime requisites for the subsequent treatment is a willingness on the part of the patient to forgo completely the use of alcohol. At times, if the situation is not too serious, this may be accomplished on an outpatient basis. Unfortunately, it often must be performed within the confines of an institution. However, it must be remembered that, although it is relatively easy to prevent an individual from drinking while he is institutionalized, the important criterion for the success of the treatment is whether or not he can maintain his abstinence subsequent to discharge. Many a patient has been "successfully treated" while he is in a hospital. The promises and guarantees given to the physician are numerous; however, a fairly large number of these patients, when again faced with the problems of ordinary living which beset them prior to their admission, resort to the use of alcohol after their discharge.

From a psychological standpoint, then, the adequate therapy of the alcoholic patient initially revolves around helping him to arrange his living schedules and routines in such a way as to provide him with a well-balanced life. Then it is essential for him to realize that he is, by virtue of his psychological and physiological construction, unable to use alcohol at all. He must be made aware of the fact that he will not be able to drink "socially," because it is an established fact that even one or two drinks are sufficient to begin the entire cycle of alcoholism again. And finally, the patient must be helped to understand more about the inner workings of his own personality through increased insight. He must be helped to understand how relatively childish his relationships with others have been, in the sense that he has been a comparatively selfish person. The relationship which the alcoholic tends to form between himself and the therapist is an extremely dependent one in which the patient is prone to make great demands upon the therapist. As one might expect, his tolerance of frustration is low and in many instances, unless his demands are immediately met or astutely interpreted, he is apt to begin again to resort to alcohol as a way out of his frustration.

It must be said here that medical and psychiatric treatment for chronic alcoholism has not been overwhelmingly successful. Any description of the therapy of this condition would be incomplete without mention of the national organization, Alcoholics Anonymous.[1] During the past few years this organization has grown to remarkable proportions and has achieved a better-than-average record in the treatment of chronic alcoholism. The organization was founded by, and is at present composed of, former chronic alcoholics. It is founded upon several ideas, one of which is that only an individual who has suffered the difficulties and tribulations of chronic alcoholism is in a position to thoroughly understand and adequately help alcoholics. A great deal of emphasis is placed upon the religious aspects of living. The members of Alcoholics Anonymous join the organization voluntarily and in so doing pledge themselves to help others who are suffering from the same difficulty. They meet at scheduled intervals and hold open discussions concerning the difficulties which they have faced. There is then set up a sort of group relationship in which each person is faced with the same problems as all the rest and each dedicates himself to trying to help the others. The membership of Alcoholics Anonymous includes both the prominent and the unknown, the wealthy and the poor. The only requirements for admission are a desire to join and a willingness to work under the group principles. Certainly this organization has done a great deal to further our understanding of and dealing with the large group of chronic alcoholics.

Another method of therapy for chronic alcoholism deserves mention under the psychological approach. This is the so-called "conditioned response" treatment. Essentially it involves the establishment of an aversion to alcohol as a conditioned reflex. There can be little argument as to the at least temporary success of such a method of treatment, even though its prolonged effects are ordinarily insufficient. In addition to this, it certainly must be stressed that the establishment of such an aversion response to alcohol does nothing to ameliorate the underlying psychopathology which led to the abuse of alcohol in the first place. This treatment involves the administration of palatable mixtures of the usual varieties of alcohol shortly following the administration of some emetic. The patient, of course,

[1] William, W. "The Society of Alcoholics Anonymous." *American Journal of Psychiatry*, CVI, 1949.

vomits and after a repeated "conditioning" is rendered averse to alcohol in any form. Ordinarily this treatment must be given in an institution and only to those patients whose physical condition is sufficiently healthy to withstand its rigors. Patients must be cured of delirium tremens, acute hallucinosis, and other signs of vitamin deficiency prior to such therapy. Their nutritional state must also be adequate. Attempts are made to condition the senses of sight, taste, and smell to alcohol during the treatment. The patient is given his drinks in ordinary shot glasses, utilizing regular whisky. The patient is encouraged to smell, look at, and also taste the whisky. He is told that the treatment will result in his developing a great dislike for liquor in any form. Prior to the giving of the whisky itself, the patient is given one of the emetics such as emetine hydrochloride. Such treatment is ordinarily given daily over a period of perhaps a week or even slightly more. By the time the treatment is near its end, even the taste of liquor is capable of producing vomiting in many patients. However, once again it must be stressed that treatment of this type is ordinarily successful perhaps for only three to six months, and in many cases even less. In order to be reasonably successful this aversion type of therapy must be complemented or supplemented by psychotherapy.

Any discussion on the treatment of alcoholism would be incomplete without mention of the drug popularly known as Antabuse which is actually tetraethylthiuramdisulfide. If patients are given appropriate doses of this drug, it has been found that they react violently to the effects of alcohol. The autonomic nervous system is thrown out of balance; the patient suffers from severe nausea and vomiting as well as palpitations and other symptoms. The theory behind the use of this drug is that its effect produces such a remarkably distasteful reaction if alcohol is imbibed that patients are thereby discouraged from drinking. The ordinary patient can be maintained on a dose of perhaps a half a gram a day after having been given a half a gram three times a day for a couple of days and then gradually tapering off to the maintenance dose. Patients are ordinarily given a carefully controlled "test" with this drug after they have been put on a maintenance dose. They are allowed to see the violence of their reaction under a controlled situation and this also contributes to their abstinence in the future.

There are several disadvantages to the use of this drug. In the first place it is not a real "cure" for alcoholism. At best it must be utilized in conjunction with psychotherapeutic interviews. It also requires the permission and willingness on the part of the patient to participate in its use. It is relatively easy for the noncooperative patient to reject surreptitiously or even regurgitate his Antabuse so that he will be free to imbibe alcohol. It is also essential that both the patient and his family realize the extreme toxic effects which can result from an excessive intake of alcohol while taking this drug. Death may result from the use of alcohol while the patient is on Antabuse. It is essential that the patient have frequent examinations by a physician which should include laboratory studies, especially those involving the status of the blood and blood-producing areas. It should be remembered that the chronic alcoholic patient is a psychologically disturbed individual whose emotional problems make him a questionable candidate for the use of such a dangerous drug. Only under the most optimal conditions in which both the patient and his family are cooperative in the treatment procedure may Antabuse be utilized as a temporary crutch while psychotherapeutic endeavors are being made.

The treatments for the more acute episodes inherent in delirium tremens, pathological intoxication, and acute hallucinosis are of importance and will be discussed here. However, it must be remembered that they are only the beginning of a much more prolonged therapeutic approach to a psychologically ill individual. Delirium tremens, as we have mentioned, is an acute severe toxic reaction in which the patient is manifestly psychotic. He is extremely fearful and agitated, and if allowed to go untreated may die during the psychotic episode. It is obvious that, first of all, all alcohol must be withdrawn. A general medical evaluation is essential in the early stages to determine the physical condition of the patient. The use of tranquilizing drugs has markedly improved our ability to prevent or diminish the exhausting effects of delirium tremens. Much of the patient's energy may be conserved by proper tranquilization, combined with the presence of a reassuring, understanding, calm attendant who is able further to alleviate the patient's anxiety. Even more important, the onset of delirium tremens can often be prevented by the proper use of tranquilizing agents in those patients who seem on the verge of this acute psychosis. It is essential, however, to remember that many of these patients have seriously damaged livers and, therefore, the use of a tranquilizer must be carefully controlled. The administration of glucose, insulin, and vitamins, although valuable, are probably somewhat less important than judicious tranquilization. Obviously it may be necessary, depending upon the patient's physical condition, to utilize other therapeutic measures such as digitalis in the presence of heart failure, or antibiotics in the case of an incipient pneumonia. High doses of vitamins are useful, especially those of the vitamin-B complex.

Pathological intoxication and acute hallucinosis are relatively transient situations in which the primary therapeutic endeavors are directed first toward preventing the patient from any further intake of alcohol and secondly calming him and preventing him from doing anything which will be harmful to himself and others. Here again the tranquilizing drugs are helpful. These often should be given by injection rather than orally to obtain more rapid results. Any further immediate treatment is ordinarily indicated by the patient's physical and nutritional condition. Often such people are suffering from other difficulties of an organic nature which require some type of treatment. The administration of large doses of vitamins is advisable. Most of these patients have an underlying personality difficulty which must be evaluated and a therapeutic regimen should be instituted aimed at the prevention of recurrence. Unfortunately such patients are often unwilling subjects for psychotherapy and prefer to continue taking tranquilizers rather than to undertake uncovering psychotherapy. The alcoholic patient is seldom deterred from returning to his previous drinking pattern by the use of medication alone, and may in fact combine tranquilizing or sedative medication with his alcohol intake. Close relatives should be advised concerning the difficulties which the patient has and urged to participate in a program which will eventually result in the patient receiving adequate help.

ACUTE BRAIN SYNDROME ASSOCIATED WITH TRAUMA

When an individual suffers a head injury the immediate as well as the eventual psychological outcome depends upon several factors. The most obvious factor is the degree and type of trauma, which, of course, regulates the amount and type of actual brain destruction that takes place. The brain, enclosed as it is in a bony structure and surrounded by cerebrospinal fluid, is capable of absorbing considerable traumatic insult without permanent injury to its structure. An extremely important factor concerning the eventual outcome of head injury is the organic condition of the brain at the time that the injury is sustained. If the individual, for instance, suffers from asymptomatic paresis or arteriosclerosis the results of the trauma are apt to be much more evident and even chronic than if these conditions are not present. Equally important is the psychological structure of the personality of the patient. All of these factors, namely the degree and type of head injury, the organic state of the brain itself, and the psychological maturity of the personality, are involved in the eventual outcome of head injuries, making proper evaluation often extremely difficult.

There is undoubtedly a tendency on the part of many physicians, as well as the courts, to attribute more importance to the effects of trauma than is warranted. It is fortunate, however, that the more recent classification of mental disorders by the American Psychiatric Association has dropped the term "traumatic psychoses" and substituted the terms "acute brain syndrome associated with trauma" and "chronic brain syndrome associated with trauma." It is comparatively rare that the trauma itself is responsible for the production of a true psychotic picture.

This section is concerned with those acute syndromes which result from trauma and which are temporary in nature. The most common is *concussion syndrome*. This indicates merely the loss of consciousness at the time of head injury and, upon the return of consciousness, the presence of amnesia for the incident itself and often for events for a few minutes prior to the accident. Concussion may or may not be accompanied by contusion. If it is not, there is no demonstrable evidence of injury to the brain structure itself. The spinal fluid will show neither pressure changes nor the presence of blood. In the presence of contusion there is evidence of actual injury to the brain structure, to a varying degree. In simple concussion the patient usually recovers consciousness within a few minutes or an hour or two and shows few if any residual mental effects. In the more severe cases, particularly in the presence of contusion, the patient may lapse into a comatose state where he will remain for varying lengths of time. Following this there may be a gradual emergence into a delirious state with slow recovery.

The type of reaction seen during such delirious states varies considerably. Often the patient shows considerable anxiety. On the other hand he may be quite confused or bewildered. Violence develops in some patients to the point where restraint is necessary. Others are extremely apathetic, listless, and unresponsive. Some patients during a delirium show a mental picture ordinarily associated with Korsakoff's syndrome. While the latter is usually associated with chronic alcoholism, it is possible to have it appear on a more temporary basis as a result of head trauma. Korsakoff's syndrome is characterized chiefly by the patient's tendency to lie. Such individuals may appear superficially happy, well adjusted, and in command of all their mental faculties. However, questioning them soon elicits severe memory defects which they attempt to cover by their ingenious fabrications. They frequently contradict themselves during a conversation and become angry if the contradictions are called to their attention.

ACUTE BRAIN SYNDROME ASSOCIATED WITH CIRCULATORY DISTURBANCE

Central nervous system tissue is particularly susceptible to impairment of blood supply. If such a disturbance is of a temporary nature, the personality distortion which results will be reversible. From a psychiatric standpoint the most important personality difficulties resulting from circulatory impairment fall within the chronic brain syndrome category and most of them are due to cerebral arteriosclerosis. However, hypertension, cerebral embolism, and especially cardiac failure are conditions capable of producing acute brain syndromes of a reversible nature. As the underlying circulatory problem is brought under control the psychiatric symptoms subside.

Case History: Acute Brain Syndrome Associated with Circulatory Disturbance

This twenty-six-year-old married female was hospitalized for cardiac evaluation. She had had three previous hospitalizations in the past seven years, all for a combination of respiratory infections and cardiac difficulties.

She had a long history of severe respiratory infections since early childhood. She had been told that she had "a weak heart" as early as the age of three. During her previous respiratory infection, which eventually became a pneumonia, she developed an edema. She had for two years prior to admission complained of shortness of breath on exertion, and along with her respiratory infections had developed, on several occasions, a palpable enlarged liver and a poor urinary output.

At the time of admission the patient was also found to be suffering from a mild attack of bronchitis, with evidence of cardiac failure. She responded poorly to treatment for the relief of the failure; she ate poorly and became quite depressed about her general physical condition.

On the evening of her seventeenth day in the hospital she was found to be in poor contact with her surroundings: she developed a blank stare and was unable to answer questions except with "yes" or "no." At times she repeated in a meaningless way such phrases as "I feel good" and "Scrub the kitchen floor." She was unable to name objects or persons in her surroundings.

By the next morning she was considerably improved and within forty-eight hours there was no further sign of disorientation and her spirits were generally improved. Her acute psychotic episode resolved itself rapidly, in other words, with the improvement in her cardiovascular status.

ACUTE BRAIN SYNDROME ASSOCIATED WITH INTRACRANIAL NEOPLASM

Personality disturbance may or may not accompany the growth of an intracranial neoplasm. Such symptoms as are present may be predominantly a result of pressure and of edema and may be relieved with surgery. If, however, the brain-tissue damage is irreversible and the personality changes remain, this condition will be diagnosed as a chronic syndrome.

Case History: Acute Brain Syndrome Associated with Intracranial Neoplasm

This fifty-two-year-old male was admitted to the hospital with a history of rather vague complaints for about fourteen months. His difficulty had begun with some complaints about visual disturbances, particularly with his left eye. He also had begun complaining of occasional occipital headaches. He visited two or three physicians without receiving much relief. He also began to develop a depression, as well as difficulty in sleeping, at about the same time. A few weeks later there was an onset of occasional vomiting. Some six months prior to his admission he spent two weeks in another hospital, where the vomiting ceased. The patient's headaches became increasingly severe and seemed present almost constantly. His depression increased and, four months prior to admission, he was given a series of fourteen electroshock treatments. He remained in a convalescent home at that time for approximately three weeks. His condition seemed to improve somewhat at the time, but once more took a turn for the worse after his return home. He began to experience vertigo and on two or three occasions had apparently fainted. He developed a difficulty with speech which resembled stuttering. He began having more generalized headaches which involved the frontal and parietal areas, as well as the occipital area.

At the time of admission the patient revealed the following neurological abnormalities: There was a nystagmus on looking to the right, to the left, and upward. The disks were choked. The left corneal reflex was diminished. There was impairment of pain on the right side of the face. Deep reflexes were increased bilaterally and there was ankle clonus bilaterally. Also, there was a Hoffmann sign bilaterally, but no Babinskis.

A craniotomy was done and revealed a cholesteatoma of the fourth ventricle. Postoperative course was uneventful and the patient was subsequently discharged markedly improved. There had been a remission of all psychiatric symptoms and the depression no longer manifested itself.

CHAPTER 19

Chronic Brain Disorders

THE CENTRAL nervous system, like any other system of the body, may have its proper function disturbed by disease, injury, or physiological malfunction. If such pathological processes produce irreversible chronic changes in the parenchymatous or interstitial area of the brain, the resulting personality distortion is more or less permanent. The symptomatology resulting from such changes may, as is true in acute brain syndromes, be of a mild or severe nature. Severe symptomatology often reaches psychotic proportions. It may be fairly localized, but is more often diffuse in nature. The type and degree of symptoms depend upon the particular pathological process which is involved. Such chronic organic brain syndromes are to be differentiated from disorders of psychogenic origin which are also of a chronic nature and include schizophrenic reactions, manic depressive reactions, and the psychoneurotic disorders. In these no consistent evidences of organic changes are to be found. Chronic brain syndromes are also to be differentiated from the acute brain syndromes, which are reversible in nature and do not involve a permanent disturbance of personality function.

There are certain psychopathological changes which are fairly characteristic of many of the chronic diffuse organic brain syndromes. A careful history often elicits the fact that there has been a slow progressive accentuation of the patient's previous personality idiosyncrasies. These may have been relatively minor in his premorbid make-up but have assumed major proportions as the pathological process continued. Suspiciousness, for instance, may progress to the point of actual paranoid delusions. A brilliant, optimistic personality may reveal progressively less restraint and optimism may reach the stage of hypomanic behavior. The individual who has ordinarily been shy becomes seclusive. As the disease process continues there is a gradual deterioration in the patient's level of adjustment. Whereas he may have been previously well-adjusted, his social behavior, mode of dress, and ability to work become impaired. There is a loss of ability to distinguish between finer points in ordinary conversation. Emotional stability is lost and affect becomes quite labile. Minor provocation is apt to produce wide mood swings. Crying, laughter, or anger, at least in the later stages of these conditions, is brought on by trivial causes. As the process continues there is a growing defect of the sensorium. The patient has difficulty with orientation, particularly as to time and place. His grasp of current affairs and general information is impaired. His memory begins to fail, often, at least in the early stages, seeming to be patchy, with areas that are retained intact and others which are lost.

The exact changes through which each individual patient will go vary with the type of pathological process and, at least in the beginning phases, with the type of premorbid personality which has been present. Initially there is an accentuation of the psychopathological features of this premorbid personality but eventually, as the organic destruction increases, the individual reaches a state of total personality disintegration and disorganization which is essentially a psychotic picture.

We can discuss here only the most common organic brain syndromes. The student should remember that any agent which is capable of producing localized or diffuse brain destruction of lasting nature is capable of producing a chronic organic brain syndrome.

The importance of chronic brain syndromes is illustrated by the fact that about one-third of first admissions to psychiatric hospitals in the United States are patients within this category. Their importance is even more evident when one remembers that these patients suffer permanent, lasting personality distortion which, although it may be somewhat improved by treatment, often results in hospitalization for the remainder of the individuals' lives.

CHRONIC BRAIN SYNDROME ASSOCIATED WITH CON-
GENITAL CRANIAL ANOMALY, CONGENITAL SPASTIC
PARAPLEGIA, MONGOLISM, PRENATAL MATERNAL
INFECTIOUS DISEASE, BIRTH TRAUMA

This category includes the various conditions resulting in permanent organic brain damage which occur before or at the time of
birth. Many of these conditions are associated with mental retardation and are discussed in Chapter 20. Examples are mongolism,
hydrocephalus, microcephaly, and congenital spastic paraplegia. Although these conditions continue to be officially coded under Chronic
Brain Syndromes, the marked upsurge in national interest in mental
retardation has led to their commonly being considered within the
area of that complex syndrome. It is for this reason that they are
discussed in Chapter 20 rather than here.

CHRONIC BRAIN SYNDROME ASSOCIATED WITH
CENTRAL NERVOUS SYSTEM SYPHILIS

Syphilis is a disease which reaches back into antiquity and has
been studied by every branch of medicine. Specialists in all fields are
acquainted with the many syndromes which this disease can produce. Psychiatrists have long had an interest in this disease because
of its ability to attack the central nervous system. The latter invasion
by the *Treponema pallidum* occurs in one of two broad ways: either
it primarily involves the parenchymatous tissue, thus producing general paresis; or it attacks the interstitial tissue, producing a meningovascular disorder. Such divisions are not rigid, since the spirochete
invades the whole central nervous system. However, there does tend
to be predominant damage appearing in one or the other of the
areas mentioned.

General paresis is the meningoencephalitic form of syphilis. It is
a type of tertiary lues and is the direct result of the invasion of the
parenchymatous tissue of the brain by the *Treponema pallidum*.
While clinical descriptions of this syndrome were written many
years ago, it was only during the latter part of the last century that
it began to be linked with syphilis. It remained for the development

of the Wassermann test in 1906 and the demonstration of the syphilis organism in microscopic studies of paretic brains by Noguchi and Moor in 1913 to finally establish the luetic etiology. Meningovascular syphilis is a type of lues in which the primary pathological processes are confined to the interstitial structures. It often proves to be more of a neurological than a psychiatric entity and not infrequently simulates neurological signs found in other conditions, thus making clinical diagnosis difficult without the aid of laboratory studies.

The advent of antibiotics, particularly penicillin, has markedly reduced the frequency of all types of central nervous system syphilis. Some forty years ago these represented more than ten per cent of admissions to mental hospitals, while at the present time they probably comprise less than one per cent. Various public-health measures have led to earlier detection of primary syphilis and the remarkable efficiency of penicillin has been instrumental in our partial victory over this disease.

The widespread use of antibiotics for the treatment of numerous other conditions has undoubtedly led to either the cure or amelioration of syphilitic disease in many individuals. Statistics can never reveal how many unrecognized cases of syphilis have been arrested in this fashion. Certainly it is true that today state hospitals admit only a rare case of central-nervous-system syphilis, whereas in the past these formed a sizable percentage of their new population.

Paresis usually has a prolonged incubation period. Ordinarily, from the time of the appearance of the initial lesion to the onset of paresis, anywhere from five to thirty years may have elapsed, but in a majority of cases it is somewhere near fifteen years. Occasionally one sees a case where the appearance of symptoms occurs in less than five years, but this is quite rare. The so-called fulminating type of paresis involves the appearance of symptomatology within one year of initial infection. The individual may first realize that he has syphilis when the diagnosis of paresis is made.

ETIOLOGY AND PATHOLOGY

General paresis is due to the invasion of the parenchymatous tissue of the brain by the spirochete of syphilis. The brain of a paretic is smaller than usual, with a widening of the sulci due to atrophy, particularly in the frontal and parietal areas. All of the meninges are thickened. The pia arachnoid adheres to the underlying brain structure so that attempts to peel it off tear pieces of brain tissue beneath. Microscopically there are vascular changes involving endothelial proliferation and capillary sprouting. Perivascular infiltration produces a cufflike appearance around the smallest vessels, and there is an infiltration of lymph spaces with an abundance, particularly, of plasma cells. Lymphocytes are also characteristically present. In addition there is evidence of varying degrees of destruction of ganglion cells which results in the distortion of the normal architecture and loss of normal lamination. There is a marked increase in glia cells. Of particular importance is the appearance of the so-called "rod cells." These are especially important because of their tendency to concentrate the iron pigment found in the brains of paretics and they are demonstrable by using a Prussian blue stain. It is possible to demonstrate the presence of *Treponema pallidum* in the brains of more than 80 per cent of paretics if the proper technique is utilized.

Meningovascular syphilis may be predominantly meningeal or vascular. The meningeal type may be acute or chronic; the vascular type may attack either the large or small cerebral vessels, although more frequently the latter. Thrombotic and obliterative changes as well as aneurisms occur. Both meningeal and vascular neurosyphilis tend to make their appearance somewhat sooner after the primary infection than does general paresis.

Several laboratory tests are of particular importance. The complement fixation test developed by Wassermann is positive in the vast majority of cases on both blood and cerebral fluid. In addition, Lange's gold colloid reaction is important. The cerebral spinal fluid reveals an increase in cells as well as in protein.

SYMPTOMATOLOGY

The onset of general paresis is often insidious and there may be difficulty in determining exactly when the process began. The patient begins to show a general change in behavior which eventually results in a progressive disintegration of his personality. He is careless about his behavior and his appearance becomes sloppy. He may develop impulsive behavior and a tendency toward sexual promiscuity and indiscretion. He loses his ability to see the finer differences between related things and his thinking becomes progressively worse. His judgment fails and his memory is impaired. As he continues to deteriorate, his speech becomes thickened and slurred and he has difficulty enunciating phrases such as "Methodist Episcopal" or "Massachusetts Institute of Technology." Neurological signs vary, but pupillary abnormalities are extremely common. These include pupillary irregularities or sluggishness, or even an absence of response to light and at times to accommodation. The Argyll-Robertson pupil appears in slightly over half of these cases: the absence of the light reflex with the presence of accommodation.

In meningovascular syphilis the symptomatology depends upon the type of blood vessels involved as well as the area. There is often interference with cranial nerves, particularly when there is meningeal involvement. Irritability, insomnia, and loss of ability to work, as well as headaches, dizziness, and focal neurological symptoms are common.

Case History: Paresis

This forty-two-year-old woman was brought to the hospital by her grown daughter. According to the latter, the onset of the present illness was approximately three days prior to admission. On this particular day the patient had gone to her employer to request time off from work to go to the hospital in the near future. Her employer acceded to her request but inexplicably the patient began to cry. The employer advised her to take a few minutes to calm herself and then return to work if she felt well enough. However, the patient failed to return to her office that day. Later in the day she telephoned her daughter stating that she was coming to visit her "sometime after dark so no one can see me." The daughter was upset by her mother's behavior over the telephone; when she tried to return the telephone call, she found that her mother had had her telephone disconnected. When the patient failed to appear at her daughter's home that evening, the daughter went to her mother's home next day, to be met by her mother's twin sister, who lived with the mother. The sister told the daughter that the patient had been sitting in her bedroom in the dark with the shades drawn without having taken off her clothes for an entire day and night.

When the daughter entered the bedroom the patient jumped up terrified, apparently fearing that two men had come for her. She told her daughter that the people for whom she worked were going to have her gassed and that some of the office girls were waiting outside for her with guns and a police wagon. The daughter was unable to calm the patient and finally the police were summoned. The police surgeon advised admission to the hospital, which required another twenty-four hours to accomplish. During this time the patient was kept at the home of her daughter where she was extremely disturbed. She was difficult to manage, confused, occasionally belligerent, and at times physically assaultive. She climaxed her stay at her daughter's home by leaping from the second-story window. Fortunately she landed in a bush, which broke her fall, and she suffered no serious injuries.

At the time of admission she appeared to be confused but superficially co-operative. She was quite suspicious from time to time but attempted to answer questions. Many of her answers proved to be illogical and at times irrelevant. She gave her age as three years older than it actually was. She said that she had been married twice, which was true, but from then on her history became increasingly incoherent. Her story of her first marriage had many contradictions in it. She elaborated a long and complicated tale of the peculiar behavior of the people at the place where she worked. She felt that they were all watching her and accusing her of misdemeanors. She felt that they were talking about her and was thoroughly convinced that they all had a plot to "frame" her for these misdemeanors. She told again how she went to her daughter's home, saying, "There was a man who said he would come there and get me. Finally, when I heard him coming, I had to jump out of the window. It didn't do me any good because two policemen were waiting for me and they brought me here and I am sure that they are going to shoot me." During the interview the patient frequently took her false teeth out and replaced them. She was oriented for person, but not time nor place. Her mood varied markedly from a seemingly euphoric attitude to a suspicious, irritated demeanor. She was actively hallucinated, often claiming that she heard a noise at the window and fearing that it was made by the same man she claimed had caused her entire difficulty. From time to time she heard a woman calling her name and accusing her of various misdemeanors at her place of work. Her memory was exceedingly poor, both past and present. She was unable to place adequately the time of her birth, the most important events of her childhood, the dates of her marriages, or even the date of the birth of her daughter. Judgment was markedly impaired. Insight was absent in that she denied that there was anything wrong with her thinking. She felt that she was somewhat run down physically and needed only a short time to rest.

Physical examination revealed normal temperature, pulse, and respiration. She was a fairly well-developed female in no apparent physical distress. She had a few contusions as a result of her jump out the window. Pupils were small, equal, but somewhat irregular. External ocular movements were intact. Reaction to accommodation was present but not reaction to light. The heart was enlarged slightly but otherwise essentially negative. The remainder of the physical examination was not particularly significant.

Originally it was felt that this patient was probably a paranoid schizophrenic. However, because the pupils did not react, a strong suspicion of paresis was entertained. Subsequently laboratory analysis confirmed the diagnosis. The Kolmer-Wassermann was positive, 32 units. Colloidal gold curve was 5554321000. Spinal fluid protein was 76 mg. per cent, Kahn positive 64 units. Subsequent laboratory studies confirmed the original findings and a diagnosis of paresis was made.

The patient was given 7,000,000 units of penicillin. Considerable improvement followed and within a few weeks the patient was able to return to the home of her daughter and resume her occupation. She subsequently moved back with her sister and until the present time has continued to make a satisfactory adjustment. There has been a marked diminution in the mental symptoms and the patient is relatively clear from a mental standpoint.

CHRONIC BRAIN SYNDROME ASSOCIATED WITH CENTRAL-NERVOUS-SYSTEM SYPHILIS (MENINGOVASCULAR)

Meningovascular syphilis is a type of lues in which the primary pathological processes are confined to the interstitial structures. It is, therefore, to be differentiated from general paresis (meningoencephalitic syphilis), in which the pathology is primarily parenchymatous. Meningovascular syphilis is often referred to as "psychosis with cerebral syphilis." Meningovascular syphilis often proves to be much more of a neurological entity than a psychiatric one, frequently simulating the neurological signs found in many other conditions and thus making clinical diagnosis difficult without the aid of laboratory studies.

Meningovascular syphilis is ordinarily subdivided into meningeal and vascular types. It must be recognized that although one or another of these particular types may predominate in a case, there is frequently seen an admixture of the two with a consequent variation in symptomatology and neurological findings. Generally speaking, meningovascular lues is apt to make its appearance somewhat sooner after the primary infection than does general paresis, often appearing in a few months to three, four, or five years.

Meningeal neurosyphilis may occur in an acute or chronic form. In the acute form there is a much slower onset than is seen in the meningococcal form of meningitis, but many of the signs are similar, including a stiff neck, headache, temperature rise, and frequent disturbance of extraocular muscles. It is of practical importance to note here that inadequate earlier treatment for syphilis seems to play a prominent role in the development of subsequent meningeal neurosyphilis. The chronic form of meningeal neurosyphilis may follow the acute form or may appear as the first sign of meningeal lues. It again is often revealed by the presence of headache, vertigo, visual disturbances with extraocular paralyses and at times localized neurological signs depending upon the particular area of primary meningeal involvement.

In cases of luetic meningitis the cerebrospinal fluid reveals an increase in cells and protein with a luetic curve on the colloidal gold reaction and positive Wassermanns on both blood and cerebrospinal fluid.

Vascular neurosyphilis, as the name would indicate, refers to those cases in which there is primarily involvement of the cerebral vessels, either large or small, although far more frequently small. A secondary result of the thrombotic and obliterative as well as aneurism changes in the vessels is an ischemia of the parenchymatous areas. Vascular syphilis often reveals its presence through headaches, dizziness, and the onset of focal neurological symptoms. The patient may awaken in the morning without any complaints, only to find that he is suffering from a hemiplegia. Depending upon the size of the vessel and the extent of involvement, there are varying degrees of interference with personality function. Irritability, insomnia, loss of ability to work, and various changes in the sensorium are apt to occur. Again there is often involvement of the cranial nerves, particularly since some degree of meningeal involvement is often present. Once again, the Wassermann on both the cerebrospinal fluid and the blood is ordinarily positive. The colloidal gold reaction shows a luetic curve and there is an increase of protein in the cerebrospinal fluid. There is some tendency toward reversibility of symptoms in this type of lues, so the ultimate degree of incapacitation cannot be judged immediately.

Case History: Chronic Brain Syndrome Associated with Central Nervous System Syphilis (Meningovascular)

This forty-six-year-old male was admitted to the hospital in a confused, disoriented state, complaining of weakness of his arms and difficulty in walking properly. A history obtained from his wife revealed the following incidents. About seven months prior to admission he had a transient episode of weakness of his arms and legs with an unsteady gait, slow speech, and forgetfulness. However, this episode lasted only a few days. Then, about six months later, he was visited at home by a group of friends and was at that time dazed and confused. This state also lasted only about two days. About a month after this, while he was watching television, he became extremely excited, fell out of his chair to the floor, and had a generalized convulsion. He was seen at that time by his family physician and referred to the clinic. At that time he was given fifteen injections of penicillin and there was some improvement in his condition. He also developed a skin reaction to penicillin. Several days later there was a transitory episode: his right arm was partly paralyzed. The next day he took an electric motor apart for no apparent reason. On the following day he slept all day. When he awoke in the evening he was hallucinated, claiming that he saw little round objects under his bed. He also saw a red dog and a cow in his bedroom. He became frightened, saying that he saw a cat clinging to his daughter's blouse. Later in the evening he had another convulsive seizure. The following day he cried, saying that he had pains in his stomach and wished that he would die. He screamed and used profanity whenever a member of his family approached him, claimed that he was being held prisoner, and apparently did not realize that he was in his own home.

That same day a friend brought him a basket of fruit which he refused, saying that it contained a bomb.

The following day he slept all day but was awake all night carrying on a conversation with former business associates he hallucinated, some of whom had been dead for years. This behavior continued for approximately three days; then he was admitted to the hospital.

This patient had been married for twenty-one years and had four children. His wife had had no miscarriages or stillbirths and was said to be in good health. The patient had a good reputation in his business and in his neighborhood until the onset of the present illness. He always had many friends and was very generous with anyone with whom he came in contact. He had been employed at the same establishment for twenty-six years.

Physical examination was essentially negative except for the following: He was lying on a bed and unable to lift his legs. There was a marked weakness of the leg muscles on testing and a less-pronounced weakness of all the muscles of his arms. Tendon reflexes were hyperactive in both upper and lower extremities. Abdominal reflexes were absent. The Babinski reflex was equivocal bilaterally. The patient could stand up with assistance, but was unable to maintain himself in a standing position. Any attempt to walk was successful only for a few steps, when he had to grasp something to remain standing. There was incoordination on the finger-to-nose test, much worse when his eyes were closed. Electrocardiogram was normal. Pupils reacted to light and accommodation.

Mental examination revealed that the patient was disoriented as to time and place. His memory was poor for recent events and he had no idea of the year or of his family doctor's name. He couldn't say where he was at the moment. He named as President of the United States a man who had been President eight years before. He was unable to name the governor of his state. His speech was slightly slurred. He had no insight into the fact that he was ill.

Laboratory findings revealed a positive spinal Wassermann, Kahn protein of 62, white cells 13. He had a positive blood serology and the colloid gold curve was 3344332000.

Treatment consisted of the administration of 9,000,000 units of benzanthine penicillin given in doses of 3,000,000 units at weekly intervals. Improvement was quite marked in the early stages, but eventually the patient leveled off and remained somewhat unstable and irritable. He died a year later from a ruptured cerebral aneurysm.

CHRONIC BRAIN SYNDROME ASSOCIATED WITH OTHER CENTRAL-NERVOUS-SYSTEM SYPHILIS

Included here are the comparatively rare cases of syphilis which do not fall within the previous two categories. The most important type included under this heading is gumma, but even that is an infrequent type of syphilitic cerebral involvement. When it occurs it is apt to simulate brain tumor, although such patients show a higher incidence of epileptic seizures. At times serious hemorrhage into the gumma may occur and yield all the signs of shock without any external evidences of bleeding. At times rupture of the gumma with seeding may occur and give rise to an acute syphilitic meningitis.

TREATMENT OF NEUROSYPHILIS

Treatment of all forms of neurosyphilis has been revolutionized since the discovery of antibiotics. Penicillin has proved to be an excellent therapeutic agent in this disease, and has almost completely displaced other methods of treatment. Some years ago fever therapy, produced by malaria organisms, mechanical means, or by foreign proteins, was commonly used. At the present time these therapies are no longer in use.

According to the U.S. Public Health Service[1] the treatment recommended for neurosyphilis is benzanthine penicillin G, 6 to 9 million units total given in 3-million units at seven-day intervals. They recommend as an alternative 6 to 9 million units of PAM given in one 1.2-million units at three-day intervals. Or, as a further alternate, aqueous procaine penicillin 6 to 9 million units given in 600,000 units daily. It is further recommended that if the cell count does not return to normal within one year, or if either the cells or protein increase during the follow-up period, further treatment is indicated.

[1] Public Health Service Publication #743, Revised July 1961. U.S. Government Printing Office, Washington, D.C. 1961.

CHRONIC BRAIN SYNDROME ASSOCIATED WITH INTRACRANIAL INFECTION OTHER THAN SYPHILIS

Invasion of the central nervous system by any organism may produce permanent organic changes. Probably the majority of such infections, exclusive of syphilis, are of an acute type and are so classified. However, a certain number of infections result in lasting personality distortion because of organic changes which are irreversible. Encephalitis epidemica is an important condition within this category, particularly since it often produces chronic irreversible brain damage resulting in severe behavior problems in youngsters. (This condition is also discussed in Chapter 5, dealing with emotional disorders in children.) At times a severe meningococcic meningitis may leave permanent brain impairment. It is of interest that the newer antibiotic treatment methods are proving a life-saving measure in certain cases of tuberculous meningitis; however, the authors have seen a small number of these cases who have continued to show marked mental impairment in spite of apparent "cure" of the active meningitic process. This situation will undoubtedly become more important as more of these cases are treated.

Case History: Chronic Brain Syndrome Associated with Intracranial Infection Other Than Syphilis

This six-year-old female was admitted to the hospital with a chief complaint of headache which had been present for approximately one month prior to admission. Two weeks before admission the patient had a bout of epistaxis. Approximately a week prior to admission she began to have projectile vomiting. Two days before she came to the hospital she began to complain of paresthesias of the lower extremities. At the time of admission physical examination showed a rectal temperature of 101°, pulse 124, respiration 28. The child was well developed, but acutely ill. Her neck was rigid. The impression upon admission was meningitis of unknown etiology. Lumbar puncture revealed a pressure of 210 mm. of water. The spinal fluid showed 326 cells, chlorides of 123 mg. per cent; another spinal tap several days later revealed a pressure of 590 mm. of water with 622 cells per cubic millimeter. Protein at that time was 170 milliequivalents, chlorides 166 mg. per cent. No acid-fast bacilli were found, but approximately two weeks later the laboratory reported that the three spinal-fluid cultures were positive for acid-fast bacilli. The youngster had been started on streptomycin, isoniazid, and p-amino-salicylic acid. She responded slowly over the next few months, so that after six months of hospitalization her symptoms of active tuberculous meningitis had all but subsided. She became more or less ambulatory but needed support.

Most conspicuous, however, was her continued marked behavior disorder which could not be handled adequately by the hospital staff. She was completely unmanageable in regard to medication, often refusing to eat or to take oral medicine. Her aggressive behavior was so marked that it was impossible to gavage-feed her. She was impulsively aggressive to anyone who happened to be near her bed. After a few months of treatment, she could smile and talk clearly, coherently, and intelligently, but would suddenly, for no apparent reason, strike out at whomever she was talking to. She was quite well-oriented and showed a good use of her intelligence. She was a very likable, friendly youngster, except for these frequent, unpremeditated outbursts of aggressiveness. Attempts were made to assign certain ward personnel to her for prolonged periods of time in an attempt to build up a better relationship, but even these people were the objects of her occasional outbursts. The slightest frustration or criticism would bring about such attacks. The patient was finally, after seven and a half months of hospitalization, discharged to her mother at home. The mother proved to be a warm, interested, loving person who made every effort to help the youngster bring her impulsiveness under control. However, five months after discharge from the hospital, it was still not possible to permit her freedom to play with other neighborhood youngsters because of these outbursts. An electroencephalogram done shortly after discharge showed marked cerebral impairment with a convulsive tendency. Incidentally, this child never did have a grand mal or other type of epileptic seizure. There has been no recurrence to date of the tuberculous meningitis, but it would appear that future improvement in the impulsive aggression of this child will probably be minimal.

CHRONIC BRAIN SYNDROME ASSOCIATED WITH INTOXICATION

Various toxic agents are capable of producing permanent damage to the brain structure. Among the more common are lead, arsenic, mercury, carbon dioxide, and illuminating gas, as well as various drugs. Perhaps most prominent, however, within this group, is alcohol. The typical example of the latter is Korsakoff's psychosis. This syndrome, originally described by Korsakoff, is in reality due to a vitamin deficiency. It is often, but certainly by no means always, secondary to the exaggerated use of alcohol. The most characteristic symptoms of this psychosis are a severely disturbed memory and a tendency on the part of the patient to cover this defect by remarkable fabrications. The patient is typically rather jovial, although at times he may become depressed or irritable. He is usually quite willing and even anxious to talk and superficially does not give the picture of being psychotic. However, upon closer attention it is found that much of what the patient is saying is of a purely confabulatory nature. He is prone to tell long and involved stories about where he has been and what he has been doing during the past twenty-four hours when, as a matter of fact, he has been in the hospital all the time. He ordinarily cannot remember the names of the attendants, doctors, or nurses and many times even of his relatives, although he is apt to greet and apparently recognize all of these people. Hallucinations are at times present. There is often found in conjunction with this syndrome an avitaminotic polyneuritis involving the neurones particularly of the extremities and at times even involvement of the brain stem. In this case the syndrome includes the so-called Wernicke's disease.

Korsakoff's psychosis may or may not follow delirium tremens. If it does so it is often impossible to tell where the delirium tremens ends and the Korsakoff begins. Ordinarily the latter may last anywhere from six weeks to three months and at times much longer, depending upon the severity of the condition at the time therapy is instituted. In some patients one finds only partial recovery with residual memory defects as well as intellectual impairment. In a large percentage of cases the condition becomes more or less chronic and irreversible.

Case History (1): Korsakoff's Psychosis

This forty-one-year-old male was admitted to the hospital after having been sent to a convalescent home as a chronic alcoholic, where he had spent approximately one month. On the night of his hospital admission he had apparently unscrewed the light bulb in his room, cut his wrist with it after breaking it, and subsequently wandered out into the street in his nightclothes. He had been disoriented and hallucinated and had talked about suicide. He was picked up by the police and brought to the hospital.

At the time of admission he was found to be poorly nourished, dehydrated, and extremely weak. His speech was irrelevant and incoherent. His general physical condition was poor and cor pulmonale was diagnosed secondary to emphysema. The patient was so ill that he was put on the critical list. However, he gradually began to improve and in four or five days became oriented as to person but still was disoriented as to time and place. He gave the date four years ahead of its proper time and yet named as President of the United States one who had been in office six years previously. He was unable to tell what hospital he was in and often called it the "medical and clerical hospital." He said that he had been in the hospital for three weeks on one occasion, three months on another occasion, and overnight on still another. He would relate that the previous night he had been out for a walk with his friends. He went on to deny vehemently that he ever drank anything: "I want that understood. I never touch that stuff." From time to time he would count the coins in his empty hand. On two or three occasions he complained that he saw snakes under his bed but said that he "saw no more than anybody else does." He explained at great length that the lacerations of his wrists, which were actually produced by cutting them with a light bulb, were the result of his girl's having rubbed her head against his wrist and scratched him with an ornament in her hair.

For the next few days the patient talked incessantly about someone being after him. He elaborated the idea that he was in prison. From time to time he kept calling for the "housekeeper" or the "waitress." At other times he wanted to know where "Joe" was, particularly at times when he wet or soiled himself. He gave his occupation as engineer, manager of a large automobile company, vice-president of a railroad, and carpenter, along with several other such fabrications. From time to time he became irritated about being kept in the hospital and said, "I'm going to the Supreme Court about this matter."

There were occasional evidences of further visual hallucinations when he saw "little tractors" on the floors and walls. He was capable of identifying simple objects presented to him but often fell asleep during an interview. His attention span was extremely short. When he could be gotten out of bed he showed a marked ataxia and walked with a broad base, pushing his feet along the floor. It was necessary to give him some support in his attempts to walk. Neurological examination revealed positive Babinskis and Oppenheims. There was diminished sensory response of his legs and a poor vibratory sense.

Treatment was essentially supportive, nutritional, and tranquilization. It became quite difficult to get him to drink water but he gradually and steadily improved. He grew somewhat more quiet and cheerful. He became continent and revealed a sense of humor that was a little bit too marked, often singing and cajoling the nurses into singing with him. He would answer questions without hesitance, although even several weeks after his admission there persisted very obvious fabrications. He was sent to the state hospital where he continued a marginal adjustment.

Case History (2): Korsakoff's Psychosis

This thirty-seven-year-old male patient was first seen by the psychiatric service through a consultation from the orthopedic department. He had been admitted to the hospital approximately one week prior to consultation, having suffered a fracture of the right leg in an unknown manner. He was brought to the accident dispensary by the police and was subsequently admitted to the hospital where the fracture was set and a cast applied. All attempts to obtain an accurate history had been to no avail, since the patient had apparently given many different histories with various conflicting data, none of which had proven accurate on further checking.

This man appeared to be a pleasant, fairly well-nourished man who talked readily to the examiner and seemed quite willing to co-operate. It had meantime been ascertained that he had sustained his fracture falling down a flight of stairs. He, however, maintained upon different occasions that he had broken his leg while skiing, while sleigh-riding, and, on one occasion he stated that it was because he was struck by an automobile. He said that he had been in the hospital some six weeks and that he was due to be discharged within a day or two. He gave the psychiatric examiner a history of having been married and having two children, although this conflicted markedly with other stories which he had given to other examiners. When he was asked to describe his wife he went into a very lengthy dissertation which became increasingly involved and filled with further fabrications. Throughout this he remained smiling, pleasant, and seemingly quite co-operative. He denied the fact that he had any difficulty with his thinking and said that his memory was excellent.

He was unable to remember the names of any of the nurses on the ward, although he had been in contact with them for approximately a week. He could not name any of the physicians who were caring for him and even misnamed the hospital. When he was asked about whether or not he had been in the last war he immediately answered, "Yes," and thereafter began a long story concerning the Army division with which he had served. He was initially confused as to how such divisions were named and only when the examiner gave him a few possible numbers of such divisions did he subsequently pick another number and give a long and extensive history of this division and his service with it. The number which he chose was one which never belonged to any division but whenever the patient was presented with this discrepancy or any of the others, he quickly continued his story in a way intended to cover up his original remarks.

Five minutes after the interview began, even though the examiner made it a point to stress his own name to the patient, the latter was unable to remember it. Again, in spite of having many of these difficulties called to his attention, he remained cheerful and seemingly convinced that there was nothing wrong with him. When asked the date, he stated that it was September 7, 1950, when in reality it was August 22, 1952.

The patient became quite friendly with many of the other patients on the ward. His talkativeness and apparent interest in everything that was going on made him a prominent figure on the ward and yet it soon became evident to the other patients that he was not able to remember most of the events which took place. There were no evidences of delusions or hallucinations. His primary defects were in the area of the sensorium with disorientation and a conspicuous difficulty with memory, both recent and remote. His grasp of current events and general information was spotty and subject to fabrications.

At the time of physical examination, the patient was bedridden, his fractures encased in a plaster cast. Neurological examination showed diminished sensation of the lower extremities below the knee where it was possible to test them. There were diminished Achilles and knee reflexes and some mild weakness in both upper and lower extremities. Laboratory studies were essentially negative. Serology, both spinal fluid and blood, was also negative.

The patient was treated with high doses of vitamins, particularly vitamin B complex, and gradual improvement resulted. It subsequently developed that about nine-tenths of the material that the patient had given as a history in the hospital was pure fabrication. It turned out that he was not married and that he had been a chronic alcoholic for many years. He had, on two previous occasions, suffered from delirium tremens. His improvement was slow and at the time of his discharge from the hospital he was transferred to the outpatient psychiatric service where a continued effort was made to watch his progress. After six months there had been perhaps 50 per cent improvement, and at the same time it was felt that further improvement would probably be very minimal. He still showed a major memory defect, although it was not nearly as marked as it had been at the time of his original admission to the hospital.

TREATMENT OF KORSAKOFF'S PSYCHOSIS

The treatment of Korsakoff's psychosis begins with the discontinuation of any further intake of alcohol. Vitamin preparations are administered, as in the other syndromes, with particular reference to the vitamin-B complex. Tranquilizers are often useful, but a careful watch on liver function is necessary. Such patients usually must be institutionalized because of their obviously psychotic status and their inability to be responsible for their actions. In those cases where the damage has not been of sufficient severity to be irreversible, improvement under a good medical regime usually begins relatively soon in the disease. There are certain patients who continue to show some residual symptoms and in whom even the administration of massive doses of vitamin preparations is of little avail. Obviously any other evidence of polyneuritis must be treated as it would be even in the absence of the Korsakoff syndrome.

CHRONIC BRAIN SYNDROME ASSOCIATED WITH BRAIN TRAUMA

This category includes the posttraumatic chronic brain disorders which produce permanent impairment of personality function. It is necessary to realize that any attempt to subdivide this category further is rather artificial in that one ordinarily finds a combination of such subdivisions. However, it is possible to list several categories into which chronic brain syndromes due to trauma may be divided. These are (1) posttraumatic personality disorders, (2) posttraumatic personality defect, (3) encephalopathy of pugilists, and (4) traumatic epilepsy.

The posttraumatic personality disorder, which has, incidentally, been given many other names, is not particularly uncommon. It is often mixed with, or at least contributed to by, an underlying functional problem which has existed long before the trauma. The individual suffers from a concussion, with or without contusion, of moderate to severe degree. Following this there is a change in personality, particularly manifested in emotional instability, difficulty in maintaining previous work adjustments, and a general loss of ability to discriminate in finer meanings. Such a patient also presents chronic headaches, irritability, vasomotor instability, and an intolerance of external stimuli, particularly those of light and noise. Such individuals often show an excessive degree of impulsiveness and have lost the previous controls over behavior which prevented action on impulse. In such cases it is not unusual to find emotional problems playing a secondary role, particularly if matters involving financial compensation are involved. Individuals suffering from posttraumatic personality disorders may show electroencephalogram changes and, if so, are sometimes improved by medication with sodium dilantin. Rorschach tests as well as other projective personality tests may occasionally reveal organic changes and be of some use in making a diagnosis.

"Posttraumatic personality defect" is a term indicating a condition in which there is a serious incapacitation in one or another area of the personality function. Apraxias and aphasias are two excellent examples. Because of vocal defects patients often present a picture simulating severe psychiatric disorders and yet they may retain most of the rest of their personality abilities. Some of these patients, however, because of the type and degree of organic involvement, gradually progress to a thorough personality disintegration, particularly if there is a concomitant arteriosclerotic or paretic involvement.

The encephalopathy of pugilists is a well-known syndrome which is commonly referred to as being "punch drunk." Such a condition results from repeated traumatic insults to the brain structure itself, and is most often seen in fighters. There results widespread damage to the cerebral tissue, particularly evidenced by numerous scattered small petechiae throughout the cerebrum. Such individuals show varying degrees of personality disintegration. There is a faulty memory, irritability, emotional instability, a tendency to grandiose ideas, and often varied neurological abnormalities. A certain degree of euphoria is frequently observed in these individuals with the result that they feel their abilities to be far beyond actuality.

Case History: Pugilistic Encephalopathy

This thirty-eight-year-old soldier was admitted to the Army hospital at his own post. He had been assigned to that station only one week prior to his admission, having just recently been inducted into the service. His immediate commanding officer had found him completely untrainable and had requested a medical evaluation. Apparently the patient, who had been a professional fighter prior to his induction, had made a heroic but completely unsuccessful attempt to master the rules and regulations of Army life. It had soon become quite evident that he suffered from a severe mental disability and was totally unfit for military training.

At the time of admission the patient complained that he suffered from repeated chronic headaches which had no relationship to his activity, the time of day, or any other factor that could be determined. As far as he was concerned this was the primary reason for his admission to the hospital and also the reason that he had not adjusted well in his basic training. He brought with him to the hospital a large portfolio of photographs and newspaper clippings which portrayed his past pugilistic career. Whenever he had the opportunity he brought out this portfolio and would show it to anyone who would take the time to look at it and listen to his long tales of his past ring battles. As far as could be determined, he had attained a few minor successes in the ring which had enabled him to accumulate the clippings which he was so anxious to show. However, he had fought for at least twelve or thirteen years and had, on many occasions, suffered severe beatings.

While on the ward this patient was a very pleasant, talkative and at least superficially co-operative man who was liked by all the ward personnel and other patients. He never showed a belligerent attitude or animosity toward anyone and seemed generally unconcerned about his plight.

Physical examination revealed a very well-developed muscular individual. His nose had apparently been broken several times and was somewhat disfigured. In addition to this he bore a few other minor facial scars resulting from his pugilistic career. He frequently grinned and seemed to be generally in a mildly euphoric mood during most of his interviews. He was anxious to please the examiner but seemed almost childlike in his demeanor. Upon closer questioning it soon developed that his memory was severely disturbed. He was poorly oriented as to time and place. He was unable to remember important dates during his life and had equal difficulty in remembering the date of his induction into the service or the date of his hospitalization. He lived on an extremely superficial plane, being primarily interested in whatever was going on about him at the moment and apparently unconcerned about the larger problems which he faced.

This patient was anxious in his childish way to remain in the Army and saw no reason for a discharge "if you can just cure my headaches." He was, on the other hand, perfectly willing to accept a discharge and seemed to feel that he might possibly return to a ring career. All laboratory studies were essentially negative. Electroencephalography revealed "diffuse cortical dysrhythmia," which it was felt was due to diffuse cortical damage. No abnormal neurological findings were present. The patient never revealed any hallucinatory or delusional material as long as he was in the hospital. He was ultimately discharged and was returned to civilian life.

Traumatic epilepsy refers to those convulsive states resulting from some type of head trauma. In almost one-quarter of penetrating head wounds a chronic seizure state is the eventual outcome. Such convulsions may or may not be Jacksonian in type, but are frequently accompanied by gradual yet progressive personality disintegration and disorganization, as is typical of many other syndromes within this category.

Case History: Posttraumatic Syndrome

This patient was first admitted to the hospital some three months after she had been involved in a serious automobile accident. At that time she had sustained fractures of her elbow, pelvis, hip, and skull. She had remained in coma for approximately five weeks and for a period of about ten days following recovery of consciousness had complained of a severe headache. There had been a noticeable personality change following the recovery of consciousness. Whereas previously she had given every evidence of being well adjusted, she now revealed considerable irritability, poor concentration, susceptibility to fatigue, excitability, and a short attention span. Her speech became thick and difficult to understand.

At the time of admission she had no complaints, seemed oriented, cheerful, and willing to discuss her situation. She was amnesic for the accident itself. Neurological examination revealed essentially normal eyegrounds and external ocular movements except for a slight lateral weakness. There was a Hoffmann sign on the left but Babinskis were not present. There was a transitory left ankle and wrist clonus with some weakness also of the left upper extremity and lower extremity. Sensation was intact. The neurological impression at this time was that there was a residuum of severe cerebral concussion with contusion and an intellectual change with partial right hemiparesis. The electroencephalogram showed "diffuse depression of cortical activity." It was felt that since the patient had improved considerably in the weeks following her accident, recovery was probable, although possibly some posttraumatic changes might be expected. She was discharged to be followed as an outpatient.

The patient was readmitted to the hospital approximately five months later. At this time the complaints involved marked personality changes and spells during which she would stare at someone she knew without recognizing him. In addition, the patient had begun to suffer with what were apparently catatonic episodes of negativism. She remained somnolent much of the time. At the time of this admission she was conscious and co-operative. She was oriented as to person but not time or place. She varied considerably in her behavior, at times being completely mute, although staring at the examiner, and at other times answering questions relatively well. Neurological examination revealed that the right pupil was larger than the left, although both reacted well. External ocular movements were normal along with visual fields. There was some relaxation of the left lower face. There was an increase in deep tendon reflexes on the left but again no Babinski. There was a slight weakness of the left upper extremity. The most obvious psychiatric findings were ones closely resembling those to be expected in a catatonic state. Negativism played a large role in this patient's behavior in the hospital. At times she responded well and at other times seemed mute, catatonic, and negativistic.

The patient was subsequently transferred to an institution closer to her home where prolonged care was available. The final diagnosis was posttraumatic syndrome following severe head injury incurred in an automobile accident.

CHRONIC BRAIN SYNDROME ASSOCIATED WITH CEREBRAL ARTERIOSCLEROSIS

The presence of sufficiently advanced arteriosclerotic processes within the cerebral vessels is capable of leading to a distortion of personality function which may eventually reach a psychotic degree. The concomitant gradual diminution of blood supply results in the slow destruction of parenchymatous brain tissue. Such a pathological sclerotic process within the brain may or may not be associated with similar blood-vessel pathology elsewhere in the body. The particular degree and type of personality distortion varies with the type, location and degree of the sclerotic process itself. As with the senile syndrome, the onset is often insidious, so that it is not easy to ascertain the exact time when such personality changes became evident. At other times in cerebral arteriosclerosis the onset is more rapid and obvious. This is especially true where there has been one or more cerebrovascular accidents. The frequency with which arteriosclerosis currently produces mental disorders is revealed in the 1951 statistics when the syndrome was responsible for more than 36,000 first admissions to mental hospitals in the United States. This is more than 12 per cent of the total admissions, second only to schizophrenic reactions.

Cerebral arteriosclerosis is of additional importance in that its incidence is highest between the ages of fifty and sixty-five, during which time many individuals reach important and productive positions in their lives. The ensuing mental deterioration cuts short their contribution to their families and to society and reduces them to a vastly inferior level of adjustment. The sociological, financial, and emotional aspects of this affliction can hardly be estimated.

ETIOLOGY AND PATHOLOGY

The psychological changes which are characteristic of this syndrome are directly attributable to the damage resulting from the sclerotic process taking place within the cerebral vessels. There is as yet no definitive and positive answer to the problem of arteriosclerosis, either as to why it occurs or why it sometimes occurs more markedly in certain locations while leaving other areas relatively uninvolved. Some patients suffering from cerebral arteriosclerosis reveal comparatively little evidence of arteriosclerotic pathology elsewhere in their bodies. However, the condition of the retinal vessels is a reasonably good index to the state of the cerebral vessels themselves.

Pathologists have certain criteria by which they identify cerebral arteriosclerosis at necropsy. They report, as with senile psychosis, that the brain is ordinarily smaller than usual and that the meninges, particularly the arachnoid, are thickened. Phagocytic cells are present, indicating the presence of the destructive process which is occurring. The parenchymatous tissue is disturbed in its normal appearance, showing fewer ganglion cells than usual; those which are seen are paler than is normal. There is also an increase of glia scattered about and, depending upon the type and extent of the sclerotic process, there are areas of fatty degeneration, destruction, and atrophy, and other evidences of damage to the blood supply. The blood vessels themselves reveal typical changes of arteriosclerosis and as a consequence appear quite prominent in cross-section. The intima is particularly involved.

In certain cases the larger vessels are primarily involved; in others, the process is most marked in the smaller vessels. In the former instance one may find a rupture of a larger vessel which occurred in a cerebrovascular accident with a consequent destruction of the surrounding area where the hemorrhage has occurred. In the latter instance the damage may be less intensive but is far more extensive. It is widespread and diffuse, but particularly noticeable in the frontal lobes.

SYMPTOMATOLOGY

The onset of symptoms in cerebral arteriosclerosis may be relatively sudden, particularly in the case of arteriosclerosis involving the large vessels. However, in many cases there is the much more gradual process one would expect to find in involvement of the smaller vessels. In the former case there may be an acute episode ushered in by a cerebrovascular accident. This, of course, often entails a period of unconsciousness. When consciousness returns there may be a residue of personality difficulty which may or may not gradually improve in the period following the vascular accident. Ordinarily the diagnosis of such a condition is not particularly difficult because of the obvious signs of the cerebrovascular accident, especially from a neurological standpoint.

The more slowly progressing sclerotic process as seen in the smaller vessels produces a gradual disorganization of personality function. This often closely resembles the onset of a senile psychosis. Ordinarily, however, the psychotic picture with arteriosclerosis comes on somewhat earlier in life. It should be mentioned that in a reasonable number of cases it is not possible to differentiate between the brain syndromes with arteriosclerosis and those of senility, so that the final accurate diagnosis can be made only at autopsy. However, there is a general tendency where such doubt exists to give preference to the arteriosclerotic diagnosis. Ordinarily in arteriosclerotic patients one finds occasional periods of confusion developing and there may be a complaint of periodic headache. Irritability increases and the memory becames impaired, usually in a "patchy" manner where certain incidents or periods of time are forgotten but other events both before and after the periods are remembered. Thinking becomes less acute and speech impaired or particularly slowed. There is a decrease in judgment and a progressive loss of interest in the individual's surroundings. Personal appearance becomes neglected and, as mentioned, the picture takes on many of the characteristics of senile psychosis. It is of some importance to remember that the onset of the syndrome of cerebral arteriosclerosis shows periods of waxing and waning in many cases: certain symptoms come and go and certain deficiencies seem to develop, only to disappear and subsequently appear again. This is in contrast to the general tendency of the senile psychotic to develop his mental deterioration progressively, without as many ups and downs.

TREATMENT

Unfortunately this large group of cases represents another enigma to the medical scientist. While it is true that many important advances are being made in our understanding of the arteriosclerotic process, it nevertheless remains that there is at the present time no adequate method for preventing or curing the process.

Generally speaking, most of what is known regarding the treatment of the senile syndrome holds true for treatment of the arteriosclerotic syndrome. Arteriosclerotics ordinarily retain a varying degree of their previous mental competence and such residual ability should be taken advantage of. Obviously good hygiene, diet, and other such measures will play an important role in the therapeutic regime. Once again, however, an unfortunate situation often develops when such patients are cared for by their grown children. The family situation becomes thoroughly distorted and much emotional conflict is generated. Such conflict obviously influences the patient's children and, what may be even more important, the patient's grandchildren, who must live in such a disturbed environment.

Another solution, hospitalization, is also unsatisfactory in many respects, since little care can be provided there other than that of a custodial type. The best answer obviously lies, as it does with the senile patient, in the maintenance of separate institutions to care for arteriosclerotic patients and to utilize their remaining abilities. Again it is essential to make them feel that they are still contributing members of at least their small circumscribed society and that they have some usefulness in that particular environment. Then it is possible for these patients to achieve a reasonably satisfactory emotional adjustment and to make the fullest use of their remaining faculties. At the same time their improved mental state allows for an improved relationship between them and the rest of their family. It is possible for families to visit such patients and, when finding them in a satisfactory physical and emotional state, thereby achieve a much better intrafamilial relationship.

There have been attempts to ameliorate the symptoms of cerebral arteriosclerosis by high doses of nicotinic acid and, at least according to some physicians, by stellate ganglion blocks, as well as the other measures mentioned in the section on senile psychosis. There is considerable doubt as to the degree of improvement that follows such procedures. At times one is encouraged, but at other times little improvement is forthcoming. Certainly, even with such procedures, attention must be paid to nutritional intake and bodily care of arteriosclerotic patients. They themselves will become much more interested in these things if their environmental condition is made more satisfactory.

Case History: Cerebral Arteriosclerosis

This patient was a sixty-one-year-old woman who was seen in consultation by the psychiatrist, having been referred by a neurologist. She had apparently been in good health until approximately six months before, when she was said to have fallen in her room. There was no demonstrable injury at that time, but after that, "she never seemed to be the same," according to her son. For a period of several months she would not eat and had to be persuaded to do so or forcibly fed. About two weeks after the fall she developed a number of ideas about herself which persisted. One of these was that her hair was coming out by the handful and accordingly she felt that she was unable to wash or brush her hair, lest it all come out. She also felt that her skin was becoming loose and wrinkled, would not perspire, and was developing "pits" which she assumed were indicative of some seriously incapacitating disease which she was unable to name. She also complained that nothing tasted right and that there was no saliva in her mouth. Therefore, as far as she was concerned, it became impossible for her to eat. She also said that her intestines were dissolving and that this was causing her to smell so obnoxious that she must keep away from people. During the interview when she was asked why all these things were happening, she attributed them to having eaten some food at a friend's house which had been kept in a refrigerator that had gas leaking in it. During the interview, incidentally, she gave no history of the fall and apparently had no memory for it.

Physical examination revealed a woman with only the characteristic skin and hair changes normally present in a person of her age She had lost considerable weight and this had to a degree magnified the evidences of senility. There was no indication that she was losing any hair beyond the normal thinning out to be expected at her age. Ample evidence of arteriosclerosis was to be seen in the retinal vessels and superficial veins and was also palpable in the brachial artery. Neurological examination revealed the following positive features: the right pupil reacted sluggishly to light, there was a minimum right facial weakness when the patient attempted to show her teeth, tendon reflexes in the right arm and leg were somewhat hyperactive, a positive Hoffmann was present in the right hand and a positive Babinski on the right, abdominal reflexes were absent, sensation was normal, and the patient was able to distinguish between a dime and a penny in either hand with her eyes closed. She complained subjectively of not being able to feel anything with her hands, but this was not demonstrable in an objective fashion.

The patient had obviously suffered a cerebrovascular accident on the left side of the brain, presumably at the time of her fall in her room about six months previously. This cerebrovascular accident was a secondary result of the rather advanced arteriosclerosis and the above pathology undoubtedly contributed to her psychotic state. Her previous history revealed a relatively good adjustment and there was no evidence of premorbid personality difficulties which would account for her present state.

CHRONIC BRAIN SYNDROME ASSOCIATED WITH CIRCULATORY DISTURBANCE OTHER THAN CEREBRAL ARTERIOSCLEROSIS

Circulatory disturbances other than cerebral arteriosclerosis classified here include cerebral embolism, cerebral hemorrhages, arterial hypertension, and other chronic vascular diseases. Cerebral hemorrhage usually results in a damage to the invaded tissue which is never completely repaired: thus these cases are most frequently chronic. The damage occurring with cerebral embolism may be compensated for but there is frequently some residue of a chronic nature. The type of personality change seen varies with the location and extent of interference with nervous system function. Associated neurological changes are usually present. Any of these conditions if severe presents a general medical and neurological problem, with the personality changes being of less immediate importance. As mentioned, there is often partial improvement of the initial disturbance but some chronic residual symptomatology is bound to remain.

Case History: Chronic Brain Syndrome Associated
with Circulatory Disturbance other than
Cerebral Arteriosclerosis

A twenty-three-year-old male had gone to another clinic complaining of edema under the eyes. According to his statement, the edema would come and go and he worried over its presence to the extent that he could no longer leave his room to go to work. He felt that the edema was in some way connected with masturbation, and he believed the swelling would disappear when he discontinued masturbation or sexual relations. He feared that if he went out and mixed with people they would notice the edema and conclude it was linked to sexual activity. As a result, he lived the life of a recluse, playing recordings and reading, oblivious to the reproaches and appeals of his parents.

History revealed the patient's father to be a sturdy, reliable worker, but an emotionally labile man at home, impatient and without any clear plan for, or sustained interest in, the patient's education or development. The mother was self-indulgent and overindulgent toward the patient. She and her husband had often quarreled over the patient's upbringing and had separated for a time when the patient was ten years of age.

Because of the patient's marked withdrawal from life and his ideas of reference and borderline delusions, he was first diagnosed as suffering from a schizophrenic reaction. Treatment was suggested, and upon the patient's refusal to undergo it, he was discharged from the clinic.

The patient continued his withdrawn existence for four years until one day he developed a severe pain in the head for which he had to be hospitalized. Studies revealed a congenital aneurysm of the right anterior cerebral artery. Following operation for its removal, the patient had a marked regression of symptoms.

When seen several months after the operation, this patient showed marked improvement. His manner was more open and cordial. He reported that he had been working for some time, liked his work, and expected to advance in it. He had lost all apprehension and discomfort over the thought that people might stare at his eyes and draw uncomplimentary conclusions from their appearance. He had become more extroverted and now spent more time with people although he still remained far from gregarious. He stated that while he no longer had keen emotional distress about his appearance, some of his enjoyment of life had lessened also. In short, his capacity for emotional feeling, for both pleasure and anxious rumination, had been diminished. At the time of the operation, a portion of the right frontal lobe had been removed. Apparently the effect of the operation had been to give the most favorable effect that this kind of surgery on the brain could induce, and it must be concluded that there was a specific relationship between the structural defect and the symptomatology. The patient continued to improve for more than a year, which was the total follow-up period possible in his instance.

CHRONIC BRAIN SYNDROME ASSOCIATED WITH CONVULSIVE DISORDER

This diagnosis is now used for those cases which have previously been referred to as "idiopathic epilepsy." The term *convulsive disorder* has in recent years gradually replaced the term *epilepsy*. For centuries there has been a certain stigma attached to the person who suffers from recurrent seizures and a tendency to attribute to such patients a hopeless prognosis. As our knowledge concerning this field has grown, it has become recognized that there is a wide variety of etiological factors which are capable of bringing on a convulsive state. Convulsions may occur in syphilis, intoxication, trauma, cerebral arteriosclerosis, and brain tumors, among other syndromes.

The complete neurological aspects of the various convulsive states cannot be dealt with here but some of the general features will be discussed. For further reading the student is referred to a textbook of clinical neurology. It is our primary purpose to discuss some of the more common personality changes which accrue in a convulsive disorder. Some observers in the past have felt that it was possible to outline with some degree of clarity the typical personality of the epileptic. However, with the advances in control of these convulsive states and also a more normal work and socialization pattern, such personality changes are not apt to be seen nearly as often.

ETIOLOGY AND PATHOLOGY

In spite of extensive research, it is still difficult to delineate some of the more basic mechanisms in idiopathic convulsive disorders. They have been referred to as a "paroxysmal cerebral dysrhythmia" by Lennox, who has done a great deal of work with the electroencephalogram in this country. The instrument was introduced by Hans Berger and is essentially a means of recording the electrical potentials of the brain by means of various leads attached in the form of small wires to the overlying areas of the skull. The electroencephalogram has proven to be a valuable diagnostic instrument in localizing various intracranial pathological conditions, as well as increasing our knowledge concerning the epileptic process. Often by varying the position of the leads it is possible to locate brain tumors or other intracranial lesions accurately. At the same time it has been found that the epileptic patient presents a characteristic pattern, obtained by the electroencephalogram, in approximately 85 per cent of cases. However, some 10 per cent of individuals without any history of epilepsy give the same pattern. An increasing amount of evidence has revealed that the use of electroencephalograms in children is not nearly as accurate, particularly from the standpoint of a diagnosis of epilepsy, as it is in adults. However, this does not necessarily minimize the usefulness of the electroencephalogram.

The electroencephalogram records a pulsating rhythmical type of electrical potential of which both the frequency and voltage are measured. There occur in the various types of epilepsy peculiarly characteristic types of encephalograms. For further reading on this particular subject, the student is referred to the various treatises involving electroencephalography. It is of some importance to remember that the electroencephalogram may produce a pattern typical of the convulsive disorders when the underlying pathology is that of symptomatic convulsive disorder, rather than being idiopathic.

There has been considerable work done involving the hereditary factors in convulsive disorders. This has been furthered by the use of the electroencephalogram, which has revealed that a far larger per cent of relatives of idiopathic epileptic patients reveal abnormal encephalograms than do the control group, where no such convulsive disorder exists in the family. This has generally led to the conclusion that a marriage between two individuals in whom there is a strong family trait toward epilepsy will yield a far larger number of offspring suffering from this disorder than will marriages where the convulsive disorder is present in only one of the marital partners' families.

SYMPTOMATOLOGY

Generally speaking, epilepsy occurs in three main forms: grand mal seizures, petit mal, and psychomotor equivalent. The convulsive disorder may appear at any time in life from infancy to old age. As has been stressed, it may be secondary to various organic pathological processes or to trauma. However, even the idiopathic variety has a relatively wide age spread. It generally does not appear for the first time late in life but may well appear during infancy, early childhood, or adolescence. The individual patient may suffer from one, two, or even all three of the varieties of epilepsy. He may occasionally begin by showing petit mal early and subsequently develop grand mal; or at times psychomotor equivalent may be the only evidence of this process.

Grand Mal Seizures

Grand mal seizures are ordinarily ushered in by the so-called "aura." This involves a peculiar sensation somewhere in the body or in the psychic sphere which the patient learns to recognize and which indicates the imminence of an oncoming seizure. The aura occurs shortly before the onset of the seizure itself. It may involve a twitching, tingling, or other sensation in a particular portion of the body, or may possibly involve some type of special sensation such as hearing, smell, or taste. Shortly following this the patient falls unconscious, often uttering the "epileptic cry," and goes into the tonic phase of the seizure. This involves a general contraction of all the voluntary musculature of the body. The epileptic cry itself is due to a titanic contraction of the chest muscles which forces air explosively outward through the vocal cords. The tonic phase ordinarily lasts a few seconds, during which the individual's respiration is interrupted. As the phase proceeds, there develops an anoxia which leads to cyanosis. Following this, the individual goes into the clonic phase, which involves rhythmic contractions of the various large groups of voluntary muscles. These occur with decreasing frequency, at the beginning every two or three seconds and gradually less often until the patient eventually comes to the postseizure coma.

During the period of clonic convulsions, the patient's arm, leg, and trunk muscles contract rhythmically in a violent fashion. Also of importance is the fact that the jaw muscles contract rhythmically; and if the tongue happens to be caught between the teeth it is often severely lacerated. There may or may not be loss of bowel and bladder control. After the seizure the patient remains comatose for a few minutes and gradually comes out of his stupor. He may or may not sleep for a period of time and slowly regains his full senses. He is completely amnesic for the event from the onset of the convulsion until regaining of consciousness.

It is of importance to remember that the epileptic convulsion, if it occurs when the individual is driving a car or is in some other precarious position, can lead to disastrous results. It is for this reason that the majority of state legislatures have prohibited the issuance of licenses to the average epileptic patient. Unfortunately, there is not always adequate concern on the part of the lawmakers as to whether the epilepsy has been thoroughly and adequately controlled.

Petit Mal Seizures

Petit mal seizures are a much milder type of disorder which may or may not alternate with grand mal seizures. They involve a momentary loss of consciousness, usually with a loss of muscular tonus. The individual may be actively engaged in some task and for a few moments assume a dazed appearance as if he is completely out of contact. Just as suddenly there is a resumption of the normal activity, as if nothing had occurred. The individual often is unaware of his momentary lapse of consciousness, but on the other hand he may become gradually aware of it. At times, particularly if the petit mal seizure lasts a few seconds, there may be a collapse of muscular control and the individual may fall to the ground, although he does not then go through the rigors of a grand mal seizure. Once again, there is typically a complete amnesia for whatever has occurred during the petit mal seizure.

Psychomotor Equivalent

Psychomotor equivalent is a condition lasting anywhere from a few minutes to many hours, during which the individual remains in command of all his voluntary faculties and yet is not responsible and has no memory. It is during such epileptic equivalents that the person may travel far from home, do things which he would otherwise never do, or behave in a way completely alien to his own personality. Such epileptic equivalent states may reach the so-called "epileptic furor state" in which the individual is primarily dominated by an unreasoning and violent rage. During such a state maniacal crimes may be committed. The person may literally succumb to his rage and often attack sadistically and brutally all those within his reach. Upon recovery of conscious awareness, the person is totally amnesic for this period. At times one finds multiple murders due to this type of condition. Particular attention should be paid in any case of extreme violence to the ruling out of the epileptic process and particularly of the epileptic furor state. Individuals susceptible to this state are probably the most dangerous persons with whom psychiatry deals.

TREATMENT

The treatment of the various convulsive disorders depends upon whether they belong to the idiopathic or symptomatic variety. Obviously, if they are symptomatic, the treatment will probably involve the underlying syndrome. The paretic who develops a convulsive disorder needs treatment more for his paresis than for the convulsive disorder; similarly, this is true for the individual with brain tumor who has symptomatic convulsive disorder; and so on.

The treatment of the idiopathic variety is both general and specific. In regard to the general treatment, it has been shown many times that a heightened emotional disturbance within the individual's life increases the frequency and severity of the convulsive state. Therefore, every attempt should be made to see that the individual's mode of living consistently remains within a reasonably normal range and that he is not constantly beset with emotional crises of one type or another. Obviously his nutritional intake and dietary habits should be controlled. Considerable evidence has been accumulated to show that a so-called ketogenic diet is favorable for the epileptic, although this may often involve emotional problems of one type or another—particularly in relation to having a new and often monotonous diet—that do not seem to make the diet worth while. As long as the individual suffering from a convulsive disorder eats a diet which is reasonable and wholesome, this would seem adequate.

Specific measures directed toward the control of idiopathic convulsive disorders involve several drugs. Bromides have been used in the past but should be used only with caution, since they tend to accumulate and may eventually result in a bromide psychosis. Phenobarbital is often used, particularly in conjunction with other drugs. It has the disadvantage of producing a typical barbiturate lethargy which is certainly not conducive to mental alertness. However, if it can be used as a complement to other drugs in smaller doses, it is often advisable. The newer drugs which are ordinarily used in this condition are sodium dilantin, which has proved quite efficient in the control of the majority of grand mal seizures, and tridione, which has proved efficient in the control of symptoms of the average individual who suffers from petit mal. It is not our intention to give a complete and encompassing regime for the control of epilepsy in terms of these medications, since such subjects are adequately covered in the average textbook of clinical neurology.

Our main purpose is to describe the various types of personality disorder that may accrue to epilepsy. The typical "epileptic personality" is less often seen today, since so many epileptics are rendered symptom-free by the new drugs available.

A certain number of epileptics, because of the severity of their condition, gradually undergo a process of mental deterioration of varying degree. This often involves, initially, loss of concern about personal appearance and external behavior. The epileptic frequently becomes irritable and easily goaded to outbursts of anger. He gradually becomes dulled and develops a general organic picture in which his thinking processes are poor, his sensorium is clouded, and his judgment is impaired. There may be a development of increasing irritability and belligerence, along with a lack of a sense of moral values and ethics. Such a personality occurs often where there is some degree of mental retardation. Incidentally, it should be mentioned that a certain number of epileptics, either by virtue of intrauterine development or birth trauma, are rendered mentally deficient along with their convulsive disorder. On the other hand, it must be remembered that a reasonable number of epileptics attain a normal or superior range of intelligence in spite of their convulsive disorder. In the past it was found necessary to construct special institutions in many states to provide for the care of epileptic patients. However, since the advent of newer drugs, as well as better methods of dealing with the symptomatic types of convulsive disorders, such institutions have become progressively less important. At the present time only a relatively small number of patients suffering convulsive disorder need be institutionalized.

There are a certain number of epileptics who reach the so-called "status epilepticus" in which one grand mal seizure is replaced by another in an unending series which leads rapidly to extreme physical fatigue and eventually may result in death. Such an individual requires heroic measures on the part of the physician to control the seizures.

Like all other human beings the victim of epilepsy has loves and hates, and possibilities of excessive narcissism and frustrations resulting therefrom. He has the same conflicts in his work and sex life; their pressure-producing tension may act as a factor in setting off attacks. In fact it has been said, and still is believed by some, that the epileptic convulsion is a symbolic expression and release of pent-up tensions which cannot find expression otherwise. Others point up the sexual as well as the regressive pattern in the epileptic seizure. At any rate, even though the brain shows its dysrhythmia, the epileptic patient should have the benefit of psychotherapy for his personal and environmental adjustment. In spite of the "organic" nature of epilepsy, patients have been greatly helped in their adjustment, their illness, and their solution of personal problems. Helping the patient to obtain or retain a job usually requires great understanding on the part of the employer and fellow employees, but the physician can be the educator who helps the community to accept the epileptic and help him become a wage earner.

*Case History: Chronic Brain Syndrome Associated with
Convulsive Disorder*

A twenty-six-year-old male was admitted to the hospital in an acute
psychotic episode. There was a strong paranoid coloring to his delusional
system. According to the history obtained from relatives at the time of
admission, this patient had had a convulsive state since mid-adolescence.
He was a chronic sufferer from grand mal seizures. Approximately two
weeks prior to admission he had become increasingly confused and had
talked irrationally. He made such statements as, "Everybody is a liar.
They're all talking about me upstairs. Satan put a hole in my head.
They're sneaking up on me." He apparently felt that his two brothers
were working against him. He showed periods of quiescence alternating
with periods of agitation, confusion, and irrationality. In his quieter
periods he was quite guilty about his actions during the more disturbed
phases. He became increasingly paranoid toward his father but would
always be sorry about this subsequently. About four or five days prior to
admission he became violent and so agitated that no one could come near
him at home except his brother. He assaulted friends and members of
his family on the night of his admission and only luck saved several of
them from severe harm.

At the time he came into the hospital the patient was oriented. However, he was violent, talking loudly, and was extremely aggressive. He
was put in restraint, at which point he was sobbing and screaming.
When he quieted down he would give long, involved circumstantial
answers to questions asked him. He was obsequious to the physicians
and nurses. His speech showed some slurring. He was at times irrational.
A week following his admission he still talked as if he were intoxicated.
He walked with a wide base and still showed slurred speech. He was
still hearing voices of his family coming out of the wall near his bed.
Neurological examination was essentially negative for cerebellar disease
at this time.

The patient's earlier history showed a normal birth and development
history with the exception of some slowness in speaking and a tendency
to stammer. He was the sixth of seven children. There was no other
history of convulsive disorder in the family. He had an eighth-grade
education and left school at the age of fourteen when he developed a
convulsive state. He had been seen in the outpatient department of
another hospital for years, where he had been given medication for his
convulsive state. He had worked irregularly, often losing his job because

of the occurrence of a seizure, which most often occurred when he failed to take his medication. He was described as having had a relatively good disposition in his middle adolescence. He had been courteous, friendly, and well-liked by most people with whom he came into contact. He did not date because he was extremely self-conscious about his seizures. He became increasingly nervous and excitable as the years passed. He withdrew from social contacts to an increasing degree and developed an excessive interest in reading. His epileptic seizures, which had been previously fairly well controlled, began to appear somewhat more frequently. He became more restless and upset about the appearance of these spells. He often became quite depressed and cried, complaining of many physical symptoms. He voiced increasing guilt about having to be supported by his family. He became more changeable in his moods, showing irritability and argumentativeness. About two weeks prior to his admission he evinced a desire to come to the hospital, but was refused admission at that time because of lack of an available bed. He became increasingly agitated during the subsequent days and finally, when his psychosis was fully developed, he was admitted in the state described above.

This patient remained in his psychotic state for several weeks following his admission. There was a general personality disintegration. He was finally transferred to a state hospital for permanent custodial care. Anticonvulsant medication reduced his convulsions to a minimum, but the personality disintegration remained fairly constant with only temporary periods of improvement. His illness had both emotional and organic aspects, as is usually true in convulsive disorders.

CHRONIC BRAIN SYNDROME ASSOCIATED WITH SENILE BRAIN DISEASE

The many remarkable advances in medical science during recent years have provided means for prolonging the human lifespan far beyond previous levels. The average age of the population is steadily rising and an increasing percentage of that population is now represented by the older age group. Antibiotics, sulfa drugs, improved surgical techniques, as well as many other medical advances, now make it possible to cure or alleviate conditions which once took a large toll in older people. Unfortunately, such advances have not been uniform in all areas of medicine, so that certain problems associated with advancing age have become increasingly common. One of these, and truly an important one, is senile psychosis, for which, at the present time, no adequate curative treatment exists.

In 1951, senile psychosis accounted for more than 10 per cent of first admissions to mental hospitals. This percentage is steadily rising and forms a serious mental health problem in our nation. The elderly person suffering from senile psychosis is often hospitalized at perhaps sixty-five years of age, and may with our improved medical care live another fifteen or twenty years. Such an individual occupies a hospital bed, requires considerable medical attention, and yet, from a psychiatric standpoint, is not a candidate for active psychotherapeutic measures.

ETIOLOGY AND PATHOLOGY

The insidious personality deterioration found in the senile psychotic results from diffuse, widespread organic damage occurring within the brain structure. There takes place a gradual disintegration of parenchymatous tissue within the brain, most marked in the frontal lobes. The brain itself, when seen at postmortem, is found to be smaller than usual with narrow convolutions and widened fissures. Blood vessels show sclerotic changes and meninges are thickened. Microscopically, the most evident change is the reduction in the number of ganglion cells and an increase in glia, often to the point of masking the normal cortical laminations. The ganglion cells appear more pale than usual. Silver stain reveals the presence of numerous sclerotic plaques. Generally speaking, the more marked all of these changes are, the more severe is the resulting psychotic picture.

Medical science as yet is unable to offer any clear and fundamental understanding of the senile process in this type of psychosis. It is generally part of an over-all pattern in the direction of atrophic changes of senility occurring throughout the body. At times atrophy is most marked in the central nervous system, but it is more often widespread. Why such changes appear at an earlier age in certain individuals while other people show only a minimum of these changes even at very advanced ages is not understood. Some degrees of such senile change are to be found in the brains of elderly people who have not shown during their lifetime a true psychotic picture.

The senile psychosis involves an insidious deterioration of all personality functions and ordinarily occurs gradually over a period of years. The earlier changes, as mentioned in the introductory section, are often those of an exaggeration of previous personality traits. The senile patient becomes progressively less able to maintain his previous standards of social behavior and work adjustment. He becomes sloppy about his personal appearance and inaccurate in his work. His range of interest narrows. The patient loses his grasp of general information and current events. Selfishness becomes more prominent, and demands made upon those in the environment are often excessive. Sleep patterns tend to become reversed, with nocturnal wanderings and excessive diurnal sleep. The patient frequently collects useless things, thereby accumulating drawers full of odd bits of paper, string, and cheap trinkets, as well as other material which is of no worth or use to him. Depression is one of the most common complaints of these senile patients and may reach serious proportions. Paranoid feelings may become particularly evident, especially where there has been a previous tendency toward suspiciousness. The senile patient is extremely sensitive toward criticism or correction. He feels unwanted and unloved and is quick to sense any real evidence of such attitudes in those around him. Emotional control becomes poor and rapid mood changes occur. In a sense, the emotional picture is a childish one with wide mood fluctuations, but varies remarkably from one patient to another. As the sensorium becomes increasingly clouded, orientation, particularly as to time and place, is disturbed. Memory is impaired, especially in regard to recent events. The patient may spend long hours recounting occurrences which took place many years ago and yet be unable to remember important events of the day before. As one talks with such patients, their tendency toward circumstantiality is evident. They talk at great length about things which they are able to remember without at the same time clearly answering questions which are put to them. Judgment is slowly impaired and the patient is an easy victim of charlatans of one type or another. Money may be spent rashly without adequate forethought. Because the changes of senility occur slowly, there are many older people who have been taken advantage of through various devious means.

Medical science has made great strides in prolonging the human lifespan, but as yet has provided no adequate means of preventing or curing the changes of senility within the central nervous system. In the absence of any specific therapeutic agent, the main efforts at the present time in regard to these patients are directed toward providing them with the type of environment in which they can lead the most useful and contented lives. Unfortunately this often cannot be achieved.

In a large number of such cases the senile person is taken care of by his own adult children. His presence in the home may become an increasing burden as well as a severe influence for the development and exaggeration of emotional conflict in the home. Such a senile patient, with his increase in selfishness, his excessive demands, his forgetfulness, and at times his paranoid tendencies, may make life extremely difficult for the grown son or daughter, particularly if there are children in the home. Such elderly people may at times reveal sexual aberrations which have never previously appeared during their lives. Their forgetfulness may become a serious matter, especially if they leave gas jets turned on or unwittingly do some other careless thing which may lead to fire or accidents.

A solution which is quite common today, but only slightly more efficient, is that of placing these patients in a mental hospital. The average state mental hospital is woefully lacking in facilities to provide adequately for the care of the average senile patient. Whatever therapy is available is rightfully directed toward the younger patients suffering from some type of condition which can be remedied. Only too frequently several wards of these mental hospitals have to be set aside for senile patients who are thereafter allowed to vegetate and sink further into their senile deterioration. It is not at all an uncommon sight in such wards to see these patients sitting quietly and rocking hour after hour, poorly clothed and having lost interest in their surroundings. They are seldom visited by their guilty children and are completely out of touch with the world around them.

A much more practical and eventually more economical solution for this growing problem in the United States will be the construction of specific institutions designed to care for these patients. Such individuals, although deteriorating, still have certain abilities, even if in lesser degree than previously, and are capable of some productive work. In various places where this has been tried it has been proven that such patients can be interested in projects of their own and can be made to feel a part of the institution to which they belong. They can, in varying degrees, contribute to their own support by constructive work, even if on a limited scale. They can be encouraged to socialize with each other and redevelop an interest in living and in associating with their contemporaries. It requires a minimum of supervision to care for such patients and in the long run a great deal of money can be saved and some prevention of deterioration can result if such institutions are provided.

The senile patient becomes obviously careless of his own dietary intake and his bodily condition. A certain amount of watchfulness, encouragement, and careful planning are necessary to see that such patients lead a reasonably well-balanced life, including the essentials of nutrition, sleep, and exercise. Particular attention must be paid to vitamin intake, and it is advisable that vitamin supplements be provided. Nicotinic acid in relatively large doses has been suggested and seems advisable. It stimulates cerebral circulation, though it does not produce the conspicuous improvement that has at times been claimed for it.

Various measures have been advocated to increase cerebral circulation in the senile patient and thereby minimize the symptomatology of his syndrome. It has been suggested and found by some to be useful to block the stellate ganglion. Others have suggested arterial shunts into the inferior jugular vein. In the main it has been our experience that widespread diffuse changes of senility are not reversible by any of these procedures, although at times some minor improvements may be noted. Such procedures are more useful in younger patients who suffer from cerebral arteriosclerosis.

Case History: Senile Psychosis

This eighty-four-year-old widow was brought to the hospital by her son. She had several grown children, each of whom had taken a turn at caring for her during the past fifteen years. However, it had finally become impossible for them to care for her in their own homes because of her personality deterioration. Her difficulty had begun approximately three years prior to admission following a fairly severe bout of pneumonia. At that time it was noted that the patient had become increasingly forgetful. She seemed to live, according to her son, "in the past." She developed some difficulty with orientation and frequently seemed completely disoriented. She often talked to herself. She would wander about the house in an aimless manner; this habit became increasingly noticeable during the night time. She napped a great deal during the day and would refuse to remain in her room at night. She was finally brought to the hospital because her nocturnal wanderings could not be controlled.

Past history revealed that she had had a grammar-school education. She had worked for a period of a few years and subsequently married. She was described by her son as having been, in her earlier years, a pleasant, talkative, stable, friendly person. There was no evidence of any remarkable psychopathology during her early or middle life. Her marriage had been happy; her husband had died fifteen years prior to her admission to the hospital. Physical examination revealed a somewhat emaciated elderly woman who showed obvious signs of old age. However, there were no gross physical defects. There was evidence of a moderate arteriosclerosis commensurate with her age.

Mental status revealed an alert, superficially co-operative individual. She had some difficulty giving the proper answers, particularly where such answers involved the use of her memory, which was seriously impaired both for far past and recent past. For instance, she was unable to give the date or year of the birth of herself or of any of her children. She was unable to remember her home address, although she had lived there for many years. She was also unable to describe what she had had for breakfast earlier in the day. She was disoriented as to time and place. Several times she mentioned her husband as if he were still living. Her judgment was poor; she seemed childish from an emotional standpoint and was easily depressed over the slightest difficulties during the interview.

During her stay on the ward she caused no great problems. It was somewhat difficult to get her to take any medication because she surreptitiously spit out her pills after the nurse had left. She was found to have collected quite a number of useless trinkets and other odd items that she had found on the ward and had attempted to hide in her drawer and beneath her mattress. She frequently dozed during the day, even at the dinner table, and was often found wandering aimlessly about during the night. The treatment plan was essentially custodial with efforts directed toward maintaining her nutritional intake and her general body health.

CHRONIC BRAIN SYNDROME ASSOCIATED WITH OTHER DISTURBANCES OF METABOLISM, GROWTH, OR NUTRITION (INCLUDES PRESENILE, GLANDULAR, PELLAGRA, FAMILIAL AMAUROSIS)

This category includes a variety of chronic brain syndromes such as those resulting from endocrine disturbances, avitaminosis, and metabolic disorders. While they are not particularly common, several of them are worthy of brief discussion.

Alzheimer's disease is a presenile type of syndrome resulting from organic brain changes somewhat similar to but not exactly like those found in senile psychosis. The most common age of onset of this condition is somewhere between forty and sixty years. The onset is often insidious, progressing in a pattern similar to that seen in senile psychosis. There is a gradual clouding of the sensorium with difficulty in memory, orientation, and judgment. These patients progress through a slow but eventually complete personality disintegration. It is not uncommon to find aphasia, apraxia, or one of other similar difficulties in such a patient. There may or may not be the slow development of delusions. A certain amount of the symptom picture depends upon the premorbid personality.

The diagnosis is often difficult to make until the postmortem findings are established. Differential diagnosis involves Pick's disease and senile psychosis. The age of onset often is of help in ruling out senile psychosis. In Alzheimer's disease the symptoms ordinarily begin earlier than they are to be expected in senile psychosis. At postmortem the brain is found to be atrophied. There are senile plaques present, but the most characteristic finding is that of the so-called "Alzheimer tangles." These tangles are really neurofibrillary, with the appearance of baskets or whorls, and have replaced the neurones. There is some evidence, as yet inconclusive, to indicate that such tangles are found in other conditions and are not necessarily specific to Alzheimer's disease. There is no known treatment for this condition.

Case History: Alzheimer's Disease

A forty-eight-year-old man was brought to the hospital by his son. The latter stated that his father had shown many serious errors in judgment over the past few months, seemed to be unable to remember many events, had episodes of confusion, and had lost interest in his work and social life.

According to the son, the patient, a widower, had been in good health until approximately six to eight months prior to his admission. At that time he had met a woman many years his junior and had begun courting her. This courtship included a number of sizable gifts of money and a trip to a nearby resort where he had apparently planned to get married. He gave the woman a large sum of cash and she was never seen again. When the patient returned a few days later, the family noted that he was confused, mixed up about dates, and unable to give a comprehensible account of what had taken place. Following this, the son began spending more time with his father and noted that the latter showed frequent lapses of memory and disregard for bills which he had always paid promptly before. On several occasions the patient even forgot to go to work. One month prior to admission the patient's firm contacted the son complaining that the patient was no longer able to do his supervisory work, that he made gross errors in judgment, was unable to give instructions clearly to his assistants, could not remember order numbers which he had known for years, and often sat and did nothing.

Examination showed that the patient was oriented for person, but not for time nor place. He seemed to believe that he was in Atlantic City (he was in Philadelphia), and gave a date some two years in the past. He was unable to do simple arithmetic and could not give a clear description of what he did at his work. He seemed to have no knowledge that the affair with the young lady was over and spoke of her in the present tense. He was quite pleasant and almost jovial in manner, reacting to all stimuli in the same manner.

Physical examination was entirely within normal limits except for the fact that he showed some slight unsureness in gait. He was hospitalized and a pneumoencephalogram was done which showed some generalized cortical atrophy, most marked in both frontal areas.

Following the pneumoencephalogram, the patient showed what seemed a rather remarkable improvement and seemed to have a much better grasp of reality. He was oriented for place although he would still miss on dates. Clinical tests of calculation and general knowledge showed some impairment. Within a period of several weeks, however, the patient relapsed to his former state.

He was placed in a private sanatorium where he presented the following picture: He was oriented for person, but never for time or place. He thought he was at a resort hotel, or at the home of a friend, or in his own home. He would read the newspapers faithfully each day but would be unable to recall what he had just finished reading. He took walks daily but despite the profusion of foliage was unable to tell, from looking at it, what season of the year it was. He had one episode lasting a few weeks when he became disoriented for person, soiled himself, and had to be fed. He recovered from this but the gradual clouding of his sensorium, with difficulty in memory, orientation, and judgment, continued.

Pellagra, the syndrome resulting from a deficiency of nicotinic acid in the diet, is capable of producing a chronic brain syndrome. Early symptoms are ordinarily rather mild and are often misinterpreted as being due to neurasthenia. They are chronic lassitude, various vague somatic complaints, irritability, and depression. If the condition persists to a severe degree, there may occur a truly delirious state of a toxic variety. Cases of pellagra are much less frequent at the present time than they were prior to the extensive use of vitamins. If the pellagra has progressed to a sufficient degree the mental damage is irreversible. If, however, the condition is recognized early and large doses of nicotinic acid as well as other vitamins are given, the condition can be remedied. The patient who suffers from pellagra has been shown to have a deficiency of the other vitamins in the B group, as well as a deficiency of ascorbic acid in many cases; therefore, attention should be given to providing therapeutic doses of these vitamins as well as nicotinic acid.

Disturbances in thyroid function, whether of hyperactivity or hypoactivity, are capable of producing chronic brain syndromes. Hyperthyroidism ordinarily produces a tendency toward rapid mood changes, with irritability as well as anxiety. There may occur in relatively severe cases a tendency toward delusional formation, but this is most prominent where the patient's premorbid personality contained dynamics making the formation of delusions possible. The symptoms mentioned, along with the other characteristic findings of hyperthyroidism, are often sufficient to make the diagnosis. At times hyperthyroid patients progress to more maniclike behavior with an extreme hyperactivity. The treatment is directed toward amelioration of the thyroid malfunction.

Hypothyroidism may produce myxedema in the adult or cretinism in the child. The tendency in both these syndromes is toward a mental slowing and dulling. The patient gradually loses interest in his surroundings and develops what appears to be a true mental deficiency. In children, if the condition exists over a sufficient period of time before it is recognized and treated, it becomes irreversible, primarily because of permanent damage to the brain tissue. The treatment is directed toward amelioration of the hypothyroidism by the administration of thyroid.

Depending upon the degree of hypothyroidism in children, there is a more or less severe general retardation in development with the appearance of a particularly characteristic facies. The body is smaller than usual and the head appears large. There is a noticeable protrusion of the lips and the mouth is usually open with the tongue protruding. The hair, especially of the eyebrows, is scanty and the skin is dry. The child shows poor muscular development, and coordination and bone growth are also slowed. This condition, if it is of sufficient severity, can often be recognized within the first few months of life. If so, the administration of thyroid leads to a remarkable improvement. If, however, it is unrecognized for a sufficient period of time, subsequent thyroid medication is only partly successful.

CHRONIC BRAIN SYNDROME ASSOCIATED WITH INTRACRANIAL NEOPLASM

Certain brain tumors, either because of inoperability or brain-tissue damage, have produced personality changes which are beyond the reversible point at the time surgery is performed, and lead to a chronic brain syndrome. Obviously the symptomatology of such a condition depends upon the type of neoplasm and the area in which it grows, as well as its extent. Many brain tumors produce symptoms through pressure and edema and if surgery is performed in time the symptoms are reversible. In such a case the diagnosis belongs within the acute brain syndrome category.

Case History: Chronic Brain Syndrome Associated with Intracranial Neoplasm

This fifty-six-year-old woman was admitted to the psychiatric service with a diagnosis of catatonic depression with deterioration. She was admitted for the purpose of electroshock therapy. The history revealed that the patient had begun to develop gradual personality changes about a year and a half previously. These included feelings of depression, irritability, and delusions of persecution. During the course of time her children noticed that the patient had some difficulty in walking, with a tendency to fall to the right. There were frequent complaints of headaches and occasional nausea and vomiting. She had repeated examinations by medical men and two-and-a-half months prior to admission had been thoroughly investigated in a hospital in another city. After six weeks, diagnosis of hypertension and involutional psychotic reaction had been made. She was put on medication and discharged.

From the time of the first hospitalization until admission to this hospital, the patient's condition rapidly deteriorated until she became incontinent of bowel and bladder, uncommunicative, confused, and debilitated. On examination the patient was found to look much older than her age. Her nutritional state was poor. Her extremities were flaccid. Both pupils reacted equally to light. There was a grade four papilledema in the right eye and beginning papilledema in the left eye. There was nuchal rigidity and teeth grinding. Her blood pressure was elevated to 148/110; her pulse was 150. There was a gallop rhythm of the heart. Pressure sores were evident behind the right ear and over the gluteal region and the heels. All deep tendon reflexes were absent. She responded to painful stimuli. A tentative diagnosis of right frontal brain tumor was made and established by further laboratory and X-ray examinations.

Surgery was performed and a large, rapidly growing glioblastoma multiforma was removed from the frontal lobe. Following surgery the patient's nutritional status, blood pressure, pulse, and sensory responses improved.

Her condition continued to improve somewhat for five months, at which time she redeveloped symptoms in much the same pattern. She then began to show evidence of spread of the tumor, portions of which had not been removed. She was hospitalized, and died two months later.

CHRONIC BRAIN SYNDROME ASSOCIATED WITH DISEASES OF UNKNOWN OR UNCERTAIN CAUSE (INCLUDES MULTIPLE SCLEROSIS, HUNTINGTON'S CHOREA, PICK'S DISEASE, AND OTHER DISEASES OF A FAMILIAL OR HEREDITARY NATURE)

This is a category in which the organic brain damage is a result of a specific pathological process, the origin or etiology of which is unknown. The three most prominent syndromes in this category are multiple sclerosis, Pick's disease, and Huntington's chorea. Multiple sclerosis is the most common of the three, but all warrant brief discussion.

Multiple sclerosis or, as it is sometimes called, disseminated sclerosis is a disease of unknown origin involving the formation throughout the central nervous system of small sclerotic plaques which occur in both gray and white matter. Since plaques are scattered throughout the brain, it is possible, particularly in the later phases of this disease, to see personality changes. Not all of these cases reveal mental symptoms, but those that do show a variety of personality changes. Early in the disease there is often an accentuation of premorbid personality traits. However, as the disease progresses, there is an increasing disorganization of personality, and perhaps most characteristic in the later phases is a euphoric state of mind with apparently complete disregard for the degree of physical incapacitation which has by that time occurred. It is difficult to outline the symptoms of multiple sclerosis accurately, since the formation of plaques takes place indiscriminately throughout the central nervous system. The syndrome may affect the basal ganglia, for instance, and produce one set of symptoms, whereas it may, in another case, affect primarily another area of the brain and produce an entirely different set of symptoms.

Pick's disease is a comparatively rare form of presenile dementia occurring characteristically in people between the ages of forty and sixty. It involves the circumscribed atrophy particularly of the frontal and temporal lobes, and, in many cases, of primarily only one side of the brain. The symptoms of this condition often are very similar to those of senile psychosis or Alzheimer's disease, and the differential diagnosis, particularly from the latter, is extremely difficult, if not impossible, until postmortem. There is a progressive personality disintegration with an increasing clouding of the sensorium and disturbance of memory, orientation, and judgment. Neither etiology nor treatment is known at present.

Huntington's chorea is a familial disease, characterized by the appearance of choreiform movements, involving upper extremities, facial muscles, and finally even the lower extremities. Involvement of the latter results in a dancing type of gait which is quite noticeable in these patients. Mental symptoms come on slowly but occasionally may even predate physical symptoms. Patients may be either euphoric or depressed, but here, as with many other organic syndromes, there is a gradual disorganization of personality. Judgment is impaired; the mood becomes unstable with irritability; there may develop an apparent lack of concern about personal appearance and habits. The patient becomes difficult to manage and unable to maintain his occupation or family duties. At times one finds a temporary cessation of the progression of symptoms, but most frequently there is a continued personality disintegration on to the point of dementia. There is no effective treatment.

Case History: Chronic Brain Syndrome, Disease of Unknown Origin (Multiple Sclerosis)

This thirty-five-year-old male was admitted to the hospital with a complaint of numbness and weakness in the right arm and leg and left hand for a period of two years. Physical examination revealed some spasticity of the involved extremities with irregular sensory disturbances. Reflexes were increased unequally. There was a positive Babinski on the right, absence of abdominal reflexes, and no co-ordination in movements of the upper extremities. The patient had a hypotonic neurogenic bladder.

Laboratory studies were essentially negative, including studies of spinal fluid. Diagnosis of multiple sclerosis was made.

This patient seemed, when interviewed, comparatively unconcerned about his physical incapacitation. He was quite happy and at times almost euphoric, claiming that he loved to be in the hospital. He seemed neither worried nor depressed about his condition. He stated on occasions that his tongue was "growing" and therefore got in his way when he tried to talk. His speech was often of a scanning type. His memory was relatively clear. His first symptoms had appeared about eighteen months prior to his admission when he had difficulty walking and would sometimes fall because his knees gave way. This was soon followed by the presenting complaints, and he finally reached the stage where he was not ambulatory at all. This also gave him little apparent worry. He felt that all of his troubles were caused by "too much aggravation from being unemployed."

When left alone this patient sometimes became noisy, obstreperous, and tried to get out of bed. He was somewhat irritable and unpredictable with the other patients. At times it became necessary to restrain him. At such periods he seemed rather confused and disoriented but subsequently his sensorium would clear up. Whenever interviewed he usually presented a picture of contentment, satisfaction, and lack of concern, in spite of the gradual progression of his symptoms, difficulty with constipation, and some physical wasting.

Chronic Brain Disorders

Mental Retardation

PART VIII

Mental Retardation

CHAPTER 20

Mental Retardation

IF WE COULD PLOT statistically the intellectual endowment of every person, we would find that the majority lies somewhere near the "normal" or "average." Extending in both directions would be progressively smaller numbers of individuals. Some would be found to be endowed with a higher than usual intellectual ability, and an approximately equal number with a lower than normal intellectual capacity. It is with these latter that we are primarily concerned here.

Mental retardation may be defined as a chronic condition manifested by impaired intellectual functioning and present from birth or early childhood. This term will be used here synonymously with mental deficiency, feeble-mindedness, mental subnormality and mental inadequacy. In general all of these terms have been used to refer to individuals who show difficulties in learning, reasoning, abstract thinking, and adaptive abilities. Since there are many factors to be considered, the criteria for establishing such a diagnosis are obviously somewhat arbitrary. In the first place, the words *intelligence* or *intellect* are used relatively freely, but even the psychologists who measure this capacity are not in clear agreement about exactly what it encompasses or represents. We use the terms "smart" or "stupid" casually, often in reference to individual actions which may be motivated by emotional factors. Many children have scored poorly in intelligence tests primarily because they suffered from marked anxiety during the testing situation. Theoretically, at least, the concept of intelligence should represent the individual's potential unhampered by emotional problems, but practically it often does not. Intelligence has been defined in Hinsie's dictionary [1] as "The capacity to understand and manage abstract ideas and symbols . . . to invent and manage mechanisms . . . and to act reasonably and wisely as regards human relations and social affairs . . ." The first of these is abstract intelligence, the second mechanical intelligence, and the third social intelligence. The average intelligence test leans somewhat more heavily on the first two of these, but the total evaluation should include the "human relations and social affairs" aspects.

Early in this century the first attempts were made to provide adequate means for measuring intelligence. When compulsory education was instituted in France, it was soon discovered that certain children did not benefit by the usual type of schooling. Binet and Simon were commissioned to devise means for determining the difficulties in these children. Out of their experiments came the earliest standardized intelligence test which was brought to this country a few years later and which has since undergone several revisions. At the present time we have fairly adequate, although by no means foolproof, methods of measuring the intelligence of children as well as of adults.

Any attempt to evaluate accurately the number of mentally retarded individuals in the United States will obviously rest upon the criteria which are used to determine mental retardation itself. For instance, estimates have varied from five million to more than thirty million. The reason for such a great variation in estimates is found in the arbitrary I.Q. levels proposed for separating "mental retardation" from the "normal" population. The American Psychiatric Association, for instance, has decided that an I.Q. of below 85 is within the mental retardation category, while the American Association for Mental Deficiency has decided upon an I.Q. of 70. This means that the disagreement involves about twenty-five million or more persons. The basic question of whether a child or adult who tests reliably at an I.Q. of 80 is mentally retarded or not is difficult to answer. Such an individual can theoretically perform at about four-fifths of the average person's capacity in those areas tested by the intelligence examination. He may be able to undertake success-

[1] Hinsie, L. E. and Shatzky, J. *Psychiatric Dictionary*. Oxford University Press, 1947.

fully many useful and remunerative jobs, but may still lag behind in "pure" intelligence as we measure it. Mental retardation is a relative term, and it is impossible to decide accurately on a cut-off point based purely on I.Q. The recognition of mental retardation increases at early school age primarily because schools require certain skills which many children have not had to demonstrate previously. The incidence of diagnosis of mental retardation again rises at draft age because many young men who have previously been functioning reasonably well are unable to pass the necessary "intelligence tests." Are these children and young people really to be labeled "mentally retarded," or is this a deficiency which only appears during periods of stress, or when we administer certain tests? It is true that about one-third of our population is statistically below "average" in intelligence. Whether we call them mentally retarded or borderline or subnormal is not as important as the fact that many of them probably could function at a higher intelligence level if their parents and society had provided them with proper medical care. There is another group of mentally retarded who by virtue of heredity, birth injury, or other unpreventable situations function intellectually below the average. This is a smaller group and includes such disorders as mongolism, hydrocephalus, and many of the more rare conditions. Largest, however, is the group of mildly retarded who have suffered from poor or absent obstetrical care, inadequate nutrition, distorted emotional environments, and inadequate intellectual stimulation.

That mental retardation is an important social, economic, and medical challenge is well illustrated by the report of the President's Panel on Mental Retardation in October 1962.[2] Unfortunately, society has lagged behind in its efforts to provide maximum care and, where possible, proper education for these people. The President's Panel suggests possible answers to some of these problems.

[2] A National Plan to Combat Mental Retardation: Report of the President's Panel on Mental Retardation, U.S. Government Printing Office, Washington, D.C., 1963.

CLASSIFICATION OF MENTAL RETARDATION

There are two general approaches to the classification of mental retardation. One concerns itself primarily with the degree of retardation, and the other with the specific etiology. While space does not permit complete discussion of these two approaches, some attention will be given to each.

DEGREE

The degree of mental retardation is currently the most common basis for classification. Unfortunately there is not complete agreement here between the American Association for Mental Deficiency and the American Psychiatric Association. Both divide these individuals according to the degree of severity of the handicap, but each does it somewhat differently. The American Psychiatric Association utilizes three categories: mild, moderate, and severe; while the American Association for Mental Deficiency uses borderline, mild, moderate, severe, and profound. Below is a comparison of the two classifications in brief form.

As can be seen from the following chart, the vast majority of mentally retarded have I.Q.'s over 50. This demarcation, when not accompanied by a more thorough evaluation, often means little but it has been used by the medical profession as well as by many state legislatures to divide the so-called "educable" mentally retarded from the "trainable" mentally retarded. The former term refers to those individuals who can master at least the rudiments of reading, writing, and arithmetic. Obviously the closer they are to the upper limits of mental retardation, the better they will be able to grasp these abstract concepts. The term "trainable" has been generally used to designate those individuals whose I.Q.'s fall below 50 and who ordinarily cannot learn the fundamentals of reading, writing, and arithmetic, but who are trainable in the basic functions of self-care and self-help. Here again, the closer the person is to the upper limits of his particular category, the more adept he will be in learning various skills.

One advantage to the A.A.M.D. classification is that a somewhat

I.Q.	A.P.A.	A.A.M.D.	TOTAL IN U.S.
85 70	Mild	Borderline	25,000,000+
70 50	Moderate	Mild	6,000,000+
50 35	Severe	Moderate	600,000+
		Severe	
20 0		Profound	200,000+

more precise estimate of potential abilities can be made. For instance, in the A.A.M.D. borderline group of I.Q.'s from 70–85 we find those individuals who are capable of going through grade school and junior high school and who even may be able to complete high school in a vocational program. They are quite capable of becoming self-sufficient, and their mental retardation tends to come to light only under conditions of stress. The A.A.M.D. group of mildly retarded whose I.Q.'s fall between 50–70 can master academic material to perhaps the fifth- or sixth-grade level by the time they reach adulthood. Usually they cannot complete high school, but do profit from special education. They are capable of learning some basic trade skills and can perform these best under supervision. The group of individuals whose I.Q.'s fall between 35–50 can learn to talk reasonably well, but do not learn to master complex social situations. They can learn only the rudiments of reading, writing, and arithmetic and their eventual mental age will be approximately 4½ to 7 years. The A.A.M.D. group of severely retarded whose

I.Q.'s are between 20–35 may develop a limited vocabulary, but require supervision throughout their adult lives. Their mental age eventually will be between about 2 and 4½ years of age. Physical handicaps are more common and those in this group usually need institutionalization. Those whose I.Q.'s fall below 20 in the A.A.M.D. classification suffer profound retardation and are in need of constant care. They do not learn to talk and often cannot walk. They show the highest percentage of physical stigmata and not infrequently die at an early age.

Mention should be made at this time of the older terms *moron, imbecile,* and *idiot.* In general, the moron corresponded to our present-day mildly retarded, the imbecile to the moderately retarded, and the idiot to the severely retarded.

ETIOLOGY

The etiology of mental retardation is complex, and many factors contribute. These may be divided broadly into socio-cultural, psychological, and somatic factors. As a rule of thumb, it may be said that the milder the degree of mental retardation, the more the socio-cultural elements are prominent. In the severe degrees of retardation the somatic factors become predominant. Relevant socio-cultural factors most often are found in the lower socio-economic groups among whom adequate obstetric and pediatric care is often lacking. In addition, there is not infrequently inadequate intellectual stimulation during the child's formative years. All of this tends to produce a higher rate of mental retardation in the lower socio-economic groups.

Psychological factors are also important in leading to impaired intellectual development. Anything which slows or distorts personality development also may well impair intellectual ability. An emotionally insecure childhood often produces excessive anxiety which in turn may interfere with intellectual potential. Psychotic and borderline reactions of childhood are examples. These children usually test far below their potentials on ordinary intelligence tests, and are not infrequently labeled as mentally retarded and at times even committed to institutions for the retarded.

Somatic factors involved in mental retardation are numerous.

They include conditions associated with infection, intoxication, trauma, disorders in metabolism and nutrition, new growths and various unknown factors. In the past many of these conditions have been described according to the physical manifestations which they produced, while others have been given the name of their discoverer. As medical advances have increased our understanding of many of these syndromes, they are now recognized earlier and also treated more effectively. Space will permit discussion of only a few of them; the interested student is referred to the material in the suggested reading list.

Phenylketonuria, often called PKU, is a metabolic disorder which results from an inability to convert phenylalanine to tyrosine. Infants with this condition usually do not show abnormal neurological signs nor gross physical malformations. If untreated, they usually deteriorate to severe mental retardation. The diagnosis is established by testing the urine for phenylpyruvic acid. This test is relatively simple and efforts have been made to expand its use to include all hospital nurseries. The early detection of PKU allows prompt institution of treatment measures, primarily dietary, which will lessen or even eradicate the retardation. Genetic factors have been shown to be involved in this condition.

Mongolism is one of the most common clinical syndromes in mental retardation and derives its name from the patient's supposed facial resemblance to the Mongolian people. The eyes are somewhat slanted, and this is exaggerated because of the increased epicanthic fold. The bridge of the nose is flattened, and the tongue tends to protrude. There is hypotonicity of the muscles, and these patients have short, stubby fingers. The degree of mental retardation in Mongolism varies somewhat, but the majority have I.Q.'s of about 30 to 50. Most of these patients are good-natured and relatively easy to manage. It has been shown statistically that a woman is slightly more apt to produce a Mongoloid child during the later years of her reproductive life than in the earlier years. Recent work has shown evidence of chromosomal abnormalities in cases of Mongolism. There is at the present time no known form of curative treatment.

Hydrocephalus is a condition which not infrequently leads to mental retardation. It is the result of an excessive accumulation of cerebrospinal fluid within the skull, usually inside the ventricular system. An obstruction somewhere within the circulating pathway of the cerebrospinal fluid is usually responsible, but at times the hydrocephalus may be a result of faulty absorption. As the cerebrospinal fluid accumulates either before or shortly after birth, the internal pressure enlarges the head, forces the cranial sutures apart, and progressively destroys brain tissue. Eventually, with markedly enlarged ventricles, the cerebral hemispheres are reduced to thin layers. Occasionally the hydrocephalic condition spontaneously arrests itself and at other times surgical intervention stops its progress. The degree of mental retardation will be proportionate to the amount of destroyed central nervous system tissue.

Cerebral palsy is a condition in which there is a developmental abnormality in some part or parts of the motor cortex of the cerebrum. This leads to a spastic type of paralysis as a result of the upper motor neuron lesion. The degree of spastic involvement varies from minimal to a major involvement of all four extremities and trunk. This condition may arise prior to birth, at the time of birth itself or subsequently. The etiology is not always known, but can be a result of mechanical birth injuries or postnatal infections or RH incompatibilities. While it is true that mental retardation is somewhat more common in children afflicted with cerebral palsy than in the normal population, such a retardation is by no means universal. These children, especially those with severe motor and speech handicaps, have difficulty in communication and often appear retarded when actually they are not. The degree of retardation is not necessarily correlated with the degree of neurological involvement.

Cretinism is a condition due to hypothyroidism and may be caused by an iodine deficiency in the diet of the mother, a small or even absent thyroid gland in the infant, or by a genetically determined enzyme defect. The symptoms, which are usually not manifest for the first few months of life, include slow growth, thickening of the subcutaneous tissue, thinning hair, relaxed musculature with protruding abdomen, and general sluggishness. Cretinism occasionally does not appear until later in childhood and then is an acquired type rather than the congenital variety. Prompt recognition of the condition and institution of thyroid medication is essential. The longer the cretinism remains untreated, the more irreversible becomes the mental retardation.

Microcephaly is a condition in which the skull circumference is seventeen inches or less. Clinically, the microcephalic seems to have a head which is pointed on top because of flattening of the occipital and frontal areas. The hair is peculiar and wiry and tends to grow low on the forehead. The skin is wrinkled, giving the patient an old appearance. Most of those afflicted have moderate or severe degrees of mental deficiency and reveal a poorly developed brain structure.

Congenital spastic paraplegia forms a sizable percentage of cases within those with early etiology. There is a wide variation in the degree of organic brain impairment and there may or may not be an associated mental deficiency secondary to this organic change. Unfortunately, because of the physical handicaps suffered by many of the children in this group, they have great difficulty in making themselves understood and may at times be misdiagnosed as mental defectives when in reality they have normal or even superior intellect.

The two remaining etiological factors within this category are prenatal maternal infections such as measles, and brain damage suffered by the infant during the process of birth. The resultant degree of mental deficiency obviously depends upon the type and severity of the organic damage which has been produced.

There are many other syndromes which are associated with mental deficiency. These include some due to disorders of metabolism, such as Tay-Sach's disease and gargoylism. Others are associated with tumors and include Von Recklinghausen's disease and tuberous sclerosis. Still others, like the Laurence-Moon-Biedl syndrome are due to unknown prenatal influences. It is suggested in the A.P.A. nomenclature that only those cases which have existed since birth and which do not show organic brain disease or reveal any prenatal cause for the defect may be properly classified within the category of mental deficiency. This concept is not adhered to by the A.A.M.D., whose classification considers retardation as the important factor, and then subdivides the various causes.

It is important for the student to realize that we already possess a great deal of knowledge about the prevention of mental retardation. Much of this knowledge has yet not been put to use on a sufficiently wide basis. For instance, mental retardation due to infection, intoxication, and trauma is widespread. Much of it is the result of inadequate obstetrical and pediatric care. From the standpoint of sheer numbers a great deal of mild and moderate mental retardation could be prevented by more broad utilization of modern medical knowledge. There are other areas of mental retardation, however, which have not yet yielded their secrets. For the most part, these are the more severely retarded children; we are only beginning to make occasional breakthroughs in this area. An example is our current understanding of phenylketonuria and galactosemia which are now recognized as metabolic disorders. An additional example is Mongolism, in which our new understanding of chromosomal abnormalities is proving useful. While prevention may still elude us in many of these conditions, treatment, if applied early, can often be profitable. In others such as Mongolism, we will have to await more knowledge before we can effectively prevent or treat.

Proper evaluation of a mentally retarded child requires not only a thorough physical examination, but also a full and complete history of the patient and his family. Various other procedures are often essential. These include psychological testing, electroencephalogram, neurological consultation, psychiatric evaluation, and special laboratory examinations. Firm and accurate diagnostic procedures may or may not be possible during early infancy or even for several years. It is as important, however, to avoid early unfounded, rigid statements to parents about "feeble-mindedness" as it is to procrastinate with unwarranted remarks that "he will grow out of it." The physician should also remember that the mental defective is subject to emotional problems just as are individuals of normal or superior intelligence.

Stress is in fact more apt to produce a psychotic or other disturbed reaction in the mental defective than in a normally intelligent person. Mental illness accompanying mental retardation presents difficult diagnostic problems. Psychotherapy may not be as efficient in the mentally retarded because of their difficulty in comprehending the abstract concepts that are ordinarily dealt with in treatment. Nevertheless, many of the retarded are responsive to therapeutic help and often respond in a gratifying manner.

PSYCHOLOGICAL TESTING

The use of psychological tests has a comparable value in the diagnosis of mental retardation to the laboratory tests used in the diagnosis of somatic disorders. They serve as a valuable aid to the clinician and, if properly administered by trained personnel, can be of great assistance. However, like laboratory tests, psychological examinations cannot substitute for a clinical examination and a wise clinical judgment.

Psychological tests fall into two main categories: those which are designed to reveal the level of intellectual functioning and which are called intelligence tests, and those which are intended to elicit emotional factors within the personality and are called projective tests.

Intelligence testing was first devised by Binet in France. The original test contained a series of problems, arranged in a scale of increasing difficulty. The various problems included those of memory, language, information, attention, perception, association, discrimination, etc. A set of problems was developed which theoretically could be solved by the child of normal intelligence at each year level. For instance, the normal child of ten could solve all of those problems at the ten-year level on the test, as well as all those below, but none in the eleven or above categories. The administration of this test, which has subsequently been revised and refined, gives a "mental age" which may then be correlated with the child's chronological age. If, for instance, a child of ten solved all the problems of the eight-year level but none above that, his intelligence quotient (I.Q.) would be arrived at by dividing 8 by 10 and multiplying the answer by 100, thus giving an I.Q. of 80. Theoretically the average I.Q. of the entire population is 100, with a spread both above and below this mean. The Binet test is based upon the assumption that intellectual maturity is reached at the age of 15 years. Using this instrument in the testing of adults, one must use the chronological age of 15 regardless of the age of the adult, and then must divide it into the mental age obtained by the patient on the test.

The Binet was a great step forward in the evaluation of intellectual functioning. It must be remembered, however, that there is still no clear agreement as to the scope of "intellect." Theoretically this concept includes the individual's ability to adapt to his environment and to plan for his future. How efficiently these abilities are evaluated by intelligence tests is debatable. Since the original Binet test was introduced there have been several revisions made, particularly the Stanford-Binet [3] revision of 1916 and the Terman and Merrill revision in 1937.[4] The Binet leans heavily upon the individual's ability in verbal performance. Various other tests have been revised which deal primarily with performance in solving various puzzles. These do not discriminate against the person who lacks a formal education or who has a language or reading handicap. The combination of verbal and performance tests is used by the Wechsler-Bellevue Intelligence Scale.[5] This test was originally devised for adults and has some advantages over the Binet for use in this age range. A subsequent downward extension of the Bellevue, the Wechsler-Bellevue Intelligence Scale for Children, or WISC, has been widely used.

A few relatively simple tests have been devised which can be administered to groups of individuals. These are particularly useful to the military services; a good example is the Army Alpha Test. These examinations are not as accurate as individually administered tests, but nevertheless, where group testing is essential, they do give some rough estimation of intelligence and tend to point out gross mental retardation.

Psychological tests have been devised for use with infants; a popular example is the Cattell Infant Scale.[6] Obviously the measurement of intellectual endowment in the very young child or infant can only be a rough estimate and is subject to more errors than tests of

[3] Terman, L. M. *The Measurement of Intelligence*. Boston, Houghton Mifflin, 1916.

[4] Merrill, Maud A. and Terman, Lewis M. *Measuring Intelligence*. Boston, Houghton Mifflin, 1937.

[5] Wechsler, David. *Measurement of Adult Intelligence*. Baltimore, Williams and Wilkins, 1941.

[6] Cattell, Psyche. *The Measurement of Intelligence of Infants and Young Children*. New York, Psychological Corporation, 1940.

older children or adults. However, there has been sufficient development of infant tests to make them a valuable addition to the psychological armamentaria. In this area, perhaps more than any other, the adequate training and good judgment of the psychologist are essential.

The projective tests are devised to reveal emotional problems and present to the subject a partially structured or unstructured stimulus which requires that he "project" something of himself in the form of a response. Such stimuli may be ink blots as are used in the widely known Rorschach Test [7] devised by Hermann Rorschach, a Swiss psychiatrist. This is a standardized set of ten cards, each with an ink blot. Some of the blots contain colors while others do not. The patient is shown one card at a time and asked merely to tell what he thinks it looks like. This is an unstructured type of stimulus and requires that the patient "project" something of himself and his inner thinking into his response. The card has no obvious or definite meaning and the patient's answers are dictated primarily by his own inner emotional life. It has been found that the patient's reactions to color or to shading, for example, are indicative of various emotional aspects of his life. Some patients react to the entire ink blot, while others use only small portions. Some show a great deal of originality, while others give more or less "popular" answers —those which have been found to be frequent in the records of many people. The use of the Rorschach requires considerable experience and study on the part of the psychologist, and its correct interpretation is a skill mastered only after such training. Various other tests of a projective type have been devised such as the Thematic Apperception Test or TAT. This is a series of cards showing different scenes with human figures and the patient is asked to tell a story about each. He is instructed to say something about what has gone before, what is going on during the picture, and what will take place subsequently. The structuring here is more obvious than in the Rorschach, but the scenes are so portrayed as to highlight the important inner emotional complexes that might otherwise not be particularly apparent on clinical examination. The Thematic Apperception Test has been extended to include a group of cards suitable

[7] Rorschach, Hermann. *Psychodiagnostics.* New York, Grune and Stratton, 1943.

for testing children; these are called the Children's Apperception Test or CAT.

Numerous other psychological tests are available, some designed to reveal specific aspects of the personality, such as the presence of visual-motor defects. While it is not within the scope of this book to discuss all these tests, mention should be made of the Bender-Gestalt, which is particularly useful in determining the presence of diffuse organic brain damage. This is a series of cards with various geometric figures which the patient is asked to reproduce on a piece of plain white paper. Many patients who suffer from organic brain damage are unable to reproduce such figures with any degree of accuracy. They have difficulty in perceiving the Gestalt or whole arrangement. Other factors, such as anxiety, may impair the patient's ability to reproduce such designs and again, the psychologist's training is important in the proper evaluation of the test results.

It should be re-emphasized that all of these psychological examinations should be used primarily as adjuncts to clinical judgment and not as a replacement for such judgment. The services of a competent psychologist are invaluable, but cannot replace an adequate history, physical examination, and evaluation of the emotional status of the patient.

TREATMENT

The proper treatment and care of the mentally retarded is based upon an accurate diagnosis, consideration of the current function and potential of the particular child, and the total family situation. Treatment plans cannot be made on the basis of the answer to a simple question, such as "Is this child retarded?" Rather, they need to be based upon such questions as, "What is the degree of retardation?" "What are the various potentials?" "What lies behind the retardation?" and "What is the total family picture which must be dealt with in the long-range planning for the youngster?" Other problems usually present themselves in the evaluation of such a child. These include the availability of community services such as special education classes, sheltered workshops for the retarded, and institutions. A proper therapeutic plan is one which is feasible in the particular situation.

One of the greatest difficulties the physician may face is the parents' unwillingness to accept the fact that their child is mentally retarded. This is most apt to occur where parents are quite intelligent and the disparity between their intellects and that of the child is great. Such parents are apt to feel guilty, unconsciously feeling at fault for producing such a child. Their guilt forces them into "medical shopping" in the hope of finding some other answer. Many well-educated parents today are acquainted with the concept of childhood psychosis, and look for someone who will tell them that their child is really psychotic rather than retarded. They feel that such a diagnosis would offer them a more favorable prognosis. Other parents, after hesitantly accepting mental retardation as a diagnosis, will seek some type of drug or other treatment that will "cure" their child. The physician's first big task is, therefore, to convince the parents that their child has limited intellectual ability and that his future must be planned around this fact.

Following the establishment of a reasonably accurate estimate of the child's intellectual and social potential, as well as his family's emotional maturity and their acceptance of the child's limitations, the physician must be prepared to offer a long-range plan of therapy. In all probability he will have to continue to play at least a peripheral role in such treatment plans. It is his responsibility to evaluate not only the child and family, but also the potential resources within the community which are available. The so-called "educable" child, usually considered to be the one with an I.Q. above 50, can often remain within the community and live in his own home. In many areas his education can be provided by special classes offered by the public school systems. Such classes are usually comprised of a smaller number of students than in the ordinary class and are taught by an educator trained in special education methods. These classes are often referred to as "ungraded" rooms. The material presented to these children is within their potential for learning and they are not in constant competition with more normal youngsters. Whenever possible, intermingling of special-education-class children and regular-class youngsters is arranged, such as at recess, lunch period, and so forth. Thus the mentally retarded children are provided with the special classroom approach which they require but without being made to feel totally different or separated from normal children.

Each state maintains institutions for the retarded which may be referred to as "schools," "hospitals," or "homes." Many of these were established years ago when our understanding of mental retardation was quite limited. They were intended for the "trainable" group, but it was not realized that some "educable" children, because of family difficulties or emotional problems, might need institutionalization, nor that certain "trainable" children could live comfortably within the community. As a result many of these large, overpopulated institutions now contain certain children and even middle-aged adults who do not belong there.

In general it may be said that no mentally retarded child should be institutionalized when it is possible within the home and community to provide him with good care and a reasonable education. Very often a mildly or moderately retarded child is institutionalized because of emotional problems within himself or his family rather than because of the retardation itself. The more seriously retarded child often requires and benefits by institutionalization. His care requires constant supervision, which is not within the capabilities of the average family. In a well-run institution for the retarded he will not only be well cared for, but will have the opportunity to reach his maximum potential.

Another point which should be stressed is that admission to an institution for the retarded is not necessarily a permanent decision. The child may, after a period of time, be quite capable of return to the home and community from which he came. It has been repeatedly proven that many young people can return home from such institutions if adequate social casework services are available to their families and to the community.

PART IX

Therapy

CHAPTER 21

Principles of Psychotherapy

THE ETIOLOGY of psychiatric disorders varies from the purely psychological to the organic and traumatic. It follows that any method of treatment, if valuable, will be based upon an understanding of the etiological process. Such treatment may be surgical, medical, endocrinological, psychological, or any combination of these. Many of the general principles involved in treatment of functional psychiatric disorders can be applied to the other conditions, but only in conjunction with the more specific treatments indicated.

Psychotherapy may be defined as the art and science of treating mental and emotional disorders and diseases through changing ideas and emotions to bring about a more favorable psychic equilibrium. Almost every physician except perhaps the pathologist uses psychotherapy to some degree, with greater or lesser skill. This includes everyone from the general practitioner to the mental hospital psychiatrist. Almost any method utilized to alleviate or remove the results of emotional conflict and improve psychic adjustment may be termed psychotherapy.

The individual in need of psychotherapy is one who has failed to meet his life situation adequately. Therefore, in considering his problems we take into account both his external situation and the structure and function of his personality. The degree of disturbance in his adjustment may vary all the way from a mild neurotic reaction to a severe psychotic state. When the incapacitation is sufficiently great it becomes necessary to remove the individual from his environment and place him in a hospital, where his activity will not bring harm to himself or others. When the incapacitation is less, he may be treated in his own environment. Certain people because of a very poor personality development are precipitated into various types of functional disorders by relatively minor environmental problems. To such poorly integrated people even the ordinary problems met by the average person are too difficult, and a neurosis or psychosis is the result. Other individuals with more mature personalities are able to withstand greater amounts of environmental pressure before breakdown occurs. For instance, it was shown in the last war that the neuropsychiatric casualty rate rose sharply after about two hundred straight days of combat. It was at this time that the excessive and continued pressure of the external situation began to disrupt even those soldiers with the most mature personalities.

It is truly amazing the degree of stress which can be withstood by the human personality if it is well integrated. In the world today such stresses are increasing. Life is complex and man must make new adjustments daily. The insecurities arising from the constant threat of war, the stress of great competitiveness in today's world, and, at least in the United States, the importance attributed to achievement all place their burdens upon the psychic adjustment. Life moves very rapidly; personality flexibility is an essential to a stable adjustment. The individual hampered by inner conflict finds himself unable to withstand the strain and begins to develop increasing signs of maladjustment. Such manifestations may be in the form of neurotic symptoms such as phobias, compulsions, or anxiety. They may be in the form of personality disturbances such as alcoholism, delinquency, or promiscuity. Constant undischarged emotional tension may on the other hand upset body physiology and lead to psychophysiologic disorders. Certain individuals find the whole affair of living to be intolerable and break with reality to become psychotic.

It is with all such individuals that psychiatry is concerned and it is for them that psychotherapy is intended. The inner problems are ordinarily the crucial ones on which the therapist's attention must be focused in dealing with the patient. For a certain small number of individuals, environmental manipulation will suffice to let them attain and maintain freedom from symptoms, but in the average case this is not true, and the therapeutic result will also depend upon attention being given the inner conflicts. For instance, a man may begin to suffer with insomnia after the loss of his job and increasing accumulation of debts. If he is reasonably normal, providing him with a new job will cure his sleeplessness. On the other hand, if he lost his job because of an inner difficulty which led to unnecessary arguments with his co-workers, then a new job will not provide permanent improvement.

The individual who is in need of psychotherapy is the one who has, as a result of his childhood years, formed a faulty personality structure which still retains many of its infantile characteristics. For instance, the patient who still has much of his childish dependency will find the adult world a difficult and frustrating place. He may openly acknowledge and freely attempt to gratify his needs by form-ing an obviously dependent relationship with various important people in his environment, such as his wife and his boss, or may continue to manifest his dependency upon his parents in an exag-gerated way. It may however be unacceptable to him to reveal to himself or to others the extent of his dependency needs and he may then attempt to deny them by assuming a characteristically inde-pendent attitude. The inner unfulfilled urges may then lead to a disturbed gastrointestinal physiology and eventually to ulcer forma-tion. Obviously the more the therapist is able to recognize the inner difficulties of patients the more rational and successful will his assist-ance be.

There are certain general principles applicable to the psychothera-peutic situation. First of all, let us discuss what is now being called one-to-one psychotherapy, which is based on a relationship between two people. The patient has come to the physician for assistance in understanding himself in an effort to reach a more mature level of adjustment. Two things are therefore demanded of the therapist: first, he must be able to correctly evaluate the patient's dynamic picture; and secondly, he must find a means of imparting this infor-mation to the patient in a way that will have meaning and will produce benefit. Unfortunately the mere intellectual explanation of the patient's pattern to him will not produce such a change. The knowledge must reach an emotional level to be of effective and lasting value. One of the greatest paradoxes of psychotherapy lies in the fact that the individual comes seeking help, makes sacrifices to obtain it, and yet his own inner defenses automatically slow up and hamper the therapeutic process. The essential point is that the patient reacts to the therapist with the only means at his command: his warped emotional pattern. He may be hostile, withdrawn, facetious, sarcastic, friendly, or exhibit any one of a multitude of other possible reactions. To the therapist the patient's emotional patterns of reaction must become a matter for consideration and understanding rather than a situation which calls forth a variety of emotional responses from the therapist. The capable psychotherapist is friendly, kind, interested, consistent, and considerate. He does not react to hostility or withdrawal with hostility or withdrawal, but rather with an attempt to understand why the patient is angry or withdrawn.

Neurotic symptoms and patterns of behavior have resulted from the individual's attempt to adjust to inner conflicts which have in turn been engendered by a pathological past environment. For instance, the child coming from a home where emotional display is frowned upon will probably set up various defenses against such an expression and will find it difficult to change them later in life. As he becomes an adult and finds most people are not like his family and there are advantages to emotional expression, he will discover himself handicapped. Yet in psychotherapy he will continue to demonstrate this very difficulty in his relationship to the therapist. Here in the controlled situation, however, he can work through the problem, find reason for its existence, and have the opportunity to learn to express emotion in therapy. Once he has learned to do this his ability to express it elsewhere in his environment will increase. It will, however, be some time before he will be able to thoroughly convince himself that the therapist will not frown upon his emotional expression in the same way his family did. He knows it very soon from an intellectual standpoint, but emotional conviction takes time.

Similarly the patient who has built up considerable hostility to a parent during childhood, but was forbidden expression of it, may have set up any one of a number of defenses to keep this hostility unconscious. He may possibly have adopted an ingratiating manner toward people of importance in his life as an additional means of preventing emergence of the anger. Within a short time after therapy begins he will have clearly manifested the same ingratiating attitude toward the therapist and there will follow a period of elucidation of the reason for this unrealistic attitude. Subsequently the way will be cleared for the hostility to emerge and for its roots to be understood. The neurotic person reacts to reality as if it were different from what it actually is. The goal of psychotherapy is to help the patient make a more realistic and therefore more mature adjustment.

PSYCHOTHERAPEUTIC METHODS

Below is a list of some of the methods utilized to accomplish the therapeutic task:

1. Persuasion
2. Suggestion, hypnosis, and hypnoanalysis
3. Confession
4. Reassurance, encouragement, and approval
5. Bibliotherapy
6. Narcosynthesis
7. Distributive analysis
8. Psychoanalysis
9. Psychoanalytic psychotherapy
10. Group therapy

Because of their essential difference from the above types of treatment certain other procedures listed below will be discussed in a separate chapter (Chapter 22, "Other Treatment Procedures").

1. Tranquilizers and psychic energizers
2. Family therapy
3. Hospitalization
4. Shock therapies
5. Psychosurgery

PERSUASION

Persuasion is a therapeutic method by which the physician presents to the patient in a more or less authoritative way the necessity for overcoming his symptoms. Inherent in the method is consider-able activity on the part of the therapist, who pushes and pulls the patient into the desired channels. While in the main this method has great limitations and is often totally ineffective there are certain instances where its application is desirable and beneficial. For in-stance, in dealing with the secondary gain from a chronic incapaci-tating neurosis it is at times necessary to apply an authoritative atti-tude of firm pressure upon the patient and to insist upon attempts to return to some type of activity. At times the infantile personality is so lacking in self-restraint and self-discipline that it needs an au-thoritative figure in the background to strengthen the very weak ego, in much the same way that a child needs a parent to help him control his behavior. With the average neurotic and personality-disorder patient, however, the method of persuasion is too superficial and its results are inadequate.

SUGGESTION

Suggestion as a therapeutic method involves utilization of a more or less illogical quality of most human beings in that they accept as valid the statements of someone to whom they attribute omnipo-tence. Suggestion is one of the most common of all psychothera-peutic approaches. Suggestibility is primarily emotional and tends to be devoid of logic. The degree of immediate success of suggestion is based upon two factors primarily. First is the innate suggestibility of the patient, his willingness to accept an idea or attitude advanced by another. This is generally greater in conversion reactions than in compulsive patients and psychotics. Secondly, there is the manner in which the suggestion is offered to the patient. The physician's position of authority enhances his ability to utilize this particular means; also he can select the way in which he imparts to the patient the idea that "what I am going to do (or be) to you is going to help you." Often his technical instruments add to his power of suggestion because of the patient's intellectual ignorance about them and his readiness to attach emotional significance to them. It is common knowledge that conversion aphonias, for instance, are often cured at least temporarily by bronchoscopy. This is particularly true if the patient is informed prior to the procedure that it will restore his voice. However, as Freud discovered early in his work with hypnosis, this method is not permanent in its results and does not change the basic personality structure.

HYPNOSIS AND HYPNOANALYSIS

Hypnosis is an extreme form of suggestion in which the subject gives up his own voluntary controls over himself and accepts a state presided over by the hypnotist. The trance is induced either by an authoritative, commanding attitude or a monotonous, repetitious, expectant attitude on the part of the therapist. The patient is usually first reassured concerning his misconceptions about hypnosis. For instance, he is told that hypnosis is really innocuous and that he cannot be made to do anything while in that state which would violate his moral code. He is told that he will not remain under the "power" of the hypnotist permanently and that even if left alone he would soon awaken from the trance without ill effects. After being reassured in this way he is made comfortable, usually asked to fix his eyes upon something which puts them in a slightly strained position, and then requested to pay close attention to the words of the hypnotist. The latter begins either to command the patient to go to sleep in a loud authoritative manner, or to repeat monotonously suggestions of sleepiness, tiredness, drowsiness, and fatigue. Within a few minutes the suggestible patient is in what resembles a sleeping state, but is still capable of listening to and answering the hypnotist and also of moving about at direction. He is awakened merely by being told that he will do so, for instance, at the count of three. While under hypnosis, dialogue can be carried on with the patient and a rapid effort made by questioning to get the patient to come to an understanding of the meaning of his symptom. The patient can then be asked if he can live normally without it and, if he acquiesces, be told that if this is so then it will be gone when he is aroused. Some physicians using hypnosis would think it preferable to suggest that symptoms will begin disappearing upon arousal and, depending upon the degree of improvement, gauge how much re-hypnosis will be required to bring about full understanding of conflict and full rejection by the patient of the symptom.

The setting for psychotherapy which hypnosis provides may diminish resistance to understanding the unconscious meaning of symptoms and a more ready acceptance of ego-strengthening statements by the therapist. All patients are not accepting of hypnosis and not all psychiatric conditions are open to the application of hypnosis. But, in certain psychoneurosis it can be of definite value as well as being more rapid than a consciously carried out, face-to-face dialogue.

CONFESSION

Confession as a therapeutic method involves the therapist's listening to the patient's accounts of things he has done or thought or felt and about which he either has, or feels he should have, guilt. It has long been utilized by religions and its value recognized by them. The individual's conscience is frequently a harsh taskmaster and its chief weapon that of guilt. The person staggering under such a load of guilt welcomes the chance to confess and take his chances on real punishment. A certain relief is felt whether the listener metes out punishment or adopts an accepting attitude. It is as if the guilty individual has aired his faults to someone in authority and thereby lessened his own responsibility. If he is punished, his guilt is at least partially assuaged. If he is not punished he feels that his sin was not as great as he had himself adjudged it. It must be stressed that confession deals only with conscious material and therefore has little effect upon the important underlying dynamics. It is often remarkable, however, in its immediate effects even if these are usually neither permanent nor productive of any basic changes.

REASSURANCE

Reassurance is a method by which the therapist attempts to impart to the patient a less pessimistic and fearful attitude toward his difficulties and to help him feel the problems are really not too serious. It is probably the most common of all psychotherapeutic approaches. The patient with palpitations due to anxiety may be fearful that he has heart disease. Such fear increases his anxiety and therefore his palpitations. The cycle is vicious and at times may be broken by medical reassurance to the effect that his heart is perfectly all right and his palpitations are only due to emotions. As with some of the foregoing approaches this does not get at the root of the original anxiety but may, particularly in the milder cases, be very beneficial. The physician assumes a somewhat omnipotent role similar to that of the parent to the child, and his reassuring words that all is well calm the patient's anxiety in a very similar way.

Reassurance can be a most appropriate part of psychotherapy to express in some way approval of the patient's ability to comprehend, his willingness to use insight and suggestions, or his courage and versatility in trying new ways of relating to job, family, or friends. It is particularly necessary in some cases to give more than the implied faith in a patient's ability to change and recover that is inherent in accepting him as a patient. To say when it seems necessary: "I believe in your ability to change" or "I have faith in your ability to succeed in such and such an endeavor" are most important gifts to some patients and aid in their progress.

BIBLIOTHERAPY

Bibliotherapy, the assignment of reading to the patient, has a limited application. As with other psychotherapeutic methods its main intent is to increase the patient's understanding of himself. Most of such insight gained by reading is intellectual and becomes emotional only if discussed more fully with the therapist. Compulsive patients tend to develop such intellectual "insight" very readily, but it soon becomes a method of resistance to real emotional insight and produces no improvement in the symptomatology. Anxious patients frequently become frightened by such reading and imagine themselves to have all sorts of psychiatric disorders. This is similar to "sophomoritis" of medical students, where in the beginning of the study of disease entities one is apt to find waves of imagined syphilis, tuberculosis, and diabetes cropping up within the sophomore class. However, there are certain worth-while books on the subject of emotional adjustment with which every physician should familiarize himself. Some of these are listed at the end of this book.

NARCOSYNTHESIS

Narcosynthesis, the procedure of stimulating production of emotional material by the use of barbiturates, was given a great stimulus during the last war. It was found that battle-reaction cases, if given the proper amount of intravenous sodium amytal or sodium pentothal, often re-enacted with great vividness traumatic battle scenes which they had been through. Great amounts of emotion were released and improvement often followed. Essentially this is a method of abreaction or reliving a highly emotional experience which originally could not be handled adequately by the psychic apparatus. Far more emotion may have been stimulated during the actual battle than could be released, and the narcosis provides an avenue of escape for this emotion. Fifteen grains of sodium amytal are mixed in 20 cc. of water in a syringe and a sufficient amount is slowly injected intravenously until the subject is quite drowsy, but still responsive to questions. Suggestions are made during this time that the subject is again in the traumatic situation and feeling as he did at that time. In the more dramatic cases the patient will go through all the original trauma, often shouting and attempting to move about, with extreme emotional discharge. Following such a procedure the patient usually sleeps for a while and then the re-enactment can be discussed with him and gradual desensitization brought about. The state reached by many closely resembles hypnosis, and at times a combination of barbiturates and hypnosis is used. Abreaction, whether of war experiences or other crucial life situations, still does not change the basic personality structure. The efficacy of the procedure is greater where the environmental trauma has been acute and severe and the personality was well integrated beforehand.

DISTRIBUTIVE ANALYSIS

Meyerian psychotherapy, psychobiology, or, as it has been termed, distributive analysis, is the therapeutic approach and school of thought originated by Adolf Meyer. His views encouraged a pluralistic approach to the cause of mental and emotional disturbances. The patient in the present is considered to be a cross-section of the long stream between birth and death. He now is the result of all that he has experienced. The organic factors, psychological factors, and environmental factors are all included in formulating the complete picture. As outlined by Strecker and Ebaugh,[1] psychobiological psychotherapy can be formulated in six steps. First, there is the *establishment of rapport* between the patient and physician. This occurs during the introductory phases when the history taking, physical examination, laboratory tests, and mental examinations are done. The patient is impressed with the interest and thoroughness of the physician and develops respect and confidence toward him. Second, there is *aeration* or ventilation wherein the patient, during successive interviews, has the opportunity of relating his problems to the physician. This may be done by direct interview, hypnosis, narcosynthesis, or a discussion of material learned about the patient elsewhere by the psychiatrist. Third comes *desensitization,* the period during which the patient is repeatedly exposed during the interviews to material to which he has shown an exaggerated emotional response. This is somewhat akin to the allergist's procedure of exposing the patient to increasing doses of a particular substance to which he has originally been very sensitive so that his tolerance for the substance grows more nearly normal. This method is said by its proponents to be the most efficient in various fear reactions. Fourth is the principle of *re-education* of the patient into more mature and acceptable means of dealing with his life situations. There is little rationale to removal of one type of pathological process without substituting a more normal type in its place. The fifth step in the process is that of *dealing with the family of the patient,* with the purpose of desensitizing them to the patient's illness and re-educating them to a more healthy method of dealing with it. And last, the patient's *physical condition* is reviewed with the goal of correcting any difficulties which may be present.

As may be seen, Meyerian psychotherapy is truly pluralistic in its approach. The individual is considered from every possible standpoint and any factor which may have had an effect upon him is included in the evaluation and therapy. However, there is usually little stress put upon the unconscious factors. This is undoubtedly so be-

[1] Strecker, Edward, and Franklin Ebaugh. *Practical Clinical Psychiatry.* Seventh edition. Philadelphia. Blakiston Co., 1951.

cause Meyer never fully accepted the principles of psychoanalysis, especially the concept of the unconscious. If we accept the existence and importance of unconscious factors, the Meyerian result will fall short of achieving a maximum of basic change. However, the sincere interest of the therapist combined with an understanding of the pluralistic approach should often lead to an amelioration of symptoms.

PSYCHOANALYSIS

Psychoanalysis, the method of research and type of therapy originated by Sigmund Freud [2] late in the last century, has contributed greatly to our present understanding of personality dynamics. Almost every school of psychiatric thought has accepted at least some of the principles outlined by psychoanalysis, and its influence is widespread in other fields outside of medicine. Freud began working with hypnosis but became dissatisfied with the results because although they were often dramatic they were seldom permanent and did not produce significant change in the basic personality difficulty.

After considerable experimentation he arrived at a method called *free association* as a means of obtaining deeper understanding into the dynamic function of mental processes. The patient is instructed to say whatever comes into his mind without regard to whether it is completely logical and rational, and even if it is embarrassing or otherwise distasteful.

In everyday life, normal conscious verbal productions are censored by the individual in order to produce logical, intelligent, coherent, and acceptable speech. Because of his position on a couch with the analyst seated behind him out of direct vision the patient is not only in a relaxed position but is not continuously watching the analyst's facial expression and appearance to see the effects of his productions on him. The fewer stimuli reminding the patient of the actual situation the more able he will be to free-associate and to allow his unconscious pattern expression.

The purpose behind the technique of free association is to reduce to a minimum conscious censorship of unconscious material. The

[2] Freud, Sigmund. *The Interpretation of Dreams.* New York. Basic Books, 1955.

patient reports his train of thought spontaneously and gradually there become recognizable various urges, tendencies, and conflicts from the area of the unconscious. The patient is enabled through well-chosen interpretations by the analyst to bring into his ego material which had previously been dealt with in a pathological manner in the unconscious. Once within the domain of the growing adult ego such problems are amenable to solution in a more efficient way. In other words, the therapeutic purpose of psychoanalysis is to bring into the conscious previously unconscious material of an infantile and conflictual nature and to enable the patient to work out a more harmonious and mature adjustment of his own needs in relation to his environment.

The phenomenon of *transference* is of importance in the technique of psychoanalysis. It is the automatic tendency of the patient to transfer to the analyst feeling which he has had in his childhood years toward important figures in his environment, particularly his parents. For instance, the man who comes from a home where his father was a brutal, sadistic, demanding person is stirred from early childhood to rebellion against this type of treatment. He has never been able to get along with his bosses, with officers while in the service, nor with any other figure of authority. Soon in the analytic situation he becomes rebellious toward the analyst, finding all sorts of faults with the treatment situation, feeling the analyst is unkind to him and even resentful of him. Thus he transfers hostile feelings of the type that he originally had toward his father to the analyst and accuses the latter of the same unfair, cruel treatment as he has suffered at the hands of his father. Meantime, of course, the analyst's attitude remains friendly and understanding so that eventually the patient can be helped to see the unreality in his feelings and behavior. Previously in his life when he has become hostile to authoritarian figures they have reacted with hostility toward him, which in turn has prevented him from recognizing his original neurotic reaction. However, in the treatment situation he has the opportunity to trace the pattern back to its origin and develop a more mature solution.

The carrying out of psychoanalysis demands not only technical and theoretical knowledge on the part of the therapist but also an understanding of his own personality. Immaturities or neurotic patterns injected into the treatment situation by the therapist's personality will prevent the patient from learning the unreality of his own reactions. For this reason every candidate for psychoanalytic training must himself undergo psychoanalysis.

This science has, as mentioned previously, contributed greatly to the understanding of the dynamics of personality function and its principles have been applied in a wide variety of fields. However, there are certain disadvantages to the procedure, not the least of which is the time element involved. Treatment by this method rarely can be accomplished in less than eighteen months and often involves two or three years, during which time the patient is seen an hour a day five days a week. Further there is the matter of the small number of psychoanalysts available (approximately 1,000 in the United States); they cannot provide orthodox psychoanalysis for more than a small number of patients. As a consequence of the time involved and the limited number of patients who can be treated by each analyst the cost of the procedure is beyond the reach of many, even though clinic situations have been established to meet a portion of this need. Psychoanalysis, originated by Freud as a treatment method for neurotic patients, cannot in its strictest sense be applied to certain other types of emotional disorders. The psychoses, for instance, are now better understood as a resut of psychoanalytic reseach, but psychotic patients do not ordinarily lend themselves well to the orthodox procedures. In recent years, modifications of the technique utilizing psychoanalytic principles have been successful with some psychotic patients; but in many respects these endeavors are still in the experimental stage.

Patients with the various types of personality disorder are difficult analytic subjects because of their tendency to "act out" excessively. This term refers to a tendency to express emotional conflicts which are present or are stirred up by the analytic situation by behavior outside the analytic hour. Excessive drinking to alleviate feelings of anxiety or inferiority instead of waiting to analyze them is an example of this.

The suitability for analysis of a patient presupposes his desire to get well, and his willingness and ability to co-operate in the procedure. Also it demands a reasonable ability to control his behavior outside the treatment situation, at least to a degree that will preclude his getting into any serious difficulty. Such control is often impossible for those with personality problems, and such individuals can sometimes be treated successfully only when confined in some type of institution where their behavior can be controlled for them. Since psychoanalysis is available to so few, it is the custom to choose patients whose potential intellectual and emotional abilities will be commensurate with the time and energy involved. There are some areas where psychoanalysis, primarily as a method of research, has proven its ability to produce results in other than neurotic patients.

PSYCHOANALYTIC PSYCHOTHERAPY

Psychoanalytic psychotherapy, as the name implies, is a psychoanalytically oriented type of treatment which has gradually evolved from attempts to provide a dynamically oriented therapy to a larger number of patients over a shorter period of time than can be provided with psychoanalysis. Various psychoanalysts, initially familar with the principles of orthodox technique, have searched for short cuts to basic personality changes that accrue in the lengthier procedure. Franz Alexander, one of the most brilliant workers in this field, has shown how, in many instances, the technical process can be shortened while only a certain portion of the total benefits are sacrificed. The purpose of this type of treatment is similar in many ways to that of psychoanalysis: namely, to make the unconscious conscious and to help the individual adjust on a more realistic level. Most of the psychotherapy done at the present time is probably psychoanalytically oriented, at least to some degree.

The results obtained from psychoanalytic therapy ordinarily do not match those resulting from orthodox psychoanalysis. Nevertheless, in many instances the improvement is quite remarkable and the individual is restored to a useful and constructive life. There are many patients who, for one reason or another, cannot undergo the lengthier procedure, but who can profit greatly from a modified treatment.

Psychoanalytic psychotherapy has been applied to individuals suffering from almost every type of emotional disorder. The majority of patients probably belong to two main types: either they suffer from one or another of the well-recognized neurotic syndromes, or they have some type of personality disorder. The efficacy of the therapy depends upon several factors. Obviously the physician who is most skilled in understanding psychoanalytic principles will be the most efficient in his therapeutic measures. Secondly, of course, is the degree of severity of the particular emotional disturbance. Another important factor which always must be borne in mind is the type of disorder from which the patient suffers. Generally speaking, the more uncomfortable the patient's particular difficulty makes him, the more likely he is to seek and utilize help. The patient who suffers from a neurosis with incapacitating and painful symptoms is much more prone to seek and utilize guidance than the individual who suffers from a personality disorder which often proves more painful to those around him than to himself. For instance, the patient who has a severe phobia which prevents him from leading a normal life and frequently precipitates him into states of panic is extremely anxious for relief, whereas the overt homosexual may be thoroughly resigned to his homosexuality and neither request nor desire any assistance.

Another factor which always must be borne in mind is the degree of secondary gain which has subsequently become attached to the illness. If the patient, by virtue of his difficulty, now receives a great deal more attention, love, and support than he had previously, it may greatly diminish his desire to return to a more mature and normal way of life. Perhaps the most obvious examples of heightened secondary gain are seen in compensation cases, where as long as the individual retains his incapacitating symptoms he receives a monetary reward which he will lose the moment he returns to a more normal life. In many instances, prior to any efficient therapy, it is necessary to deal with the secondary-gain factor.

Most of the basic principles in psychoanalytic psychotherapy are similar to those in psychoanalysis. The phenomenon of transference is one of the most important. As we have explained previously, transference is the ever-present tendency to transfer to the therapist emotional attitudes which were previously present toward important figures earlier in the life of the patient, usually the parents.

Much of the efficiency of psychoanalytic psychotherapy depends upon the correct handling of the transference. The patient with his unconscious conflicts distorts his relationships to others and will distort unrealistically the one toward the therapist. It is of extreme importance that the patient be helped to see where his emotional attitudes toward the therapist have departed from reality and how these distortions stem from earlier difficulties in his childhood. Also it is important for him to see how these same transferred emotional attitudes are present with others in his current life outside the therapeutic situation. In order to bring the transference into relief, it is essential that the therapist present a friendly, consistent, and understanding attitude toward the patient. Whereas the phenomenon of transference occurs everywhere in the patient's life, it is only in the therapeutic situation that he can learn to understand it, because elsewhere in his life other individuals counterreact to the patient's unrealistic emotional attitudes. The patient who becomes bitterly resentful of or remarkably enamored of the therapist can be helped to see the unreality of these attitudes only if the therapist has maintained his proper attitude.

This subject brings us to another important area of this type of therapy as well as of psychoanalysis, the so-called "countertransference." This term refers to the emotional responses of the physician during the course of treatment. It is safe to say that the less the physician knows and understands his own personality, the more his own countertransference will interfere with the efficiency of the procedure. As an example, the insecure therapist may almost overwhelm the patient with friendliness and positive overtures purely as a result of his own inner insecurity, in an attempt to achieve a positive relationship. On the other hand, such an insecure therapist may react with unrealistic hostility to any insinuation on the part of the patient that the treatment is inadequate. Egocentricity on the part of the physician may lead him to encourage and welcome signs of overattachment and dependence by his patients. Anxiety on the part of the therapist about certain areas in his own life may well lead to his mishandling of discussions by the patient of similar areas. Generally speaking, it is not the purpose of psychotherapy to enhance and magnify transference, but rather to help the patient understand it as soon as it has reached proportions where he can be helped to see it. The moment that unrealistic countertransference is introduced into the therapeutic situation by the physician, all hope of helping the patient see his own disturbed emotional atmosphere has been lost.

One often sees the phenomenon known as "transference neurosis" in psychoanalysis or in psychoanalytically oriented psychotherapy. This term indicates that the patient has transferred his essential conflicts to his relationship with the therapist and has thereby lost most of his previous symptoms. His adjustment seems to be almost miraculously improved after a very few visits. And yet his relationship with the therapist remains on its previously disturbed level. In theory at least, much of psychoanalysis revolves around the solution of this transference neurosis during the therapeutic process. It might be said that the patient uses the therapist as a parent in the way that he used his parents originally. However, the therapist, because of his added knowledge and understanding, serves as a better parent than the original and helps the patient to achieve what he should have achieved during his growth period. It is important that the therapist recognize that the sudden and dramatic dissolution of symptoms may only herald the onset of transference neurosis and that unless the patient is given understanding in this area the cessation of therapy will only bring about a recurrence of the original problem in the patient's life.

Resistance is the term given to the various intrapsychic forces within the patient which seem to retard and prevent his rapid and smooth achievement of maturity during treatment. While it is true that the patient has come, ordinarily, of his own free will and has made many sacrifices in order to obtain psychotherapy or psychoanalysis, nevertheless it is found that once the process is begun, many of these resistances are encountered. For instance, the stubborn and obstinate patient may spend a great deal of time disagreeing with anything the therapist says. It soon becomes obvious that he is not considering whether the therapist is speaking the truth, but is only considering the necessity of disagreeing with him. One is reminded in such instances of the four-year-old child who, whenever he is asked to do something, immediately says no without much

regard as to whether or not the proposed action will be to his benefit. Resistances vary remarkably. Tardiness to appointments, forgetting appointments, inability to remember what has been discussed
are some examples. The patient is ordinarily unaware of the meaning of such things, since if he were aware of them he would obviously not allow them to continue. Their true meaning must be
interpreted to him and very often such interpretations must be repeated many times before a true understanding results.

Dreams

Dreams form an important part of psychoanalytic psychotherapy,
just as they do in classical psychoanalysis. Freud called dreams "the
royal road to the unconscious." His monumental work, *The Interpretation of Dreams,* was first published in 1900, yet still remains
one of the most comprehensive and useful treatises on this particular subject. Freud was the first to take dreams out of the supernatural or pseudo-scientific realm and find a real place for them in dynamic psychology.

A dream is a hallucinatory experience occurring during sleep.
The portion of the dream which is remembered upon awakening
is called the *manifest dream content.* The manifest content, however, only represents the end product of a rather complicated series
of psychological events. In order to understand these events we
must first return for a moment to our discussion of the various mental components. We showed there how the unconscious contains
various instinctual urges which are constantly striving for discharge.
Those which have been found unacceptable for one reason or another are kept unconscious by the ego through its various mechanisms of defense. However, during sleep the ego loses contact with
reality and diminishes the vigilance with which it pursues its other
activities. This means that unacceptable instinctual urges which have
been seeking gratification are now faced with a less rigid censorship by the ego.

With this state of affairs in existence one of two things can occur.
Either the ego can arouse itself into wakefulness, reassume all its
duties, and put into effect the full measure of its mechanisms of defense and maintain the unacceptable instinctual impulse in the un-

conscious, or it may allow hallucinatory distorted expression of the impulse in a dream and thus permit sleep to continue. In a sense one might say that the function of dreams is to allow the individual to continue sleeping and in "successful dreams" this is what occurs.

Since the ego is not completely out of the picture even during sleep, the expression of an instinctual impulse in a dream must be sufficiently distorted to be unrecognizable. We refer to this unconscious and unacceptable instinctual material as the *latent dream content*. The various mechanisms by which this material is changed into the manifest or remembered dream content are called, in sum, the "dream work."

We often find that a dream contains elements of some occurrence or thought of the previous day which may have been quite trivial. This thought or occurrence is used by the ego as a sort of vehicle to carry the unconscious elements of the dream. Because of the lack of reality-testing functions at the time in the ego, all sorts of distortions are possible.

Dream work utilizes certain so-called mental mechanisms. The latter are various psychological processes by which psychic energy is handled. A certain number of these are utilized by the ego and are called mechanisms of ego defense. These have been discussed in Chapter 3. Others are mechanisms of expediency in conserving and dealing with psychic energy and are well illustrated in dreams.

For instance, *symbolism* is a common mental mechanism seen in dream formation but also occurring commonly during waking life. An excellent example of the latter kind of symbolism is the American flag, which although in fact assembled pieces of colored cloth, represents a great deal more to people in this country. In dreams, experience has gradually shown a tendency on the part of the mind to use certain things as symbolic of certain other things. It has been found that these situations, actions, or objects occur in the dreams of many people and frequently are not accessible to the usual free-association type of technique, which elucidates the other portions of the dream. However, after all the other portions are clarified in the usual manner, the resultant "circumstantial evidence" points to a definite symbolic meaning of the remaining portion. Whereas it has been shown that the so-called symbolic elements of the dream do ordinarily represent the objects which we have come to expect, nevertheless, this certainly cannot be taken as a universal or unbroken rule. The remainder of the dream must be first understood and only then can the presumably symbolic elements be considered as such. For instance, it is frequently found in dreams that long pointed round objects are symbolic of the male genital. Likewise, various receptacles into which something is put often represent the female genital. It cannot be too thoroughly stressed here, however, that one should never jump to conclusions in the use of a knowledge of this type of symbolism.

Another mental mechanism often seen in dreams is that of *condensation*. This is a mechanism where several factors are literally condensed into one expression which really represents them all. An example of this mechanism is seen in the following fragment of a dream reported by a young man in psychotherapy: "I dreamed I saw coming down the street this strange man whom I had never seen before, but whom I immediately disliked very much. I felt like crossing the street. He was a rather tall man, bald-headed, with a large mustache. His clothes were in poor condition and badly needed pressing."

In the process of discussing his various thoughts about this dream, the patient remembered several men whom he had known and none of whom he had liked. Each had a particular characteristic represented in the man in the dream. One wore a mustache, another was noted for his height, a third was bald-headed, and the fourth had always been notoriously careless about his clothes. The patient for various reasons had harbored dislikes toward each of these men and in his dream had condensed them all into one figure. This type of mechanism is typical of unconscious mental activity and therefore is represented clearly in dreams which stem from this portion of the mind.

In many dreams we see an example of another mechanism called *displacement*. It involves the displacing of importance or feeling from the situation to which it belongs to a more trivial one. This mechanism is discussed more thoroughly in Chapter 3 under the mechanisms of ego defense. As it occurs in dreams, displacement usually involves exaggeration of a particular portion of the dream which in the manifest content would appear to be the most important element. However, during therapy when a dream is dissected and better understood, it is found that some seemingly trivial incident in the dream really represented by far the most important psychological element.

In view of the fact that dreams contain a wish element in the form of an inner urge, the existence of anxiety dreams or nightmares must be further explained. The wish element remains valid but it is necessary to remember that not all unconscious wishes can be accepted into the conscious mind without giving rise to anxiety. This anxiety is often engendered in the ego by fear of superego disapproval. If the wish expressed in the dream is contrary to superego dictates and if the distortion of this wish is insufficient, anxiety arises within the ego. If this anxiety reaches a certain level, the dream is literally unsuccessful and the individual awakens, at which time his ego defenses can again be put into full operation. Dreams of the death of a close relative are often in this category. The dreamer harbors a certain amount of resentment toward the relative but is unable to tolerate this hostility on a conscious level because of the guilt that it would engender. When it is graphically portrayed in the dream, anxiety results and the dreamer often awakens. The dream, incidentally, does not mean that there exists an active or powerful desire on the part of the dreamer for the other individual to die. The unconscious operates on an "all-or-none" principle. Where hostility exists, it will find its way, if it can, into a dream in a "total" form, rather than a mild or partial form. Should such hostility become conscious during the waking hours, it probably would lead only to a mild rebuke or criticism of the other person, but when bottled up in the unconscious, it retains its more primitive form.

In psychoanalytic psychotherapy, the patient cannot achieve as complete an understanding of his dreams as is accomplished in psychoanalysis through free association. The ability to grasp and understand the underlying meaning of the latent content of dreams varies markedly from one individual to another. Some are capable of uncovering the hidden meanings of dreams with very little help, while others have great difficulty in making any sense out of the seemingly distorted manifest content. The patient in therapy is asked to present all the ideas and thoughts that he can about his dreams. The therapist, with his understanding of the patient's dynamics as well as of the situation in therapy, is capable of learning a great deal about the unconscious processes. A warning should be made against a "wild interpretation of dreams." One must always bear in mind that the interpretation cannot be very much deeper than the patient's present understanding of his problems, if it is to be useful to the patient. For instance, the patient who dreams of the death of his mother cannot be told bluntly, "You wish your mother were dead." During the dream itself, the patient probably experienced a good deal of anxiety stemming from his superego's inability to accept such a hostile wish about his mother, so the therapist must take the approach of explaining to the patient that, while he certainly does not consciously wish for his mother's death, perhaps he has a certain amount of resentment toward her, which is then expressed by the "all-or-none" principle in his dream. Such an explanation is much more acceptable to a patient and does not increase resistance to an uncongenial thought or wish.

Technique of Interpretation

The technique of interpreting various things to patients is an ability that can only be obtained through constant practice. It is similar to the process of becoming proficient at doing appendectomies. One can read many books on this technique and listen to many lectures on the subject, but such knowledge must be supplemented with practical experience. So it is with interpretations in psychotherapy. One must learn to gauge scientifically, as well as intuitively, the proper form and time of the interpretation. Generally speaking, one is apt to be interpreting either a defense of some type or some conflict from the unconscious. Ordinarily the interpretation of an unconscious conflict before most of its defenses have been removed is useless. The patient must initially be helped to see where he is defending himself unrealistically against some inner conflict. Following his understanding of these defenses, the conflict can then come closer to the surface where its final interpretation will be of use. Again it must be mentioned that there are wide variations in the ability of patients to understand and to utilize interpretations.

A good example of defense interpretation preceding the uncovering of unconscious conflict lies in the patient who is markedly over-attentive and oversolicitous to her mother because of unconscious hostility. To interpret this hostility initially would be useless and the patient would either react with anger and leave therapy or would be thrown into a panic of guilt. She must be first helped to see that her present method of dealing with her mother is an unrealistic one. She must be helped to see that her oversolicitousness has no real foundation and must be made to be somewhat curious as to where such an attitude may have arisen. She must be helped to see that no human could possibly have this attitude on realistic grounds. As her relationship to the therapist improves, and she becomes less fearful of his criticism, she is more able to accept the idea that her present attitude results from an underlying hostility to her mother. Another example lies in the man who is constantly belligerent and aggressive, which attitude is a defense to cover up an inner feeling of inadequacy and insecurity. To interpret the latter attitude to the patient originally would again result in failure. He must first be shown that there is no realistic reason for his belligerence and aggressiveness. Following this it becomes easier for him to tolerate an interpretation and an understanding of his inner feeling of inadequacy.

Termination of Therapy

The termination of therapy theoretically comes at a point when the patient has gained insight into the majority of his conflicts and has resolved them sufficiently well to form what is called an "object relationship" to the therapist, rather than the transference. The term *object relationship* merely means that the patient now relates to the therapist as he really is rather than having him cloaked in an aura of previous figures from the childhood environment. For therapy to be considered successful the transference situation must be resolved so that the patient is no longer dependent upon or showing other unrealistic residual attitudes toward the therapist. He should have achieved a more mature and independent level which is no longer colored by his defensive attitudes against inner childish conflicts. The therapist should assure the patient that ego growth must continue throughout life and that insight is never complete enough to remain completely static. The patient should be encouraged to return to the therapist when and if a situation arises which he feels he does not understand. At the same time, he should be encouraged not to return for each small difficulty which arises.

GROUP THERAPY

Group therapy involves the treatment in a group and by one therapist of several patients with emotional disorders. The pressing need during the last war for more psychotherapy lent great stimulus to the technique of group therapy, which has the obvious advantage that more individuals can be given help at one time. Most workers prefer to have a group of from six to ten patients. It is advisable that the therapist see and evaluate each individual prior to his being assigned to the group; frequently individual therapy is carried on in conjunction with the group treatment. The patients are given an explanation of the purpose of the treatment situation and are encouraged to bring their own problems into the group for discussion. The more aggressive and outspoken patients tend to be most active in the initial sessions, but as time goes on the more timid and shy are able with some encouragement to participate. As each individual reveals more and more of his neurotic structure various group pressures are instrumental in helping him to gain a better understanding.

The therapist's prime role in group treatment is as a sort of catalyst. He is often looked upon at least unconsciously by the various members of the group as a parent figure and interesting sibling rivalry situations are liable to develop between patients. All of these, however, sooner or later become subjects for discussion and understanding. Many patients who have difficulties in socializing are greatly benefited by group therapy. Obviously this type of treatment has its limitations. Not every type of patient is suitable. The task of the therapist is not an easy one, since he must keep in mind the dynamics of each individual member of the group, keep the treatment procedure moving along, and yet at the same time not adopt such an authoritative attitude as to rob the group of its natural spontaneity.

QUALIFICATIONS OF A PSYCHIATRIST

There are certain qualities that a psychiatrist should possess in order to effect best possible results with psychotherapy. One of the most important is a genuine liking for people. This is not found as often as one would think. Nine out of ten persons, if asked whether they like people, would probably answer "yes." However, undoubtedly they would be overlooking either their lack of interest in children, the modicum of sympathy or understanding they have for the problems of older people, or even the marked prejudices they hold against people of other races or nationalities. They might, further, be unaware of their prejudices against the opposite sex or their unsolved parental resentment. A "liking for people" carries with it an awareness of many facets of living, including rich and satisfying experiences which serve as a reservoir for understanding. "Liking people" will not cure a patient suffering from a neurosis, but it does help to establish rapport and to extend some of the necessary buoyancy, encouragement, and inspiration which form a part of psychotherapy.

It is important that a psychiatrist have lived with, worked with, or otherwise come in contact with a cross-section of people from every walk of life. To know and understand the thinking and mannerisms of a laboring man helps to establish a relationship with him more quickly. To know and feel at home with the scholar, the aesthete, or the fun-loving extrovert gives versatility and the understanding so necessary for empathy.

A good psychiatrist is a person who understands the stresses and strains of living as well as its pleasures. To have done humble work even briefly as well as to have lived luxuriously; to have known privation, grief, frustration, disappointment, illness, and discomfort, as well as to have known happiness, is part of the wider understanding that the psychiatrist should have. To have participated in sports and be aware of envy and jealousy as encountered in competition; to have known loneliness and boredom, all of these are necessary for a better understanding of the complicated signs of illness in psychiatric patients and for understanding what the patient is trying to impart.

It will be helpful if the psychiatrist has seen how people live, work, and enjoy themselves in other parts of the world. He should be as well read as possible in all areas of knowledge. If he likes and is well acquainted with poetry and imaginative literature he will have more with which to serve his patients. It is advantageous to have worked and lived in situations that place the psychiatrist in the role of leader as well as follower.

A psychiatrist, like a physician in any other sphere of medicine, needs to have a capacity for the tolerance of anxiety within himself. Just as a surgeon must operate courageously and take certain risks to save lives, so must the psychiatrist have the courage to undertake difficult cases and undergo the risk that all will not turn out well. To always choose the safe and easy course is no more conducive to good results and success in psychiatry than it is in any other field of medicine.

The psychiatrist, possibly more than any other specialist, must be verbal, articulate, and able to communicate readily and well. He must have imagination and versatility of expression. He must have tact and must have mastered a careful phraseology. Bluntness or a poorly chosen word can easily alienate a patient and hinder therapy. The psychiatrist should be able to talk at the patient's level whether the patient is a day laborer, a poorly educated housewife, or a highly intelligent professor.

Not only is it important to master the refined art of communication with the individual patient, but the psychiatrist has an additional obligation in the field of preventive medicine. The education of the public depends on him. It is how he expresses himself, presents himself in public, on the platform, radio, or television, that determines whether people will seek psychiatry or avoid it. Many people still regard psychiatry as a luxury and have little understanding as to the meaning of mental illness or mental health. When they suffer pain they are not so particular about their doctor's words and manner, but when they discover maladjustment in themselves their decision to get help for it may depend a great deal upon the ability of the psychiatrist to communicate his message properly.

That the psychiatrist must be as free of prejudices as possible and be willing to learn is almost too obvious a statement. The sick patient does not always have a distorted imagination about himself and his surroundings. When a patient protests that he is not being treated considerately enough, it may be that he is showing the evidence of a deprived childhood. Yet he may have a bona fide complaint. The road to human understanding is a two-way thoroughfare, and the psychiatrist who focuses entirely upon the neurotic shortcomings of his patient and ignores the role of his own personality in the therapeutic interaction will surely fall short of giving the most help.

The psychiatrist should always be ready and willing to explain his work and his methods to his colleagues, taking their quips and jokes (and even insults, as sometimes happens) with equanimity and good humor. He should keep up with activities and advances in other fields of medicine as much as possible. It must be remembered that some people are still unsure about psychiatry and feel uncomfortable in the presence of a psychiatrist. They often attribute to him more knowledge and clairvoyance than he, of course, possesses. To cover their own anxiety or embarrassment, they feel compelled to tell the latest joke about the psychiatrist or in some way comment upon his skill as a crystal gazer or allude to the emotional instability which the psychiatrist must possess to be attracted to this field of medicine.

Many psychiatrists avail themselves of Freudian psychoanalysis as part of their training to make up for some of their defects in self-knowledge and to enable them to better identify with others and achieve a greater maturity. While this is not a mandatory part of training it is a unique and highly desirable method of condensing some of the personality change and growth so necessary for the practice of psychotherapy. The psychotherapist is dealing with heavy responsibilities most of the time and needs wisdom, seriousness of purpose, and integrity of a high order.

Psychiatrists must be content with results which are obtained slowly and often undramatically. Psychiatry does little that is quick, flashy, or dramatic, and satisfactions of this kind are not as frequent for the psychiatrist, or for the patient and his family, as in most fields of medicine and surgery.

Above all the psychiatrist should be an optimist, not the overbearing, back-slapping type, but one who has a calm, sustained, and quiet belief in the capacity of every individual to improve.

EXAMPLES OF PSYCHOTHERAPY

The authors have found in their experience that the average medical student is interested in the fundamentals of psychotherapy, but feels himself somewhat at a loss when presented with a patient who seems to require this particular form of treatment. For instance, junior and senior medical students often begin their service on psychiatry just after they have come from the medical service where, statistics agree, probably more than half of the patients that they have seen are suffering from emotional rather than organic disturbances. Yet when they are faced with these same patients in psychiatry, they seem confused as to what to say and do. It is as if they feel that Mr. Smith, who came to the medical clinic complaining of tachycardia, and whom they referred to psychiatry, is now a new and strange person when he is seen in the latter department. In his original visits to the medical clinic, they did very well in taking a complete history of his present illness and even touched upon his family background. This was followed by a complete and competent physical examination which revealed no evidence of organic disease, but did show an obviously anxious and neurotic individual. They referred him to the psychiatric clinic with the vague notion in their mind that since he suffered from no organic ailment, he belonged in the realm of the psychiatrist. As fate would have it, they now have the responsibility of continuing with his care! This particular situation may not occur too frequently in medical schools, but it certainly is a valuable one if it does, for the physician in practice should not have to refer every case he sees with emotional disorder to a psychiatrist. He should be equipped to give such a patient a reasonable evaluation, and if the difficulty lies within his scope, a well-rounded type of therapy. For this reason, we will try to give a few case examples of actual patients who have been seen in psychotherapy.

Prior to doing this it may be well to say a few words about the efficiency of psychotherapy. This is one of the most disputed subjects among both psychiatrists and nonpsychiatric physicians. The latter particularly feel that the psychiatric treatment is long, tedious, and questionably efficient. Their accusations are not always easily answered, because it is difficult to evaluate the results of psychotherapy due to the numerous variables which are present. Undoubtedly for this reason the literature does not contain many statistical summaries of the efficiency of psychotherapy. Innumerable variables such as the length of the illness, the diagnosis, the severity of the condition, the motivation which the patient has for getting well, the secondary gain from the illness, the reality factors which the patient would have to face if he were to get well, the intelligence of the patient, and his ability to relate to the therapist must be considered in such a study.

As if these factors were not enough, there remains the difficult question of how to measure properly the degree of improvement which the patient has achieved. This cannot be done with the laboratory tests that are available, for instance, with the diabetic. Who is to evaluate the degree of stress which the patient after therapy should be able to tolerate? And how long a period after therapy should elapse before a "cure" is claimed? These are extremely difficult questions to answer. In cancer, for instance, a period of five years is usually considered as a statistical evidence of cure, but are we justified in using this particular measure for emotional problems? Pursuing the subject further, we may legitimately ask whether amelioration of symptoms should be considered a "cure" or an "improvement." It is often easy to eradicate a conversion paralysis with one hypnotic session, but the patient is still of conversion type, prone to develop a recurrence of his paralysis or other new symptoms under sufficient stress.

The human psyche is an extremely complicated thing and years of formative experience have produced in an individual certain traits of character and types of defense mechanism. It is the goal of psychotherapy to give him as much understanding as is possible under existing conditions and to alleviate his symptoms as far as can be accomplished as well as to minimize the chances of recurrence. Our goals must often be varied to meet the conditions of the patient's life. However, it is reasonable to say that compared with other branches of medicine, psychiatry stands respectably high in the scale of therapeutic success. Certain conditions are easily helped— as is true also, for instance, in internal medicine. However, some require chronic care, and others are rarely if ever helped.

With these factors in mind, we will discuss a few specific cases of therapy. The student should remember that, although we have mentioned several types of therapeutic approach, it is rare that one finds a single type utilized in an individual case. More commonly we see a combination of methods used on the basis of an understanding of the dynamics of a particular case and the needs of the individual patient. The latter must be stressed, since rational use of the various methods is much more efficient than a hit-or-miss rather rigid type of therapeutic approach. The more the therapist understands the dynamics and needs of his patient, the more apt he is to be able to help the patient understand and improve his emotional status and reach a higher degree of maturity.

Case History (1)

This thirty-four-year-old married woman, mother of two sons, presented a multitude of complaints, most of which were phobic in nature. The symptoms had been present for about two years. The final symptom which precipitated her visit to the psychiatrist was of one week's duration. It was that of dizziness whenever she attempted to talk to anyone while she was standing up. She had had many phobias in the past. She had feared eating anything because of the possibility of becoming nauseated. She had had a definite fear of heart disease for several months and when this diminished it was replaced by a phobia of leukemia. Most of her difficulties had begun following a robbery two years previously in the store which she and her husband owned. During the process of being questioned about the robbery by detectives, she had developed a fear of being alone in the store. In addition to this she subsequently feared going out on the street alone. As her many fears developed, she was forced into a very limited type of existence and her husband was immobilized to a large degree because he was required to stay with her.

The patient had been married for thirteen years and she and her husband had operated a furniture store for most of that time. She felt that their marriage had gone reasonably well, at least up until the time of the robbery. Since then, her increasing symptoms had injected considerable difficulty into their marital life.

Her family history revealed that her father had died when she was four years of age. Her mother was still living and had had to work most of the patient's life. Following her father's death, the patient had lived with her maternal grandmother until her mother had remarried when the patient was sixteen. The grandmother had been an unstable person, prone to temper tantrums and frequently a sufferer from what must have been psychophysiological illnesses. At the time of her mother's remarriage, the patient had gone to live with her own mother and step-father. The mother was a demanding person with whom the patient had never gotten along particularly well. There was one younger brother whom the patient felt had always been preferred by the mother.

During the first interview, the patient revealed that her mother routinely came to visit her on week ends and that it was at these times particularly that she was upset. She said that her mother was demanding of attention both from the sister-in-law and from the patient, but that the sister-in-law did not feel obligated to give such attention, while the patient did. She freely admitted that she was not particularly close to her mother and at the same time gave little evidence of feeling any degree of overt hostility toward her.

This was most of the informative material gained from the patient during the interview. Most of it she had volunteered herself, but the rest of it had been elicited by further questioning by the therapist. The patient was reassured by the therapist that the condition from which she suffered was not an uncommon one, and that ordinarily it was amenable to help. Prior to coming, she had been quite concerned about her difficulty and felt that in all probability it was both a condition new to medical science and was incurable. She gained considerable reassurance out of the initial interview, both from the friendliness and interest of the therapist and also his statement that such conditions had been alleviated in other people.

On her second interview the patient came in to say that she had been out unaccompanied two times since her first visit. She said that she was still quite anxious and, as she described it, "pushed inside." She said that she had not been bothered by her fears since her first visit, but she was still somewhat concerned about being alone anywhere except in her own home. She then went on to discuss her childhood when, she said, she had had few friends, although she had always desired many more. She had always felt that she was not liked as a child because she was not particularly good-looking. It was interesting that she had always gotten along better with boys than she had with girls. This subject started her talking about her marriage. She said that whenever she attempted to go out with some of her women friends, her husband objected and usually told her mother about her having gone out. The mother then gave the patient "the dickens."

She said that she found she could feel somewhat better if she gave vent to her anger by working that much harder around the home. This led her to talking about her mother who, she said, had had little time for her as a child. She said that her brother had always been sick and her mother had spent a great deal of time with him. The patient herself had read excessively as a child.

During this second interview, the examiner adopted the attitude of being quite pleased that the patient had felt better since her first interview and reassured her that she would probably continue to improve as she began to understand more about her own feelings. He attempted to show her that her present personality difficulty was the result of the environment in which she had lived and grown up and that the feelings that she had encountered in her earlier years were important in helping develop an understanding of the feelings which she had lacked all these years.

She was encouraged to discuss her relationship with her mother and her husband. The examiner recognized clearly the degree of hostility which she had toward both, but made no comment about it as she began to discuss them. He was careful not to let her give vent to more hostility than she would be able to tolerate and was quite accepting of the complaints which she made about both her husband and mother.

For instance, at one point the patient said that the mother always beat her rather than her brother. She said that her brother had always been a "bone in my throat." It was quite evident during this interview that the patient had a good deal of hostility toward her mother, because of the innumerable complaints which she verbalized toward her. From her own description, it was easily grasped that her mother and grandmother had been somewhat rejecting of her during her earlier life and that this rejection and lack of love had stirred considerable hostility in her. However, it was also evident that she had never been able to consciously recognize the degree of this hostility and that its unconscious existence was contributing greatly to her problem. She had been far too guilty to recognize the anger toward her mother and, therefore, most of it had been relegated to the unconscious. The examiner discussed with her in a general way how it is possible, and as a matter of fact, commonplace to love a parent and yet have certain feelings of irritation toward that parent because of the demands which are made. She was helped to see that her feelings toward her mother were not as unacceptable as she had previously thought.

On her third visit, approximately a week later, the patient said that she had been upset for two days following her last visit, but had subsequently felt a good deal better. She said, "You upset me." She had had difficulty with the idea that she was annoyed with her mother and said, "It's all right to feel that way about any mother except mine." In the discussion that followed, she began to realize that the degree of difficulty which her mother had had earlier in life, while very real, could not be expected to prevent her, the patient, from having feelings of annoyance. She then went on to say that the only dreams that she could remember were those of fighting with her mother. She said, as an example of the difficulty with her mother, that someone had once given her something that was particularly nice and which she had made a great fuss over, but her mother had been very irritated that the patient had even taken the gift. The patient then went on to tell the therapist that most of her symptoms had diminished remarkably.

She continued to discuss her guilt about her resentment toward her mother. She was quite concerned that she herself might turn out to be similar to her mother. She said that she used to be able to dislike people strongly without any difficulty, but recently had had a great problem in doing so. The examiner again discussed with her the fact that, as a result of her growing resentment about her mother's interference in her marriage, she had attempted to repress all evidence of any resentment toward anyone, lest her resentment toward her mother become obvious to her.

At her next interview about a week later, the patient revealed considerable improvement. She said that she felt quite a bit better because "I have talked a good deal of it out." She said that her mother had come as usual on the previous week end and that she herself had gotten along much better with her mother than she ever had before. This was primarily because she had given vent to her annoyance in small matters whenever her mother had attempted to dominate her marital situation. She then went on to discuss her two sons. She said that the older one had a difficulty similar to her own and that he was beginning to "hold everything in and even be jealous of his little brother." She had become increasingly aware that this older boy was harboring considerable jealousy of his younger brother, but that he was fearful of letting it out because of the guilt involved and the fear that she would disapprove and punish him.

This led her to a discussion of her resentment toward her brother because of his having gotten everything during their childhood. She said that she herself was always rather frightened when her brother was angry with her and had never been able to retaliate against him with her own anger. She began to realize that she had always been rather irritated with his superior position and was envious of him. This led into a discussion of her relationship with her husband. She began to bring forth some of the resentment about her husband's tendency to dominate her and also his tendency to go along with her mother in complaints about her.

The examiner listened in a friendly way to all her complaints about her mother, her brother, and her husband. He attempted to help her see that by being dominated by various people, she had accumulated hostility which, if it was completely repressed, was capable of causing the symptoms she had.

On her next visit, a week later, the patient came in to talk about her irritation with her husband, particularly in regard to his dominating attitude around the home. She went on to say that she did not like to argue with him and that she had usually given in to him, but she was beginning to realize that this was a source of some of her difficulties. She had been reading a book on child rearing which had been recommended to her by the therapist, and was beginning to recognize more clearly some of the difficulties which her children were having. A good deal of this hour was spent in discussing various ways and means of improving her relationship with her children as a mother, and in attempting to show her how to help her husband understand his role as a father. She had felt fairly well since her last visit, but was still aware of a certain number of difficulties.

A week later when she came, the patient began the interview by stating that she had been feeling quite well. Her children were away at camp and were apparently enjoying it. She said that she had begun to wonder whether her attachment to the physician and to the therapeutic process was responsible for keeping her feeling well and she was somewhat concerned about this because, if it were true, she was fearful of stopping treatment. She then went on to say that her husband had told her that she was cured and should now stop. She herself was a little dubious about this and felt that her husband proposed it because he was jealous of the therapeutic situation. She said that on one occasion when she had developed some gynecological difficulty and had gone to a gynecologist, her husband had become very angry with her. Here again she expressed more hostility to her husband for some of his dominating and authoritative ways.

The following week she reported that she had been feeling fine. She said that she recognized that she had not as yet grown up completely, but that she felt that she was beginning to make progress. She went back over much of the material that had been discussed previously; most of her resentment was centered around her mother, brother, and husband, along with a certain amount of residual guilt about this resentment.

The next week she reported having continued to feel well. She was becoming more concerned about her husband's asocial attitude and desired very much to encourage him to become more social. There was some discussion of sexuality. She said that she had had little sexual education and the discussion in the therapeutic hour was somewhat embarrassing to her. She had always felt that one should not enjoy sex, because if one did it indicated basic badness. The fallacy of such an attitude was pointed out to her and she began to see that her original impression had been erroneous.

On her next visit, she said that she had been upset for two days following her last interview. She thought that perhaps this was because of the discussion she had had during that interview and said, "Nice girls don't discuss sex with anybody." Once again the subject was entered into in a rather more thorough manner, and it was pointed out to her how unrealistic some of her views regarding sexuality were. Obviously she had considerable guilt over the possibility of enjoying any sexuality. She then hesitantly admitted that she had begun to enjoy sexuality a bit more in the past month.

It must be mentioned that a certain amount of her increased sexual enjoyment was undoubtedly due to a transference phenomenon. However, if handled properly, this type of improvement can be made permanent.

On her following visit a week later, the patient said that she had been quite well and had been completely free of all of her fears for the past three weeks. She said that she felt a desire to "try it on my own." There followed a general discussion of her difficulties, much of which had been covered previously. The interview was ended with a suggestion that she see the therapist again should she wish more assistance or were she troubled by any recurrence of her original difficulty.

Discussion

This is a fairly typical case of phobic reaction. The general dynamics are similar to those that have been previously discussed in Chapter 9 on this syndrome and will not be gone into in any detail here. Instead, an attempt will be made to show some of the thinking the therapist had in regard to this individual and the techniques he utilized in order to assist her.

In the initial interview, when the patient presented as her chief complaints several phobias, the examiner assumed that she would probably fall within the general classification of phobic reaction and would therefore suffer from the essential conflicts found in this syndrome. He assumed that she had a certain ambivalent attitude and had attempted to deal with her hostility by relegating it to the unconscious in order to escape guilt. During the interview he attempted to discover where in her earlier life she could have built up such an ambivalent attitude and why she had such difficulty with her hostility.

From her description of her mother, it became clear that the mother had been a very demanding and rather unloving individual toward whom any child would have had a certain amount of hostility. It was evident, too, that the mother had preferred the brother and the patient had been very envious of him.

As the patient described these two individuals rather accurately, she showed less hostility than one would expect to find toward a situation of this type, and therefore the examiner assumed that her own guilt had made this hostility unacceptable to her. He knew then that the result was that she had developed numerous phobias which were outer projections of her inner fears.

The examiner began to see that—and this is typical of many of these patients—as her husband had added more of a demanding and authoritative attitude to her already overburdened personality, the final outbreak of her acute symptoms had occurred. Subsequent to her initial anxiety, she had begun to develop anxiety about this anxiety; this had then become a vicious cycle. The therapist by his tolerant, understanding, friendly attitude had helped her ventilate many of her feelings. As is true of the ordinary phobic, she formed a quick, superficial, and friendly relationship to the physician. This particular relationship had unconscious undertones to it which psychoanalysis labels "transference." This phenomenon is nothing but the transference of emotions to the therapist which had previously been felt toward important figures in the patient's early life.

In this situation, we might postulate an overidealization of the father who had died when the patient was four, and therefore might additionally postulate the "transfer" to the therapist of positive feelings which she had fantasied toward this departed father. Certainly she tended to make the therapist an omnipotent figure, at least in her unconscious, and felt that his interest and his knowledge were almost magical things to assist her in getting well.

Another important process occurred in this patient which ordinarily happens in a psychotherapeutic process. She gave to the therapist the role of superego; in other words, if the physician condoned the resentment which she held toward various members of her family—then it became more acceptable to her than her own superego had been able to allow. As she gradually brought forth more of these feelings and found in the therapist a friendly, accepting, and understanding attitude, she became more and more comfortable with her feelings and had less need for her phobic symptoms.

It is interesting that one of the complaints often made about psychiatrists is that they teach patients to become hostile to various members of their families. This is an obvious fallacy, since the psychiatrist's only duty is to bring forth to consciousness previously repressed emotional material, and therefore allow the patient to make conscious, rational, logical decisions about its handling. In this particular case this occurred. The therapeutic results are not remarkable and are certainly obtainable by the general practitioner if he is willing to spend some time and effort learning the fundamentals of these difficulties and in working with these fundamentals with the patient. In this particular patient her relationship with her mother was improved as a result of her becoming aware of her hostility. She could then, in minor instances, show her resentment in an ordinary way without letting it gradually build up to an explosive point or to a point where her symptoms became necessary.

Case History (2)

The following case is presented as an example of how at times circumstances may necessitate setting limited goals in psychotherapy. Such things as the patient's degree of illness, intellectual limitation, home setting, or family resistance may require less than complete treatment.

A twenty-year-old student came to therapy rather reticently, having been referred by an internist. She had consulted the latter because of anxiety attacks which she had been suffering for the past few weeks.

These were manifested by palpitations, excessive perspiration, a sense of fear, "butterflies" in her stomach, and tremors. During her initial interview, she told the therapist of her visit to the internist and the symptoms for which she had gone to him. She said that her mother was in the menopause and suffered from anxiety and various hypochondriacal sensations and was, all in all, quite a problem for the patient. The patient said that her mother resented her being in technician's training and "pulled spells to get me out." She was an only child, and was living at home while in training. She elaborated her mother's difficulty by saying that the maternal illness had been a prominent family problem for many years and that she herself had always assumed a great deal of the care and responsibility for her mother during these illnesses. She evinced absolutely no resentment at having had this additional burden, nor did she seem to be irritated at her mother's resentment of her choice of career, or even her mother's attempts by illness to get her to give up this career. The family was a rather rigid one from a religious as well as a social standpoint. Her father, she said, had always been quite concerned about her mother and had given in to her mother in most matters. He did not seem to be nearly the dominating personality in the family that her mother was.

The patient had been developing anxiety attacks over a period of time. She had had some brief anxiety spells earlier in her life, particularly at examination time. She had always been an honor student in school and her conduct had been far above reproach. She made it plain to the therapist that she had always told her parents "everything." She gave the impression, as she described the situation, that she had almost compulsively felt the necessity of reporting each small incident in her daily life to her mother and father, but particularly to her mother. She rarely lost her temper, but on the occasions when she did it was apparently quite a violent outburst followed by considerable guilt. She painted a picture of a family in which any show of emotion was considered to be not nice. She herself had adopted this attitude and firmly clung to it in the initial interview.

She said that her father had always been "cool and cut off from me." She had often made overtures to gain his affection or attention, but her mother had always come between them and had been quite jealous of her affection for her father. In response to questions she said that as a child she had shown considerable temper, particularly with her mother and rarely if ever with her father.

Near the end of the first interview, the therapist pointed out to the patient that he thought he could help her if she would be willing to spend a few interviews with him in an attempt to work out some of her feelings about the problems which faced her. He made little attempt in this first interview to give her any understanding at all of her resentment toward her mother, which had become fairly obvious through her earlier descriptions. He sensed that she had an extremely rigid conscience or superego, and that the guilt he would stir up by such interpretations would be intolerable to her and she undoubtedly would not return.

On her second visit the patient said that she had done considerable thinking about what she had said during her first interview, and had come to the conclusion that her mother really did not have the right to dictate to her as much as she had done. She said that she had been somewhat guilty about feeling a certain amount of resentment toward her mother for this authoritative attitude. Further, she was "irritated" with her mother but still found herself unable to behave in any other way than she always had with her mother. The therapist at this point followed the patient's lead and encouraged her to realize the ubiquitousness of irritation and assured her that there was really no reason for her to feel this degree of guilt.

It was obvious to the therapist at this time that he still faced the primary problem of an extremely severe superego and a rather tenuous relationship with the patient, who viewed him warily because she sensed that his flexibility was in reality a threat to her.

On her third visit a week later the patient reported that her mother had been less authoritative and demanding, therefore she had had little if any chance to give vent to her irritation. This to the physician seemed to be somewhat of a rationalization rather than a realistic statement or evaluation. However, she went on to say that she had decided to go to a movie that night with her girl friends. It was her night off and ordinarily her mother would have verbalized her resentment at the patient's going anywhere else, but on this occasion did not do so. The therapist felt that perhaps the patient's slight increase in her own understanding had been transmitted to the mother, who had therefore been more careful in asserting her authoritative attitude.

Following this discussion, the patient mentioned that she had always been bothered by uneasiness when she was alone with men. This had been true both in social circles and in her professional work. In response to the therapist's questions she said that she had been aware of this even during the therapeutic session. Here the therapist thought in terms of the transference situation. The patient had always attempted to make overtures to her father for affection and approval, but had been discouraged by her mother's jealousy and her own subsequent feelings of guilt. Therefore, when she was alone with any man, including the therapist, while stimulated in the direction of positive feeling, her guilt made its appearance and discouraged the feeling, making her feel uneasy. The therapist did not feel that it was propitious at the moment to bring this insight to the patient's attention because of the possibility of guilt, particularly about her positive feelings toward her father. He merely encouraged her, told her that it was perfectly all right to like him and that there was no objectionable feature to it.

On her fourth visit the patient reported that she had been suffering a good deal of anxiety and that she had felt mixed up and confused. She said that she had not even been able to go to church and get "straightened out" as she had previously. The therapist felt that it was now possible to discuss with her the rather rigid and severe standards to which she had subjected herself as a result of her earlier life. She was helped to see how she was more inflexible than the other technicians she knew. She was helped to see how, although others could enjoy many things, she herself felt guilty in any situation which involved any instinctual gratification. Gradually the discussion involved her mother's personality and how her mother had never really enjoyed much of anything and yet she, the patient, was taking her mother's own pattern as an example of how to live. By now her attachment to (including respect for) the therapist had become sufficiently strong for her to tolerate this new insight without becoming excessively guilty.

At her next visit, a week later, the patient reported that she had been feeling much better. She had not been home during the whole week but had stayed in the room which had been assigned to her at the hospital quarters. There had been a few minor arguments with her mother by telephone concerning her not coming home. However on each occasion she had stood up for her own rights, and although she had felt somewhat guilty, she had thought more about her last interview and had not been too upset. She was still primarily concerned about her inability to feel comfortable with men.

During her next interview, the primary discussion rotated around the fact that she was soon to finish her technician's training. She recognized that although she had used her training as an excuse to remain in the hospital many evenings, she would now have to face this problem with her mother. She recognized that her mother knew that she could now move home, and although she did not want to do so, she was rather bothered by the guilt that would be engendered if she did not. The therapist pointed out to her· that the important element was not whether she lived in the hospital or at home, but whether she could handle her own feelings toward her mother and assert her own rights and privileges if she were to live at home.

On her next visit, the patient reported that she had been home the previous evening and during a talk about her future career, her mother had an attack of palpitations and headache. She had tried to explain to her mother the realistic reasons for her remaining in the hospital, but her mother had persisted in the attack. Following this, the patient had felt considerable guilt and was still in doubt as to what her future course should be. Again the therapist pointed out to her that the important feature was not where she lived, but whether or not she was able to handle her relationship with her mother.

On her last visit a week later, the patient reported that she had decided to live at home following her graduation. She said that she had been feeling quite well and that she felt capable of handling the situation with her mother. However, she had decided that because of her mother's difficulty, she herself should be available to meet emergencies. She said that she would prefer to suspend therapy for a period of time and call the physician if she felt that she needed more help.

Discussion

The therapist felt from the first interview onward that this young lady was a typical example of a compulsive personality. She presented a rather rigid, perfectionistic demeanor. She had always been an over-conscientious and hard-working girl, closely attached to her parents and totally unable to express any resentment toward them. Her particular difficulty lay with her mother, who was demanding as well as over-protective. The mother utilized the martyr attitude, which is one of the most malignant maternal patterns known. Every time the patient attempted to express hostility or achieve independence, the mother resorted to developing some illness, which of course stimulated an excessive amount of guilt in the patient and prevented her from achieving any constructive goal. The therapist recognized that this patient was as yet not psychologically prepared for any thoroughgoing therapeutic procedure. He therefore set a lesser aim of producing some amelioration of symptoms in the hope that during the ensuing months the patient would recognize more clearly some of the benefits of therapy and return. Essentially, in the family in which she had been raised, all instinctual gratification was considered sinful. The patient had developed a rather rigid superego which prevented any instinctual gratification. She forbade herself the expression of hostility as well as heterosexuality.

In this particular case, the limited goal of therapy was achieved and the patient became a symptom-free compulsive personality, who undoubtedly, without the benefit of future therapy, would achieve a limited adjustment. She might well produce excellent work in her particular field, but nevertheless would not achieve any full pleasurable heterosexual (genital) type of existence. It was explained to her in the last visit that her improvement, while satisfactory to her, was not complete and that if and when she should desire more help the therapist would welcome her return.

CHAPTER 22

Other Treatment Procedures

PSYCHOTHERAPY, while an important and basic ingredient in the armamentarium of the psychiatrist, is by no means the only treatment procedure available to him, nor is it always the procedure of choice. The characteristic picture of the psychiatrist seeing his patient in his office once or twice a week represents only a part of the total therapy of psychiatry. The fact that there are more mental hospital beds in this country than all other types of hospital beds combined indicates the tremendous importance of the emotionally and mentally disturbed patient. As is evident from the Joint Commission's [1] *Action for Mental Health,* discussed more thoroughly in Chapter 23, the whole concept of the care and treatment of the emotionally and mentally disturbed person has changed radically since, and even during, the last ten years. The tranquilizing drugs, the concept of the smaller state hospital, the day-care center, family therapy, and other such relatively recent innovations have revised the philosophy of the care and treatment of the psychiatric patient. It has become increasingly apparent that not only all physicians, but also members of other mental health disciplines will have to be trained in increasing numbers and will have to shoulder the burden of the treatment of this large group of individuals.

If one considers the various types of treatment available other than those mentioned in Chapter 21, there are six broad additional categories which deserve discussion. These by no means represent the total of available treatment for the psychiatric patient, but they do

[1] Joint Commission on Mental Illness and Health. *Action for Mental Health.* New York, Basic Books, Inc., 1961.

encompass the broad areas involved. They are: (1) chemotherapy (tranquilizers and psychic energizers), (2) family therapy, (3) hospitalization, (4) group therapy, (5) shock therapy and (6) psychosurgery.

The discussions which follow under separate sections should not be construed to indicate that these various modes of therapy are used individually and not in combination. The needs and problems of the individual patient and his family will of course determine which method or methods will be utilized. For example, a hospitalized patient may be receiving individual psychotherapy as well as group therapy. Another patient may be receiving tranquilizers and, at the same time, participating in family therapy.

TRANQUILIZERS AND PSYCHIC ENERGIZERS

Man's search for relief from the anxieties, worries, and discomforts of life is probably as old as he himself. He has tried in every age and in every society to find means to decrease his level of tension and to elevate his mood. He has tried many medicines, some empirically and some with a basis of physiologic understanding. He has distilled alcohol since the beginning of time. He has chewed cocoa leaves, drunk coffee, smoked marihuana, swallowed barbiturates and amphetamines, and even injected morphine. While many of these substances have long been known to produce the desired effect, at least transiently, they have also produced problems of no small magnitude. Morphine not only reduces pain and diminishes apprehension and anxiety, but unfortunately when used injudiciously leads to addiction, thus producing far greater problems than it might have solved. Alcohol first attacks superego functions which leads to a false sense of well-being and omnipotence. The vengeful return of the superego the next morning, however, leads to the well-known hangover. The chronic and excessive use of alcohol leads once again to more serious disorders than might have been present in the beginning.

As psychiatry became increasingly aware of both the complexity of emotional and mental disorders and the slow pace of effective treatment, the search for some magical pharmaceutical cure for anxiety and mental symptoms gained impetus. Physicians have long been prone to write a quick prescription rather than listen to the patient. Obviously it would be a boon to them if a medication could be found which would reduce the symptoms of psychosis, allay the anxiety of neurosis, and perhaps even diminish the acting out of the individual with a personality disorder. In 1953 with the introduction of the tranquilizing agents it was hoped that we had found the road to this panacea. While it is true that we have found a road, it is not without its barricades, pitfalls, and detours. The expansion of the use of tranquilizing and energizing drugs during the last ten years has been remarkable. While it has produced benefits, it has also brought with it problems of toxicity and other new problems which we have not faced before.

The so-called tranquilizers comprise a group of drugs which were originally heralded and are still advertised as reducing tension and diminishing anxiety without producing drowsiness or other soporific effects. In essence, as the name would imply, these preparations are supposed to produce peace of mind. It is paradoxical that in spite of the widespread use of these drugs relatively little is known about the details of their physiological action. They are prescribed not only by psychiatrists, but by most other physicians, and new preparations appear on the market frequently. Scientific studies of these new drugs are sometimes hasty and poorly designed. One tremendously important factor, the placebo effect, is not infrequently neglected.

A placebo is a physiologically inert drug which the patient believes has a medicating effect, and the placebo effect is the change reported by the patient as a result of taking such a substance. Certain pharmacological preparations have demonstrable physiological effects and yet produce other unexpected effects because of the placebo value inherent in the suggestions of the physician and the beliefs of the patient. The highly suggestible individual, such as the hysteric, not infrequently experiences a diminution in anxiety or other uncomfortable symptoms as a result of taking almost any kind of medication, if he is told that it will make him feel better. There are other individuals who are much less suggestible and in whom the placebo effect is small. There is still another group who tend to react negatively to suggestions by the physician and often manage in one way or another to feel worse after taking medication.

The tranquilizers, however, do have physiological effects. They vary in potency and in their effectiveness in various syndromes. Space does not permit a detailed discussion of all the tranquilizers and their various effects and pharmacology, but a general review of the main types would be useful. It is possible to divide them into four general categories: the phenothiazines, Rauwolfia alkaloids, diphenylmethanes and the propenediols.

The phenothiazines include drugs with such trade names as Thorazine, Sparine, Compazine, Trilafon, Pacatal and Phenergan. Chlorpromazine, the first of this group to be used extensively, was introduced in 1952. It has proved particularly useful in the treatment of the schizophrenic. These drugs cause many psychotic patients to lose some of their most disturbing symptoms, such as agitation, destructiveness, and even hallucinations and delusions. State hospitals have found these preparations particularly useful, not only in diminishing the number of patients who present serious management problems, but in enabling the discharge of many who would otherwise have to remain in the hospital. Neither these nor any other drugs really cure schizophrenia. The patient who improves to the point that he may leave the state hospital because of these drugs still presents many of the features of the schizophrenic. His relationships are still not mature and his affect is usually still blunted. If he is to remain in the community he usually has to continue to take the medication. Unfortunately, the cost of the drug over a long period of time is high, and if the patient cannot afford to buy it, he may have to return to the hospital. Some states are beginning to make allowance for all or part of the cost of the medication. Such a plan, of course, is much less expensive than rehospitalization. The phenothiazines do have an element of toxicity. Leucopenia and agranulocytosis occur at times, as do liver damage and jaundice. Parkinsonian symptoms may appear, but usually stop when the drug is diminished or withdrawn. Convulsions and somnolence are other evidences of toxicity.

Of the Rauwolfia alkaloids, Reserpine is probably the best known. The tranquilizing effect of this group of drugs requires a longer period of administration than is true for the phenothiazines. The depressant effect is also somewhat greater and, therefore, it has gradually become more popular in the treatment of mania and somewhat less so in the treatment of schizophrenia. As with the phenothiazines, toxic effects may occur in the form of extrapyramidal symptoms, but additional possible side effects are lethargy, depression, nasal congestion, and bradycardia.

The diphenylmethanes include such proprietary preparations as Frenquil, Atarax, Benadryl, and Suavatil. Most of these drugs have antihistamine qualities and many of them have been used for this purpose since their introduction. In general they have been used much more with neurotic patients than with psychotics. They have somewhat fewer toxic effects than the previous two groups. At times they produce drowiness and rarely leucopenia.

The final group of tranquilizers are the propenediols. They are represented by such preparations as Tolserol, Miltown and Equanil. Like the diphenylmethanes they have a previous pharmacological history, but in this case as muscle relaxants. With the discovery that such muscle relaxing drugs also had the effect of diminishing anxiety, new preparations were evolved which emphasized the tranquilizing effect. In general, this group is not particularly toxic, although symptoms such as diarrhea, diplopia and hypotension occasionally occur, particularly when the drugs are administered in large doses. Convulsions may at times occur during withdrawal. This group of drugs generally has been used more successfully with neurotic individuals than with psychotics. Here again is a group of drugs somewhat less toxic than the phenothiazines, but in a sense somewhat less potent in their actions.

Psychic energizers is the name given to a heterogeneous group of stimulating drugs which are presumably of use in the relief of depression. Some of these, such as Benzadrine and Dexadrine are amphetamines and produce hyperexcitability. Others are amine-oxidase inhibitors, such as Tofranil and Marsilid. In general, if used excessively, the amphetamines can lead to convulsions and the amine-oxidase inhibitors to liver damage and hypotension.

It is really difficult, if not impossible, to evaluate accurately the over-all usefulness of these drugs. The depressed individual may or may not respond favorably to their use and when he does, we are not always certain whether a placebo effect has played a part. Milder neurotic depressions can be dealt with satisfactorily by psychotherapy. Some serious psychotic-like depressions at times respond to these energizers; at other times they may require electroshock treatment.

It should be emphasized that tranquilizers and psychic energizers are by no means cure-alls for mental and emotional disturbances. Certainly they have made a tremendous impact on all of medicine, and undoubtedly new preparations will continue to appear on the market. In general it may be said that particularly the phenothiazines have been of value in reducing the number of hospitalized schizophrenic patients and in making many of those who must remain in the hospital more manageable. The long-continued use of such drugs, however, carries with it risk as well as expense, and they should be administered only under careful, watchful medical care.

Probably the most widespread use of tranquilizers has been made by nonpsychotic individuals suffering from neurotic symptoms or other vague emotional complaints. The prescription of tranquilizers appears to be a quick and easy solution for both physician and patient, and often leads to a continued dependence on medication. Unfortunately it also usually means that no attention is given by the patient or physician to improving the anxiety-producing situation or the patient's neurotic methods of dealing with intrapsychic conflict.

Perhaps a parallel can be drawn between the production of antibiotics and that of tranquilizers. When they first appeared, antibiotics were assumed by many to be the cure for all infectious diseases. It was soon discovered that they were not only ineffective against viruses, and only partly effective against the entire spectrum of bacteria, but they also produced occasional serious toxic effects. New antibiotics rapidly appeared, each with great promise. Their injudicious use not only sensitized some people, but failed completely to help others. So it has been with the tranquilizers. They hold considerable promise, but they can be misused and can produce toxic effects. Our knowledge of the actions of these various drugs will improve, but it is essential that the physician remain cautious in their use and that he acquaint himself thoroughly with the patient's physical and mental status and make every effort to deal with all aspects.

FAMILY THERAPY

Family therapy is a relatively new concept in the field of psychiatry. Until approximately 1950 the psychiatric treatment of the patient involved a relationship between him and the psychotherapist with only peripheral contacts of the physician with other members of the family. It was assumed that only by this route could a meaningful relationship develop between physician and patient which would eventually enable the patient to learn more about his own inner psychological problems. However, it became gradually more evident that this one-to-one relationship did not accomplish its goal in every case. There were many situations in which other family members were obviously contributing to the illness of the patient, whether this contribution was conscious or unconscious. It became evident, in other words, that there often existed a sort of family psychopathology which needed to be treated in a group situation. The emotional problems of family members other than the patient had traditionally been dealt with by the social worker, but such an arrangement often left many loop-holes. The social worker might well become almost totally concerned with the problems of the parents of a disturbed child while the psychiatrist was focusing exclusively on the child himself. Neither therapist would necessarily view the total picture. The possibility then arose of seeing the entire family in such a case and of having one or even two therapists deal with the total family situation.

One of the other factors leading to the development of family therapy was the growing awareness that the "patient" who was either brought or who presented himself to the psychiatrist was often not the sickest member of the family. Those who have worked in residential treatment centers for children have long recognized that the child brought for in-patient care is not necessarily the one who most needs help. It remained however that new techniques needed to be developed if an entire family was to be seen in therapy by one or possibly two therapists. It was no longer possible only to evaluate matters of transference and countertransference between therapist and patient, but in addition to utilize some aspects of group dynamics and of group therapy. The psychiatrist could no longer operate as a totally neutral figure on whom his patient transferred earlier important emotional investments. It now became necessary for the psychiatrist literally to see the family in action and to develop an increased awareness of total family dynamics.

It must be borne in mind that when a patient is presented to the psychiatrist, particularly if he is a child who is brought by the family, the other family members do not usually anticipate becoming patients themselves. However, if given sufficient understanding of the procedure to be undertaken, the majority of families will be willing to participate. It is at this juncture of family therapy that the psychiatrist often fails or succeeds. If he can explain to the various family members what he intends to do and why, they will often support his efforts and join with him. If, however, he conducts this crucial interview in an unintuitive or authoritative manner, they will often resist his suggestions.

In general, then, it became gradually more evident that this traditional one-to-one relationship of psychotherapy did not do everything necessary for refractory cases. Typical examples were found in psychotics, the various personality disturbances in family members, alcoholism, and at times drug addiction and delinquency. The patient who is greatly self-centered, who has little feeling for others and who exercises poor discipline over his moods and behavior often fares much better when other members of the family join in the treatment sessions. Such an effort enables the therapist to observe the family members interact with each other and gives much more information than it is possible to obtain from the patient alone. When such a patient is interviewed alone he may distort the picture of the behavior of other family members, especially as it affects him. When brought together in therapy, however, it is possible to gain a more realistic insight into the manner in which family members impinge upon each other.

The technique of family therapy is difficult and best undertaken only after the therapist has thoroughly developed his skills in individual psychotherapy. The treatment of a total family by one therapist or even by co-therapists should not be thought of as a time-saving device enabling fewer therapists to treat more patients. Certainly not all families are good candidates for this type of treatment, and only the most well-trained and intuitive therapist can determine these factors. Family therapy does not always proceed rigidly along the lines of weekly visits with the total family. It is entirely possible that the therapist may decide that at some period during the treatment one or another of the family members will need individual sessions. Here again it is not possible to lay down rigid ground rules for such treatment, and only the therapist's intuitive understanding of the entire family dynamics, as well as the individual problems of each member, will enable him to make proper decisions.

Case History

A fourteen-year-old boy was brought to the child psychiatry clinic by his parents, who complained that he was doing poorly in school, that he had few friends and that he seemed afraid of many things, including new situations, competitive games, and being in the house alone. He was an only child who had apparently had a relatively uneventful childhood until age ten, at which time he had suffered a compound fracture of one arm as a result of an automobile accident. He had subsequently been subjected to considerable orthopedic surgery, and it was from this time on that the parents had begun to notice his difficulties.

The family history revealed the fact that both parents had been married previously. The father had been widowed and the mother divorced. Neither had had any children. When they married, they had not planned on raising a family, but they had a son, and both claimed to have been quite happy. The mother was a rigid, controlling, and overprotective woman who had always worried lest some harm come to her son. She had been unwilling to allow him even the normal freedoms of a child and had intently watched every detail of his daily life. The father was a passive man who worked two jobs, thus keeping him out of the home most of the time. He seemed less concerned about the son's problems than did the mother.

After the initial work-up involving detailed family history and interviews with the child, as well as psychological testing, it was decided that family therapy might prove helpful.

During the following sessions the boy often complained that his mother watched over him far too closely and that his father paid too little attention to him. The father meantime stated that he worked many hours a day and, therefore, was not well acquainted with the boy's difficulties. The mother repeatedly castigated the father about his lack of interest. She seemed to feel that if he played a more active role she would be less overprotective. It soon became evident in the course of treatment that the boy, although resentful of his mother's overprotection, did everything he could to encourage it. It also became increasingly clear that the father worked two jobs because he found life at home difficult and felt he was excluded from the almost symbiotic relationship between his son and his wife. The most refractory member of the trio was the mother, who had great difficulty in recognizing her own contribution to the family psychopathology. It became possible to show her some of her own problems when the father began to play a more active and masculine role and she was unable to accept this. At the same time it was possible to show the boy his mixed feelings about gaining independence as his mother began to give it to him, and he found difficulty in accepting it.

This family continued in treatment over a period of nine months at weekly intervals. The eventual solution was reasonably satisfactory, although by no means perfect. It is probable that had the child been seen by one therapist and the parents by another, there would have been a longer period of resolution of conflicts. This was certainly an entire family problem, and one which in this particular case lent itself best to family therapy.

It is to be stressed that family therapy is not intended as a method preferable to individual psychotherapy in all cases. Its use is limited to those cases where the more orthodox approach would be hampered by interlocking family psychopathology which cannot be worked out by individual therapists. It also is useful where the "primary patient" is not the most disturbed, but the latter can be brought to treatment only if the entire family participates. This type of treatment can be carried out only by the most skilled therapist and cannot usually reach the degree of personality changes in patients that can be attained in individual psychotherapy.

HOSPITALIZATION

When most of the large psychiatric state hospitals of our country were constructed, the prevailing philosophy was that of custodial care for the mentally ill. Patients, for the most part, were sent to these hospitals when their illness seemed to preclude their ability to adjust to community living. If and when they became sufficiently improved, they were discharged; when such improvement did not take place, they remained for years. As the enormity of the problem began to impress physicians, legislators, and others, newer methods were devised for dealing with such individuals. In the first place, it became evident that early recognition and treatment would be of value in preventing prolonged later hospitalization. This led to recommendations for, and establishment of, child guidance clinics and community mental health centers. This movement has recently received national Congressional attention and the number of such centers should increase rapidly in the ensuing years.

Advances in modern medicine have led to a prolonged life span, which has also increased the number of senile patients being sent to state mental hospitals. Many plans have been devised for improved care and treatment of such patients. The state hospital is geared primarily toward the treatment of the mentally ill, but has gradually become a custodial institution for a large number of senile patients. Proposals have been made and institutions have been established specifically for the care and treatment of these older people. Active psychotherapy is less important with this group than others. They do need a supervised, orderly, and well-planned routine which allows them to be constructive to the extent of their limited capacities. In such elderly people the greatest need is often to combat feelings of uselessness and helplessness. If they can be given suitable and pleasant tasks commensurate with their abilities, their entire psychic status often improves.

A further innovation in the care and treatment of the mentally ill is that of the day-care center. There are many people suffering from a variety of psychiatric illnesses who can live at home while treatment is undertaken in a well-supervised, therapeutically oriented day-care center. In such institutions psychotherapy as well as occupational therapy, recreational therapy and other treatment approaches are available. Conversely there are some patients who are capable of continuing with their occupations while spending their evenings and nights in a hospital situation.

Another impressive improvement in our care of the mentally ill is the establishment of psychiatric facilities in various general hospitals. Here again it is to be stressed that the care is not custodial, but is active and oriented toward returning the patient to his own home and community as rapidly as possible. The care of the psychiatrically ill in the general hospital has as an important asset the lack of segregation and isolation so prominent in the state mental hospital. Other advantages are the avoidance of the legal commitment procedures necessary for admission to some state hospitals; the absence of stigma, which often makes the patient and his family more willing to accept the recommendation for necessary hospitalization; and the opportunity for the psychiatrist to work more closely with physicians of other specialties.

As is explained more thoroughly in Chapter 23, the recommendations for future state hospitals contain the concept of the smaller institution. Many of our state hospitals now have literally thousands of beds. They are often located in isolated areas which make family contact difficult and, in addition, make it harder to obtain a professional staff. These state hospitals are in operation, however, and will in the foreseeable future continue to be utilized.

The large number of mental hospital beds and of mentally ill patients means that physicians are constantly making decisions about when a particular patient should be removed from the community and placed in an institution because of his psychiatric disorder. In general it may be said that hospitalization in a mental institution becomes necessary whenever an individual reaches a state where he is potentially dangerous or unable to be responsible for his behavior toward himself or others. Such a decision, however, cannot be made without an adequate study of the patient and his circumstances. Not infrequently the physician overreacts in the direction of immediate hospitalization when a more careful evaluation of the situation would enable him to institute reasonable outpatient procedures. This tendency represents a sort of attempt to get rid of the patient because he is difficult to understand, does not respond immediately to suggestion, or displays a combination of symptoms that are frightening to the physician. It does remain, however, that a certain number of individuals are sufficiently disturbed to require removal from society and placement in an institution.

Current psychiatric philosophy strongly advises that every institutionalized patient be given a maximum of therapeutic attention in order that he may return to the community as soon as possible. Unfortunately in reality many of our state hospitals have too many patients and an insufficient staff so that they become essentially custodial institutions. The majority of them, however, are making every effort to increase the size and effectiveness of their staffs and to utilize all possible methods of therapy. Perhaps typical would be the "total push" method described by Myerson[2] and Tillotson.[3] This involves the careful planning of most of the patient's waking hours so that he is involved in one or another kind of scheduled, useful, and therapeutically oriented activity. He is encouraged to participate actively in recreational therapy, occupational therapy, group activities, and other such organized efforts. Included, of course, is psychotherapy of whatever type seems most advisable. At times, and where appropriate, this is an uncovering type of treatment, while at other times it is primarily supportive in nature. The psychotic patient often tends, if left to his own devices, to retreat farther and farther away from the real world. In the "total push" method he is literally pushed, cajoled, and helped into a better contact with reality. Obviously such a treatment procedure requires a staff which is well-trained and numerically adequate.

The state hospital or other mental institution utilizes tranquilizers, electroshock, and hydrotherapy as are appropriate in each individual case. Generally speaking, most state hospitals have increased the freedom given to their patients. It is obviously necessary that there be certain wards which are "locked" for the patients' own protection. But much of a typical state hospital is "open" and the patients have relatively free access to the grounds, the snack bars, and other such areas.

The mental institution also retains close ties with the community

[2] Myerson, A. "Theory and Principles of the 'Total Push' Method in the Treatment of Chronic Schizophrenia." *Am. J. of Psychiatry*, XCV, 1939.

[3] Tillotson, Kenneth J. "Practice of the 'Total Push' Method in the Treatment of Chronic Schizophrenia." *Am. J. of Psychiatry*, XCV, 1939.

and with the families of its patients. The social work staff makes every attempt to help the families of patients better understand themselves as well as the patient's illness. Treatment wherever possible is oriented toward returning the patient to his own family. The institution also maintains an active outpatient clinic which serves not only as a community mental health center, but also as a resource where discharged patients and their families may continue to receive help.

GROUP THERAPY

Group therapy is a treatment approach in which a number of individuals are gathered together at regular intervals for psychotherapeutic help under the direction of one or occasionally two therapists. Some people attach an even broader meaning to this term and extend it to include such "groups" as Boy Scouts, sewing circles and altruistically oriented fraternal groups. While it is true that members of such "groups" probably gain from these "therapeutic" experiences, we are not dealing here with group therapy in such extensive terms. We are primarily concerned with those groups which are set up with treatment as their goal and, more especially, those under the direction of trained mental health personnel. Such groups may be homogeneous or heterogeneous, that is, they may be made up of individuals with similar difficulties, or patients with markedly dissimilar problems. Groups are composed of either children or adults. It is often erroneously assumed that group therapy is an easy avenue for treatment of many more patients by fewer therapists. Unfortunately, only a selected number of individuals are good candidates for group therapy, and, not infrequently, individual therapy is a necessary adjunct to group treatment.

Group therapy attained its widest acclaim during World War II when many servicemen in large military installations were suffering from emotional problems. Further impetus was added when, following the war, there were still far too few therapists to treat the number of emotionally disturbed who required help. Many experiments were made involving the size, make-up, and type of therapeutic approach to be used.

It is possible to present only a summary of the current status of group therapy and some of the principles involved here. There is still much we do not know about the group process itself, and the whole area of group therapy is in a constant state of flux. It may be said that most group therapists prefer a group comprised of about six to ten individuals. Complete and thorough evaluations are done on each individual prior to their introduction into the group, and the therapist has had the opportunity to interview at length each of the prospective participants. Some group therapists prefer a mixture of syndromes, while others would rather treat individuals who suffer from similar problems. For example, when groups are formed in an institution for addicts, each member of the group will have at least one similar problem, that of addiction. However, when a group is formed in a psychiatric clinic, it may be comprised of individuals having a variety of difficulties. In the latter case, the more aggressive often take the lead in the beginning and inadvertently help the more passive members eventually to make their contributions.

The group therapist operates somewhat differently from the individual psychotherapist in that he cannot give each member of the group the complete attention he would a single patient. Group members will vie for his attention and will often compete with each other in a situation similar to that of siblings within a family. As mentioned previously, the group therapist should be thoroughly trained in individual psychotherapy prior to taking on a group. He cannot be completely passive in the face of group interaction, nor can he be autocratic if he is to succeed in his task. Rather he must understand the various interplays of group reactions, such as when one member may begin to evince considerable hostility to another member who has attempted to dominate the group. As the process moves forward, many new insights are gained by group members from remarks of other members, rather than from those of the therapist.

Choice of patients for group therapy is difficult. Often they are chosen because they react poorly to individual psychotherapy alone and can be led to greater understanding of themselves only through interactions with others in a group. This is a complex process and one which requires considerable training and experience on the part of the therapist. Group therapy is being carried on currently by psychiatrists, psychologists, and social workers and certainly has a place in the armamentarium of all of the mental health disciplines.

Following are a few examples of the types of patients who have been found to benefit from group therapy. While not an exhaustive list, these examples will illustrate some of the general principles involved in determining the usefulness of group therapy.

Heterogeneous adult group: Certain patients with particular types of aggressive or passive problems may have difficulty in gaining useful insight in a one-to-one therapeutic relationship. If they are made part of a group in therapy, pressures exerted on them by others of their group often enhance their ability to see some of their own problems. For example, a more aggressive group member may gain additional understanding of himself when several other members join together and point out his aggressiveness.

Homogeneous adult group: Certain clinical syndromes such as alcoholism have frequently proven refractory to individual psychotherapy. In certain instances these patients participate more actively and willingly in treatment if this is done in a group comprised of others suffering from the same problem. Alcoholics Anonymous has, among other things, a sort of group therapy orientation. There may or may not be a professionally trained group therapist present.

Delinquents: These youngsters are often difficult to reach by individual psychotherapy. Not infrequently, however, it is possible to bring them into a group therapy situation with considerable benefit to individual youngsters. Social group workers have been particularly adept in this area.

Parent groups: Child guidance clinics and other such agencies have, over the years, experimented with group treatment of parents of emotionally disturbed children. Here again the group's ability to share their similar problems with each other often stimulates more active participation in the whole treatment process. Many of these parents will also need individual treatment at some point.

Family therapy: Therapeutic work with the entire family is discussed earlier in this chapter. It is unique in that it is a group situation, but contains both children and adults.

SHOCK THERAPY

The various types of shock therapy used today had their origin in the work of Sakel,[4] who found that the production of coma by large doses of insulin had a beneficial effect upon schizophrenic reactions. He originally used insulin as a physiological antagonist to adrenalin, which he felt caused excited states seen in the withdrawal states of drug addicts. He found that insulin improved these confused, delirious, and excited states and made the patients more cheerful and comfortable. He therefore decided, on the basis of this knowledge, to utilize insulin on the excited schizophrenics he saw. His original work was published in 1933. In 1935, von Meduna,[5] working with the idea that schizophrenic reaction and epilepsy rarely occur together, evolved the method of convulsive therapy using metrazol. Actually his initial assumption was not true, since schizophrenic reaction and epilepsy do occur together from time to time. The majority of shock treatments used today are a direct outgrowth of these two pioneer methods.

Insulin shock therapy has for the most part disappeared from psychiatric treatment. It was by far the most difficult to utilize of the shock treatment procedures and involved the administration of doses of insulin sufficient to produce coma. Over the years it has begun to be apparent that this is a not particularly effective, but relatively dangerous type of treatment, and it has largely been abandoned by psychiatric centers.

As mentioned previously, the convulsive therapies began with the introduction of metrazol seizures for the treatment of mental diseases by von Meduna. Originally he had used camphor in oil for the same purpose but had found the disadvantages too great. Even with metrazol, these disadvantages were still large. Particularly

[4] Sakel, M. *The Pharmacological Shock Treatment of Schizophrenia.* New York. Nervous and Mental Disease Publishing Co., 1938.
[5] Meduna, von, L. J. *Die Konvulsiontherapie der Schizophrenie.* Halle. Carl Manhold, 1937.

unfortunate was the time interval between the injection of the drug and the onset of convulsion with its loss of consciousness, perhaps 15 to 30 seconds. During this period the patient felt a sense of impending doom and was often in a state approaching panic. In 1938, Cerlitti and Bini [6] in Italy demonstrated that such convulsions could be produced with an electric current. This method of electroshock has since supplanted pharmacologically produced convulsive methods, and is not only much safer, but spares the patient the intolerable interval between application and loss of consciousness. Of no minor importance is the fact that fewer patients resent, and therefore refuse, treatment.

Electroshock therapy is administered utilizing a machine which regulates the duration and the amount of current. Electrodes are placed ordinarily upon the temporal regions of the scalp and a current of 200 to 1600 milliamperes is used for a period of from one-tenth to five-tenths seconds. This current produces a grand-mal type of seizure with an initial tonic phase followed by a clonic phase. The patient recovers gradually, passing through a confused period and slowly regaining consciousness in a way that is similar to that seen in an epileptic. Electroshock is given from about three to six or even seven times a week. It is often used in combination with various tranquilizing agents, using the EST only when the tranquilizers alone are insufficient. The number of shock treatments is kept at a minimum to produce the improvement necessary to allow tranquilization and/or psychic energizers and psychotherapy to be effective.

Electroshock does have contraindications, chiefly cardiovascular disease, recent operations or fractures, active tuberculosis and pregnancy. However, many of the former contraindications are reduced in seriousness by the use of muscle relaxants such as succinylcholine. Such a preparation markedly attenuates muscular contractions. This type of convulsive therapy preferably is administered in a hospital by experienced operators and assistants. Necessary equipment and medication for the handling of emergencies should be immediately available. There are instances when the risk of electroshock is con-

[6] Cerlitti, V. and L. Bini. "L'Elettroshock." *Arch. Gen. di Neurol. Psichiat. e Psicoanal.*, XIX, 1938.

siderable because of the age or physical condition of the patient and yet this must be weighed against the debilitating effects of the disease from which the patient suffers. The hyperactive, manic patient, who is literally wearing himself to death and who responds to no other form of therapy, may be a candidate for electroshock in spite of the risks attendant to this type of treatment. One of the most common complications of electroshock, namely a fracture of the dorsal or lumbar vertebral bodies, is seen much less frequently when the muscle relaxants are used.

It remains somewhat of a mystery as to why electroshock produces improvement in certain patients. Early speculations presumed that the psychological impact of the sudden loss of consciousness produced in this particular fashion had a marked impact upon the patient's personality organization. It has become more probable as our knowledge of brain physiology and biochemistry has improved that the electroshock does alter the function of some of the deeper portions of the brain in ways which are not yet well understood.

PSYCHOSURGERY

The procedure of prefrontal leucotomy or lobotomy was introduced in 1936 by Egas Moniz.[7] It is based on the view that the frontal lobes play a dominant part in the production of mental disorders and that interruption of the various association pathways and their connections, particularly between these lobes and certain nuclei in the thalamus, will alleviate a mental disorder. Since the first attempts in this direction, there have been many procedures devised, based upon similar principles. In all probability, these attempts will continue until every portion of the brain has been surgically approached with this goal in view. At the present time, the chief methods utilized are lobectomy, topectomy, leucotomy, and thalamotomy. The surgical techniques involved vary from intricate procedures performed by skilled neurosurgeons to questionable "operations" done in the comatose state following electroshock.

Psychosurgery has enjoyed progressively less acceptance and utili-

[7] Egas Moniz, Antonio. *Tentatives Opératoires dans le Traitement de Certaines Psychoses*. Paris. Masson et Cie., 1936.

zation during the past ten years. There are still rare instances in which an intractable and presumably "incurable" severely agitated, depressed, or almost psychotically compulsive patient may be a potential candidate for this type of treatment. Since the destruction of central nervous system tissue is permanent, the choice of cases for these procedures is a matter for careful consideration. In general these operations have, at least in the experimental stages, been limited to psychotic patients on whom ordinary procedures, including shock therapy, have been unsuccessful. Occasionally they have been tried on obsessive-compulsive neurotics, as well as on some patients with behavior disorders who have failed to respond to treatment of any other type. However, surgical procedures on the brain designed to modify the course of mental illness are not recommended in any but the most exceptional cases. We have been so understaffed and so unimaginative in our treatment of mental illness that we should for the present take a conservative position on psychosurgery and develop other techniques more fully.

CHAPTER 23

Mental Health and Community Psychiatry

MENTAL and emotional illnesses are one of the major problems in our society today. An increase in our understanding of these conditions has brought with it not only improved methods of treatment, but also an increased awareness of the necessity for better mental hygiene in our society. The statistics concerning the prevalence of psychiatric disorders have made a disquieting impression upon many people. More than one out of every two hospital beds in the United States today is occupied by a mental patient; one out of every ten persons will spend some part of his life in a mental hospital. The cost of mental illness is approaching four billion dollars a year in the United States, if one includes both the expense of the hospitals and the loss of earnings and federal income tax revenue from the hospitalized patient. When we consider the prevalence of the lesser emotional difficulties, the problem becomes even more formidable. About half of the average general practitioner's patients suffer from some form of emotional difficulty and about 30 per cent of hospitalized medical and surgical patients have emotional problems which contribute in measurable degree to their illness. No statistics, however, can reveal clearly the unfortunate effect which these people have upon their environment, nor can such figures show what problems they will present to their friends and families. Such statistics do not take into account the many millions of people who do not come to the attention of physicians, but who are still doing an unsatisfactory job as parents or workers because they are having difficulties in getting along with those with whom they work and live. There are still others who live totally unproductive lives and who are either parasitic or predatory in their relationships to the rest of society.

Action for Mental Health,[1] a report of the Joint Commission on Mental Illness and Health, published in 1961, is the most modern, comprehensive report on the state of our national mental health. As its title implies, it also includes strong recommendations for action. In 1955 the Mental Health Study Act, enacted by Congress, directed the Joint Commission on Mental Illness and Health to "analyze and evaluate the needs and resources of the mentally ill in the United States and to make recommendations for a national mental health program." The final report is available and should be read by everyone interested in the subject of mental health. In addition the Joint Commission has published several monographs dealing with the major facets of mental illness and mental health, each of which concerns itself with our present knowledge about a particular field. (A complete listing of these monographs may be found in the Bibliography.) The basic report itself, along with the monographs, provide guiding principles to various local and federal agencies.

It would be impossible in a book of this nature to review all of the findings and recommendations in *Action for Mental Health*. It is, however, of such importance that a summary of some of the conclusions should be presented. The report points out that our future progress in this field depends upon the solution of three major problems: (1) manpower, (2) facilities, and (3) costs.

The summary of the Recommendations for a National Mental Health Program are presented under the subheadings of "Pursuit of New Knowledge," "Better Use of Present Knowledge and Experience," and "The Cost." Under "Pursuit of New Knowledge," the report states:

The philosophy that the federal government needs to develop and crystallize is that science and education are resources—like natural resources

---

[1] Joint Commission on Mental Illness and Health. *Action for Mental Health*. New York, Basic Books, Inc., 1961.

—and that they deserve conservation through intelligent use and protection and adequate support. They can meet an ends test, but not a means test and not a timetable or appeal for a specified result. Science and education operate not for profit, but profit everybody; hence, they need adequate support from human society, whether this support comes from wise public philanthropy or private.

In this context, the summary lists eight specific recommendations dealing with increased support of mental health research by both the federal and state governments. It stresses the need for basic research to receive a greater quota of the funds than in the past, in contrast to applied research. It suggests greater efforts by the National Institute of Mental Health in investing in, providing for, and holding the young scientist in his career choice. It points out the need for the establishment of mental health research centers or research institutes, and a general diversification of grants from the standpoint of varied interests, subject matter of research and branches of science involved.

In "Better Use of Present Knowledge and Experience," the summary starts with the following policy statement:

In the absence of more specific evidence of the causes of mental illness, psychiatry and the allied mental health professions should adopt and practice a broad, liberal philosophy of what constitutes and who can do treatment within the framework of their hospitals, clinics, or other professional service agencies, particularly in relation to persons with psychoses or severe personality or character disorders that incapacitate them for work, family life, and everyday activity. All mental health professions should recognize:

A. That certain kinds of medical, psychiatric, and neurological examinations and treatments must be carried out by or under the immediate direction of psychiatrists, neurologists, or other physicians specially trained for these procedures.

B. That psychoanalysis and allied forms of deeply searching and probing "depth psychotherapy" must be practiced only by those with special training, experience, and competence in handling these techniques without harm to the patient—namely, by physicians trained in psychoanalysis or intensive psychotherapy, plus those psychologists or other professional persons who lack a medical education but have an aptitude for, training in, and demonstrable competence in such techniques of psychotherapy.

C. That nonmedical mental health workers with aptitude, sound training, practical experience, and demonstrable competence should be permitted to do general, short-term psychotherapy—namely, treating persons by objective, permissive, nondirective techniques of listening to their troubles and helping them resolve these troubles in an individually insightful and socially useful way. Such therapy, combining some elements of psychiatric treatment, client counseling, "someone to tell one's troubles to," and love for one's fellow man, obviously can be carried out in a variety of settings by institutions, groups and individuals, but in all cases should be undertaken under the auspices of recognized mental health agencies.

The report in this section goes on to point out the need for encouragement in recruitment and training as well as the support of education in the mental health professions. It deals further with the need for support and establishment of community mental health clinics for both children and adults, as well as for general hospital psychiatric units. Concerning the care of chronic mental patients, the summary states:

No further State hospitals of more than 1000 beds should be built, and not one patient should be added to any existing mental hospital already housing 1000 or more patients. It is further recommended that all existing State hospitals of more than 1000 beds be gradually and progressively converted into centers for the long-term and combined care of chronic diseases, including mental illness. This conversion should be undertaken in the next ten years.

Special techniques are available for the care of the chronically ill and these techniques of socialization, relearning, group living, and gradual rehabilitation or social improvement should be expanded and extended to more people, including the aged who are sick and in need of care, through conversion of State mental hospitals into combined chronic disease centers.

An important aspect of this subsection is covered in the following paragraph concerning "Aftercare, Intermediate Care, and Rehabilitation Services." It states:

The objective of modern treatment of persons with major mental illness is to enable the patient to maintain himself in the community in a normal manner. To do so, it is necessary (1) to save the patient from the debilitating effects of institutionalization as much as possible, (2) if the patient requires hospitalization, to return him to home and community life as soon as possible, and (3) thereafter to maintain him in the community as long as possible. Therefore, aftercare and rehabilitation are essential parts of all service to mental patients, and the various methods of achieving rehabilitation should be integrated in all forms of services, among them day hospitals, night hospitals, aftercare clinics, public health nursing services, foster family care, convalescent nursing homes, rehabilitation centers, work services, and ex-patient groups. We recommend that demonstration programs for day and night hospitals and the more flexible use of mental hospital facilities, in the treatment of both the acute and the chronic patient, be encouraged and augmented through institutional, program and project grants.

Under the subsection entitled "The Cost," the report makes some rather startling recommendations. It states: "Expenditures for public mental patient services should be doubled in the next five years—and tripled in the next ten." In further explaining how such funds should be expended and why they should come from both State and Federal sources the summary makes the following points:

1. Bring about any necessary changes in the laws of the State to make professionally acceptable treatment as well as custody a requirement in mental hospitalization, to differentiate between need of treatment and need of institutionalization, and to provide treatment without hospitalization.

2. Bring about any necessary changes in laws of the State to make voluntary admission the preferred method and court commitment the exceptional method of placing patients in a mental hospital or other treatment facilities, and to emphasize ease of patient movement into and out of such facilities.

3. Accept any and all persons requiring treatment and/or hospitalization on the same basis as persons holding legal residence within the State.

4. Revise laws of the State governing medical responsibility for the patient to distinguish between administrative responsibility for his welfare and safekeeping and responsibility for his professional care.

5. Institute suitable differentiation between administrative structure and professional personnel requirements for (1) State mental institutions intended primarily as intensive treatment centers (i.e., true hospitals) and (2) facilities for humane and progressive care of various classes of the chronically ill or disabled, among them the aged.

6. Establish State mental health agencies with well-defined powers and sufficient authority to assume overall responsibility for the State's services to the mentally ill, and to coordinate State and local community health services.

7. Make reasonable efforts to operate open mental hospitals as mental health centers, i.e., as part of an integrated community service with emphasis on outpatient and aftercare facilities as well as inpatient services.

8. Establish in selected State mental hospitals and community mental health programs training for mental health workers, ranging in scope, as appropriate, from professional training in psychiatry through all professional and subprofessional levels, including on-the-job training of attendants and volunteers. Since each mental health center cannot undertake all forms of teaching activity, consideration here must be given to a variety of programs and total effort. States should be required ultimately to spend 2½ per cent of State mental patient service funds for training.

9. Establish in selected State mental hospitals and community mental health programs scientific research programs appropriate to the facility, the opportunities for well-designed research, and the research talent and experience of staff members. States should be required ultimately to spend 2½ per cent of State mental patient service funds for research.

10. Encourage county, town, and municipal tax participation in the public mental health services of the State as a means of obtaining Federal funds matched against local mental health appropriations.

11. Agree that no money will be spent to build mental hospitals of more than 1000 beds, or to add a single patient to mental hospitals presently having 1000 or more patients.

As can be readily seen from the above quotations, both medicine and psychiatry are being called upon to increase their efforts in the direction of the management of mental illness. This report gave considerable impetus to what has been referred to as social or community psychiatry—that is, the application of what has been already learned by the investigation of causes, as well as through the treatment of mental illness, to communities and social groups. Training in both medicine and psychiatry has over the years tended to emphasize the physician's care and treatment of the individual patient. Although physicians who have responsibility for many individuals at the same time in institutions or hospitals have developed concepts of the handling of such large groups, the tendency to think of one patient at a time remains.

Psychoanalysis, for example, developed as Freud pursued increasingly intensive studies of individual patients. He greatly enlarged our knowledge of the function of the human psyche, but he left this branch of psychiatry with the tradition of a close intensive study of one patient by one physician. Freud did occasionally write on broader social problems, as have other analysts since, but the basic teachings, however, in both medicine and psychoanalysis have remained oriented toward the individual patient.

During recent years there has been a growing demand from society and its various institutions for assistance from psychiatrists in the areas of community and social problems. At the same time psychiatrists have turned to other professionals in attempts to be of help and to broaden their own knowledge. Educators want to know how they can refine their pedagogical techniques in the light of modern psychiatric knowledge. Theologians are becoming increasingly aware of the importance of the psychiatrist's contributions. Penologists are turning to the psychiatrist for advice as are other large agencies and community institutions. Since psychiatric knowledge is an integral part of the behavioral sciences, it is natural that these people turn to the psychiatrist for help, and that he both teaches and learns from them.

Psychiatry today finds itself in a position somewhat similar to that of general medicine a few decades ago when public health became a national concern. Tuberculosis, venereal disease, vitamin deficiencies, infant mortality, and other similar problems faced early public health physicians. They could no longer think only of the individual patient, but had to broaden their perspectives to include the entire community. They had to find ways of educating the public in the newer knowledge concerning these conditions, for only by public awareness and acceptance could they hope to gain their ends. Through education they had to remove many prevailing prejudices and distorted beliefs.

Psychiatry's position today, however, also differs from that of the early public health physician. A great deal of effort has already been expended to "popularize" psychiatry and the need for broader application of psychiatric principles. Demands for psychiatric service have mushroomed throughout the country. Many people hold an image of an almost magical branch of medicine which should have the answers to many as yet unsolved problems. A few examples may illustrate this. It has been known for many years that the alcoholic is an emotionally disturbed individual. While this is true, if every alcoholic in the United States were suddenly to appear asking for psychiatric treatment, there would be insufficient professionals to treat this group, even if all other mentally and emotionally ill people were ignored. Similarly, it has been shown that our prisons have a large percentage of seriously disturbed inmates who desperately need psychiatric help. Even if such help should be asked, the shortage of mental health personnel would make it impossible to meet their requests.

As mentioned in *Action for Mental Health,* several courses of action will have to be augmented in order to meet the current needs even partially. There is a great need for additional psychiatrists and other trained mental health personnel. There is need for more thorough training of all physicians and medical students in the basic fundamentals of psychiatry and their applicability to community and social organizations. There is room for much greater effort in the area of prevention, which will succeed only with an enlightened public.

Psychiatric training programs during recent years have placed increased emphasis upon giving their trainees a better knowledge of community and social agencies, and to a somewhat lesser extent this has also been true of medical education in general. The current trend is to make professionals more aware of sociological principles, of group dynamics, of public health, of community resources, and other similar broad concepts. Such additional training does not carry with it any diminution in the care given the individual sick patient, but does, however, make the physician more aware of the broad aspects of social problems and the extreme importance of preventive measures.

The identification and definition of illness, either physical or emotional, is always dependent upon comparison with established norms. Mental illness, affecting social behavior as it does, needs particularly to be evaluated in reference to average—that is, "normal"—behavior for the individual's milieu. While psychiatry as a profession has always been aware of the necessity to measure the individual's relative health or illness by the yardsticks of socially acceptable behavior in his own culture, the measure of normality for larger social groups requires a broader sociological understanding than has been prevalent within the profession heretofore. What we Americans would think of as a "normal community" might be abnormal in an entirely different culture. Child-raising principles vary remarkably from one culture to another, and even from one socio-economic level in our own culture to another. What then is the psychiatrist to decide concerning the boundaries between individual and community mental health and illness?

To take one small example from our own educational system, the average teacher usually comes from a middle-class family and has attended college. She may, however, be assigned to a school serving a much lower socio-economic group where the youngsters have been taught different principles of behavior than she. Without an understanding of the mores of the children's own social background, the teacher may find herself falsely interpreting "acceptable" behavior. In fact, if these children were suddenly to adopt her mores, they would be ill-fitted to their own environment. The same may hold true for the psychiatrist who takes into therapy a child of very different social background. The physician would prefer, in all probability, to see the youngster adopt his own concepts and to internalize middle-class values, preferring to see the child move upward within our social structure. He must realize, however, that the child's assumption of his own values may not prepare him for the social adjustment problems within his own subculture.

With these thoughts in mind, let us attempt to define some of the differences between emotional health and emotional illness. In general, the mentally healthy individual is able to love in a heterosexual manner. He is able to work effectively, efficiently, and with pleasure. He is relatively free of neurotic or characterological incapacitations, and he is a willing and active participant in the affairs of his fellow men to the benefit of his community. Conversely, the mentally ill person tends to love poorly or cannot love members of the opposite sex. His work is often drudgery or he labors ineffectively. He may have neurotic or characterological symptoms or problems which diminish his capacity to a noticeable degree. Lastly, he is usually uninterested in his fellow men and plays little role in their combined efforts toward the community well-being. These distinctions appear reasonably clear, but obviously require considerable refinement. Actually the fine line between emotional health and emotional disturbance is frequently difficult to detect and define. There exists no individual who is completely mature. What is considered adequate behavior in one society, culture, or socio-economic level may not be appropriate in another. Many other similar questions indicate that we cannot adequately define mental illness or mental health, but only recognize tendencies in one direction or the other.

Space permits brief discussion of only a few of the areas in which a psychiatrist may be asked to consult. These are areas of community psychiatry and certain general principles hold true for all of them. Each, however, presents certain unique challenges.

SCHOOLS

Our schools today represent by far the largest single area of community endeavor by our society. Tremendous expenditures of money, time, and energy are devoted to the maintenance of our various school systems. While each of these may still be inadequate, they nevertheless represent one of the largest undertakings which our society has assigned to itself. Of further importance is the fact that schools exert great influence over the developing personalities of our youth. If a particular school system is poor, society will eventually suffer; and conversely, if the school system is good, society will eventually benefit.

Education itself has undergone many revolutions over the years. It began, of course, as something available only to relatively few young people. As the value of education was increasingly recognized, it spread to include larger segments of youth. Techniques of education have varied from conservative to liberal. In our own country we have gradually come to the idea that every child deserves an education commensurate with his capacity. In more recent years additional attention has been paid to the education of the mentally retarded as well as the emotionally disturbed child. Advanced training courses have been instituted in schools of education to train future teachers in the principles of understanding and educating these children.

The psychiatrist has been called upon to play an increasing role in consultation to educators and to school systems. He has been asked to advise not only in broad matters of school-system orientation, but also in the handling of individually disturbed or retarded children. A typical present-day situation would involve a community which has decided to establish special classes for the retarded or the emotionally disturbed child. The school board and other administrative officials seek advice from professional personnel who have dealt with these youngsters in other settings. When the psychiatrist is called upon to lend assistance to the establishment of such a program, it is essential that he have not only some knowledge of the children in question, but also that he understand how a school system operates and how a teacher functions.

Certainly it should be obvious that the school can well serve as a location for the early detection of the emotionally disturbed child. This early detection should then lead to prompt, effective intervention by whatever mental health agency is available and appropriate. Much work has been done in recent years on this problem of early identification of the emotionally disturbed child. The entry into school is a big event in the life of the small child. He is often subjected at this point, for the first time in his life, to a relatively structured situation, out of his immediate home environment. It is possible through observation and testing to detect those children who are having more than their share of emotional difficulties and often possible to take remedial measures promptly. If such youngsters are allowed to continue without help through several grades of school, ultimate success in therapy then becomes much more difficult. The task of early recognition of emotional problems is one which falls naturally upon the educator, and psychiatry's most important contribution here lies in disseminating its knowledge to teachers and administrators.

These and many other aspects of the whole educational system are important areas for psychiatric participation. Here we would use the word psychiatrist in a very broad sense to include the participation of any well-trained physician who is capable of understanding the emotional problems of the child.

One of the problems which faces every psychiatrist or other physician who is called upon to serve in an advisory or consultant capacity to a community agency involves a definition of what his role is to be. To use the present example of schools, there are many tasks to which the psychiatrist might address himself. He could conceivably be a member of the school board, or a member of a scientific advisory board to the school itself. He might be a consultant to a special-education program, or serve on the staff of a school of education. All of these tasks have different requirements for the physician or psychiatrist. Because of the shortage of psychiatric personnel, the physician or psychiatrist is often called upon to see individual disturbed youngsters and to make simple practical suggestions. While this is a legitimate function, it is not that of a consultant practicing community psychiatry. The latter is primarily involved in helping those who administer and who teach to do a more adequate job. He attempts to influence the over-all philosophy of such administrators and teachers toward better mental health principles in an effort to remove old prejudices and outmoded practices which are deleterious to the mental health of growing children. At the same time, his is not the job of administering the school system, nor of revising the curriculum of the individual school.

The average teacher may have anywhere from thirty to forty children in her class. She has the responsibility for the education of these youngsters during the particular year they are in her class. If she serves under an oppressive board of education which allows little freedom, her work is apt to be performed poorly. If she herself is rigid and intolerant of normal childish exuberance, she will also perform poorly. The psychiatrist consultant can contribute in several ways. He may help to influence the board of education to adopt more modern views of education, including the newer concepts of mental health. He may hold inservice training programs for teachers. He may at times see individual youngsters and use the findings to help all the teachers in the group attain a better understanding of such children.

Most school systems in the United States, particularly in larger communities, now have some form of counseling service available to youngsters and their families. Such counselors may be psychologists or social workers, and may be called guidance counselors, visiting teachers, or some other term. Such individuals obviously exert considerable influence over the mental health of the youngsters in the schools in which they serve. Unfortunately they are usually in short supply and are overworked. Sometimes they have adequate backing from the school administration, while at other times they do not. Here again is an area in which a psychiatrist can be of considerable assistance. He may hold inservice training programs for such personnel, or consult in other ways which will enhance their own skills and morale.

Example

A psychiatrist who served as a consultant to a school system of a city of 100,000 became concerned about the number of children with school phobias and the length of time they were out of school. In talking with the teachers in one of his seminars, he found that they had become discouraged in their attempts to deal with these children. Parents were often refractory to the teacher's suggestions about bringing the child to school or seeking psychiatric help. Local physicians often wrote medical excuses for the children at the parents' request. The school administrative personnel gave the classroom teachers little backing in dealing with the parents. At the teachers' request, a joint meeting of the educators and the local county medical society was arranged and material on school phobias was presented by a panel. The panelists included a teacher, a physician, a school principal, and the psychiatrist. The various groups began to understand not only the cause and proper methods of handling this condition, but they also began to work more effectively together. The psychiatrist had served as a "catalyst" in this undertaking and had helped clarify the problem as well as having brought some of his knowledge of personality problems to the other professions.

THE LAW AND CORRECTIONAL INSTITUTIONS

Forensic psychiatry has existed since the very inception of psychiatry itself. The history of the law shows that men have long concerned themselves with certain people in society who show aberrant and criminal behavior. During the Middle Ages, most criminals were considered simply as bad. If the individual who committed the criminal act was obviously insane, he was conceived of as possessed by demons or devils. One of the cornerstones of legal psychiatry was the McNaughton Rule, originally formulated in England in 1843. McNaughton was a Scotsman who developed a paranoid delusion that the Tory party was persecuting him. In an attempt to strike back by killing the Prime Minister, he shot and killed the Prime Minister's Secretary. At the trial the defense presented medical testimony that the accused was insane, and the judge charged the jury that if they found the defendant was suffering from an insane delusion so that he did not know the difference between right and wrong, and if he did not know the consequences of his act, then they should find him not guilty by reason of insanity. McNaughton was sent to a mental hospital where he died in 1865. The trial caused considerable furor. From subsequent judicial discussions came the McNaughton Rule which states: ". . . to establish a defense on the ground of insanity, it must be clearly proved, that at the time of the committing of the act, the party accused was laboring under such a defect of reason from disease of the mind, as not to know the nature and quality of the act he was doing, or, if he did know it, that he did not know he was doing what was wrong."

This rule has had widespread application in England and in the United States. In 1954 Judge David Bazelon handed down the Durham Decision. In essence, this rule states, "An accused is not criminally responsible if his unlawful act is the product of mental disease or defect." Both lawyers and psychiatrists have argued pro and con for years regarding the usefulness of the McNaughton Rule and the Durham Decision. To further complicate matters, there is recognized in many legal jurisdictions the concept of the irresistible impulse. In essence, this refers to an individual with a mental disorder which enables him to know the nature and quality of the wrong which he is committing, but which irresistibly compels him to commit the act anyway.

Another important medico-legal area concerns the punishment of those who have been convicted of criminal acts. The moral concept of punishment has led at times to acts of extreme cruelty, while at other times, punishment has been accompanied by some efforts at rehabilitation of the criminal. In our own society today, the general tendency is to send criminals to prison for periods of time presumably appropriate to the seriousness of their crime. The concept is that such punitive measures will lead the criminal to reconsider the unacceptability of his acts and thus to reform his behavior. It is also assumed that such punishment of apprehended criminals will serve as a deterrent to others who might have the impulse to commit the same crime. Unfortunately, as is well known, this whole philosophy does not work out particularly well. Harsh and even sadistic punishment does not reform the criminal. The antisocial person who is incarcerated in an ill-kept, poorly run prison will only become more resentful of the society which put him there and will await his opportunity to further act out against it.

Both legal and correctional fields have begun to accept newer ideas, many of them derived from psychiatric knowledge, in regard to the determination of guilt and to appropriate measures of punishment as well as rehabilitation.

While it is impossible here to detail all of the intricacies of forensic psychiatry and correctional measures, a few of the more important aspects can be mentioned. First of all, it is essential that the physician or psychiatrist who plans to undertake medico-legal work should be acquainted with some of the fundamental principles of law; it is also essential to understand that the so-called expert physician witness comes to court to present his findings and not to usurp the role of the lawyer or the judge. He not infrequently has to

understand three separate "languages": his own psychiatric terminology, the language of the law, and finally the language of the
laymen who comprise the jury. The psychiatrist cannot speak as
a lawyer, nor can he always reduce his concepts to extremely simple,
nontechnical language. His is the difficult task of presenting in an
accurate, effective way his own findings in a manner which can be
understood by those on whom the decisions will eventually rest.
When and if he is asked questions to which he cannot give accurate answers, he must be honest in his replies. The question of
whether an individual is actually mentally ill or not may range from
the obvious to a fine question of interpretation. There are many
degrees of mental and emotional illness which can lead people into
antisocial behavior. It is the psychiatrist's primary task in the legal
area to interpret his findings to those who will make the decision.
It is not his final responsibility to make the judicial decision himself.

The role of the psychiatrist in the field of corrections is perhaps
somewhat more clear. There is a growing realization in enlightened
circles that excessive punitiveness by society against lawbreakers results neither in the rehabilitation of the individual criminal nor in
any real saving to society. A sizable percentage of the inmates of
penal institutions can be rehabilitated if proper measures are instituted, while unscientific and sadistic treatment of these individuals
only perpetuates their acting out. The psychiatrist has a real opportunity in furthering the more modern penal attitude. This is another
area, however, in which considerable judgment, tact, and understanding are required of the psychiatrist. He cannot move into a
correctional institution which has for years functioned in a rigid,
punitive manner and expect to change it immediately. His is a task
of becoming accepted as an important and respected member of the
institution and one whose judgment is to be trusted. To gain such
a position requires time and effort spent with all levels of personnel
from the warden down to the inmates. The psychiatrist may have
to begin with inservice training programs to develop a degree of
understanding of human personality and, perhaps even more important, to make the staff feel that they have a useful task to
perform.

There are many potential contributions the psychiatrist may make in the areas of law and corrections. He may teach as a member of the faculty of a law school. He may serve as a consultant to a prison, or develop training programs for law-enforcement officers. There are areas of community psychiatry where the psychiatrist is helping those directly involved with legal and correctional matters to understand better the functioning of the human personality both individually and in groups. It is unfortunate that many psychiatrists avoid courtroom appearances whenever possible because they fear they will be made to look ridiculous either by their own lack of legal knowledge or by the difficulty of presenting complex human thought processes in simplified, clear terms. They also avoid invitations to consult in penal institutions because they realize that the solutions to the practical and philosophical problems of penology are largely unknown to them. Only by a more active social psychiatric orientation will this branch of medicine eventually be able to make its proper contribution to these fields.

Example

A psychiatrist was asked to serve as a consultant to a juvenile court and soon found that meting out punishment to adolescent offenders was the main activity of the court. Little attention was being paid to the families of these youngsters, and almost no attempt was being made to utilize other community agencies which might be of help. The attitude of the court workers was a punitive one and they felt that these children were able to understand only discipline. The judge cooperated with the suggestion of the psychiatrist and arrangements were made to add a psychologist and a social worker to the court staff. Regular meetings of the entire staff were initiated and findings of the professional mental health team were presented and discussed. Such concepts as brain damage, mental retardation, psychosis, and family patterns were clarified. Court workers became interested in trying to understand their cases and seek out ways to help them. The recidivism rate diminished, and the morale of the court workers improved.

CHURCH

We know that people with emotional problems are most apt to turn first for advice to their clergymen, rather than to any other professional person. Clergymen of all faiths have themselves during recent years become increasingly aware of the usefulness of mental health principles in dealing with their congregations, and have turned in greater numbers to psychiatry for assistance with their training programs and with their day-to-day work. While religion and psychiatry have not always existed comfortably with each other in the past, there is ample evidence that the older prejudiced conflicts are diminishing. Psychiatry, after all, is a science and religion is a belief. There may be many areas of overlap between the two, but certainly there need not be conflict. As modern clergy and church workers have become increasingly acquainted with psychiatric principles, they have seen the need to add this type of knowledge to their own religious work.

One example might be found in the Sunday school. In altogether too many instances a Sunday school teacher has been chosen solely on the basis of her willingness to serve and her devotion to the church. While these two factors may be important, they do not always include the necessary ingredients of a good teacher. The early experiences of children in Sunday school set the ground work for their later views toward religion as do early experiences in other areas. A wholesome attitude results from a proper introduction to eating, sports, work or anything else. A distorted introduction leads to a distorted response, usually either the same or the opposite of the original. If the Sunday school teacher is chosen for her warmth and ability to deal with children as well as her knowledge of religion, she will exert a markedly positive influence upon youngsters. Conversely, if she is a rigid and unintuitive person, she may well impart either a negative attitude or a copy of her own distortions toward religion to the children with whom she comes in contact.

Psychiatrists are often being called upon to teach in schools of theology, and courses in pastoral counseling are appearing in the curricula of many such schools. These in no way diminish the spiritual content of theology, but rather add scientific knowledge about human development and personality function. Every student theologian whose own understanding of human beings is thus enriched will be capable of doing a far better job after his graduation.

In 1956 the National Institute of Mental Health underwrote some pilot programs in theological education, and material from behavioral sciences was introduced into the curricula of three divinity schools. Such a move illustrates the importance of improving the understanding by the student theologian of the development and function of the human personality.

Emotional disturbances often are focused on conflicts in religious belief, and it is important to the psychiatrist to have an adequate understanding of many religions, as well as to be able to impart his understandings and skills to the clergy.

Example

A psychiatrist was asked to serve as consultant to the ministers of a Protestant church in a moderately large city. One of the first duties he was given was assisting in the preparation of some evening courses the church wanted to offer to adults and teen-agers. He was initially warned by several of the ministers that although sexual education for adolescents was a much discussed idea and was being carried on in some church groups, their particular denomination would not tolerate anything but a much attenuated version. He was told that the parents would be upset if frankly sexual material was presented to the teen-agers, and that even the parents themselves would rebel against the minister and whoever taught such courses.

The psychiatrist met several times with the ministerial group and attempted to convey to them the reasonable, and yet accurate way in which this material could be presented to the young people. He also met with the leaders of the adolescent group and they discussed their own ideas about what their group wished to learn. He showed several films dealing with the topic to leaders of the parent and adolescent groups and invited their discussion and suggestions. The entire response was favorable, and the course material was presented in a series of evening meetings. It was not only given to the adolescents, but similar presentations were made to the adult classes which were geared to their own requests.

The psychiatrist had served as a "community psychiatrist" by bringing an increased understanding of certain psychiatric concepts to a larger group and had succeeded in improving the group's attitude toward an important topic. He found other assignments equally challenging and continued to bring modern psychiatric knowledge to bear in areas where it would benefit many people.

RESEARCH

The psychiatrist today has at his command a large amount of knowledge concerning the function of the human mind, the growth and development of the personality and the various diseases and illnesses which may beset it. He has included in his armamentarium a variety of procedures ranging from intensive psychoanalysis to supportive treatment and from hospitalization to tranquilization. Today's psychiatrist compared to his counterpart of one hundred years ago is remarkably knowledgeable and effective.

Even now, however, we are not really winning the battle for mental health in the sense of producing a noticeable diminution in the extent of emotional and mental disorders. While it is true that certain conditions are seen less frequently because specific treatments have been found for them, others are becoming more numerous. For example, classical cases of general paresis are disappearing from the scene as it was years ago, while at the same time, the state hospitals are struggling with a steadily increasing number of elderly patients with senile psychoses. The changing social picture and developing recognition are factors in the increased number of individuals who become patients. Medicine has been successful in controlling, in some instances almost eradicating, many diseases such as typhoid, malaria, and poliomyelitis. Why then are we not similarly successful in the whole area of emotional and mental illness?

There are probably two major reasons for this: (1) the modern knowledge which we already possess is by no means being put to its maximum use by society, and (2) there is much that we do not yet know and which remains to be discovered if we are to be successful. The many glaring problems which currently face us are ample evidence that the battle is far from over. The existence of a high divorce rate, the hundreds of thousands of new cases of schizophrenia each year, the prevalence of alcoholism and the widespread incidence of psychosomatic disorders are only a few examples.

Research in psychiatry, as in general medicine, has pursued many different avenues, of which some have proved fruitful and others, initially promising, have yielded little of lasting value. One of the main tools of research in psychiatry which has continued to withstand the pressures of time and which still is adding to our knowledge of the human personality is psychoanalysis. Freud's writings, in themselves quite extensive, have been used as foundations on which further concepts have continued to develop. Journals of psychoanalysis, national and international, continue to present new findings in depth psychology. Psychoanalytic concepts are used in the work of sociologists, anthropologists, social workers, and psychologists, especially.

The growth of new knowledge concerning the physiology of the central nervous system has also been remarkable. Neuro-anatomy and neurophysiology have contributed to our increased understanding of the function of the nervous system. Some of the most recent advances involving the structure of the cell, its protein arrangement and metabolism, will certainly lead eventually to the development of more effective treatment for many conditions. The discovery of the spirochete of syphilis and the meningococcus were epochal events in the history of psychiatry and medicine, but they may well be eclipsed by advances which will develop from our current research. Psychiatry is in a position of great challenge. As *Action for Mental Health* states, "What is needed in mental health research is a balanced portfolio." This will include increased attention to basic research, long-term research as well as short-term projects, and a willingness to tackle new ideas and new departures in addition to the pursuit of older routes which have only been partially explored.

The most obvious enigma in the field of mental illness is the complex which we call schizophrenia. We do not really know what causes this disorder or group of disorders. It would appear that certain environmental factors, particularly early in life, are strong contributing agents. Nevertheless, we know also that many children live through similar situations without developing schizophrenia. We know that the paranoid schizophrenic is quite different from the simple schizophrenic or the catatonic. We know that many schizophrenics show marked regression, but we are not always certain why this takes place. The work of Spitz[2] and others has shown

<hr>

[2] Spitz, René. "Hospitalization, An Inquiry into the Genesis of Psychiatric Conditions in Early Childhood," in *The Psychoanalytic Study of the Child*, Vol. I. New York. International Universities Press, 1945.

the importance of early maternal deprivation on faulty ego growth, but such deprivation does not inevitably lead to schizophrenia. We know that the administration of certain drugs such as lysergic acid produce temporary symptomatology quite similar to that of the schizophrenic, but the specific physiological actions of these drugs remains unclear. Our knowledge of the genetic factors in other diseases is increasing, and at times signs would seem to point toward the genetic origin of schizophrenia. However, one can also postulate that a schizophrenic mother would be more apt to produce a schizophrenic child by virtue of her own inability to provide adequate mothering. We do not know why schizophrenic rates in a given population remain relatively constant, apparently uninfluenced by powerful social factors such as war, famine, depression, or repressive types of government. We know that such factors markedly influence the incidence of depression or neuroses, and are led to ask why they do not similarly influence the rate of schizophrenia.

In terms of treating the schizophrenic, a variety of approaches have been found partially successful. A few years ago electric shock and insulin shock treatment were widely used, less so since the advent of tranquilizers. The latter, however, really do not cure schizophrenia, but only dampen or mask certain of the gross symptoms. Many interesting research projects are currently underway in both childhood and adult schizophrenia and should provide us with valuable new information. However, it is doubtful that there will be a "breakthrough" in this syndrome as there was in poliomyelitis since it is quite probable that more than one factor will eventually prove crucial in the etiology.

Mental retardation is another area in which considerable research has already been done and in which valuable discoveries have been made. It remains, however, a continuing problem in our society and one to which we have only partial answers. Here again we have the situation of knowing certain things which could be better applied and not knowing others to which we are seeking answers. We know now much more about the various metabolic disorders and are learning about some of the complexities of the genetic problems in mental retardation. However, the mildly retarded, who form the greatest single portion of this group, are by no means dealt with adequately. We have considerable knowledge of the various social and emotional factors which are important in producing mild mental retardation, but this knowledge is only infrequently applied in society. The lower socio-economic group, for instance, produces a proportionately greater number of cases of mild mental retardation. The most important etiological factors in this group are those of emotional deprivation, social disorganization, and a lack of adequate medical care. While we recognize these causative factors, we do not seem able to find ways and means of correcting them. We know that many of these children are unplanned and unwanted, but progress in family planning has been least effective in the levels which most need it. As with schizophrenia, the questions are twofold. First, how do we apply knowledge we already have in a better fashion, and second, how do we seek further knowledge through basic research?

New developments in research are being made by a number of mental health research institutes, many of which are attached to university medical centers. Basic research, as contrasted to clinical research, has always had to struggle for its share of support, since those responsible for the allocation of money to mental health research have often preferred to support those programs which seem to promise quick clinical results. Perhaps we should learn from our experience in nuclear physics, where basic research concerning the nature of matter was instrumental in the eventual development of our current and practical knowledge. The same holds true for basic research in psychiatry. These programs may seem to offer little of practical value, yet it is through this type of investigation that some of our important new knowledge will be gained. The mental health research institute associated with a university center has available to it the combined talents of many individuals from a variety of disciplines. Close liaison between such people, while at times dealing with highly theoretical considerations, may eventually lead to a marked increase in our knowledge about mental health and mental illness.

Some idea of the extent to which the Federal government promotes research in this area is to be found in a publication of the U.S. Department of Health Education and Welfare entitled *A Sum-*

mary of the Research Grant Programs of the National Institute of Mental Health 1948–1961. The report notes that "The total number of grants awarded in the fiscal year 1961 was over 30 times the number awarded in 1948; during the same period the amount awarded increased over 80 times." From a very modest beginning the growth of the National Institute of Mental Health has been remarkable. In 1961, 1,286 grants were made totaling $30,492,081.00. There is every indication that the expansion of NIMH will continue and also that state governments will increase their support of mental health research.

Bibliography

History of Psychiatry

Adler, Alfred. *The Practice and Theory of Individual Psychology.* New York. Harcourt, Brace & Co., 1929.

Beers, Clifford. *A Mind That Found Itself.* New York. Doubleday, Doran and Co., Rev. ed., 1948.

Brill, A. A. *Freud's Contribution to Psychiatry.* New York. W. W. Norton & Company, 1944.

Freud, Sigmund. *The Standard Edition of the Complete Psychological Works of Sigmund Freud.* 24 vols. New York. The Macmillan Co., 1953– .

Hall, J. K., et al. *One Hundred Years of American Psychiatry.* New York. Columbia University Press, 1944.

Jones, Ernest. *The Life and Work of Sigmund Freud,* Vols. I, II, and III. New York. Basic Books, 1955.

Jung, C. G. *Contributions to Analytical Psychology.* New York. Harcourt, Brace & Co., 1928.

Jung, C. G. *Psychological Types.* New York. Pantheon Books, 1959.

Meyer, Adolf. "The Psychobiological Point of View," in *The Problem of Mental Disorder,* by N. Bentley and E. Cowdry. New York. McGraw-Hill Book Co., 1934.

Zilboorg, Gregory, and G. W. Henry. *A History of Medical Psychology.* New York. W. W. Norton & Company, 1941.

Personality Development and Structure

Abraham, Karl. *Selected Papers on Psychoanalysis.* Vols. I and II. Basic Books, 1953 and 1955.

American Psychiatric Association. *Diagnostic and Statistical Manual of Mental Disorders.* Washington. American Psychiatric Association, 1952.

Bowlby, J. *Maternal Care and Mental Health.* WHO Mimeograph Series No. 2. Geneva, 1952.

Deutsch, Helene. *The Psychology of Women,* Vols. I and II. New York. Grune and Stratton, 1945.

Draper, G., C. W. Dupertais, and J. L. Caughey. *Human Constitution in Clinical Medicine.* New York. Paul B. Hoeber, Inc., 1944.

English, O. S., and Gerald H. J. Pearson. *Common Neuroses of Children and Adults.* New York. W. W. Norton & Company, 1937.

English, O. S., and Gerald H. J. Pearson. *Emotional Problems of Living.* Third Ed. New York. W. W. Norton & Company, 1963.

Frank, L. K., et al. *Personality Development in Adolescent Girls.* Child Development Publications, Vol. XVI, No. 53, 1951.

French, T. M. *The Integration of Behavior,* Vol. I. Chicago. University of Chicago Press, 1952.

Freud, Anna. *The Ego and the Mechanisms of Defense.* New York. International Universities Press, 1957.

Freud, Sigmund. "On Narcissism," in *Collected Papers,* Ed. by Ernest Jones, 5 vols. New York. Basic Books, 1959.

Freud, Sigmund. *The Problem of Anxiety.* New York. W. W. Norton & Company, 1936.

Freud, Sigmund. *The Psychopathology of Everyday Life,* in *The Standard Edition of the Complete Psychological Works of Sigmund Freud.* 24 vols. New York. The Macmillan Co., 1953– .

Freud, Sigmund. *Three Contributions to the Theory of Sex.* New York. In *The Standard Edition* . . . op. cit.

Kallmann, F. J. *Heredity in Health and Mental Disorder.* New York. W. W. Norton & Company, 1953.

Menninger, Karl. "Outline for Organizing and Recording Data." *American Journal of Psychiatry,* February, 1952 (published in separate form by Grune and Stratton, Inc.).

Outline for the Study of the Mental Patient. Philadelphia. Temple University Medical School, Department of Psychiatry.

Ribble, Margaret. *The Rights of Infants*. New York. Columbia University Press, 1943.

Saul, Leon J. *Bases of Human Behavior*. Philadelphia. J. B. Lippincott Co., 1951.

Saul, Leon J. *Emotional Maturity,* Second Ed. Philadelphia. J. B. Lippincott Co., 1960.

Senn, M. J. E. *Symposium on the Healthy Personality*. New York. Josiah Macy Foundation, 1950.

Child Psychiatry

Aichhorn, August. *Wayward Youth*. New York. Viking Press, 1935.

Allen, F. H. *Psychotherapy With Children*. New York. W. W. Norton & Company, 1942.

Alt, Herschel. *Residential Treatment for the Disturbed Child*. New York. International Universities Press, 1960.

Bender, Lauretta. *Child Psychiatric Techniques*. Springfield, Illinois. Charles C. Thomas, 1952.

Berlin, I. N. *Bibliography of Child Psychiatry*. Washington, D.C. American Psychiatric Association. 1963.

Chess, Stella. *An Introduction to Child Psychiatry*. New York. Grune & Stratton, 1959.

Eissler, Ruth, Anna Freud, Heinz Hartmann, and Ernst Kris, editors. *The Psychoanalytic Study of the Child,* Vols. I–XVII. New York. International Universities Press, 1945–1962.

Erikson, Erik. *Childhood and Society,* Rev. Ed. New York. W. W. Norton & Company, 1963.

Finch, Stuart M. "Psychosomatic Problems in Children." *The Nervous Child,* Vol. IX, No. 3, 1952.

Finch, Stuart M. *Fundamentals of Child Psychiatry*. New York. W. W. Norton & Company, 1960.

Freud, Anna. *Introduction to the Technique of Child Analysis*. Washington. Nervous and Mental Disease Monographs, 1928.

Freud, Anna, and Dorothy T. Burlingham. *Infants Without Families*. New York. International Universities Press, 1944.

Gerard, Margaret. "Enuresis, A Study in Etiology." *American Journal of Orthopsychiatry,* January, 1939.

Gesell, Arnold. *The First Five Years of Life.* New York. Harper and Brothers, 1940.

Gesell, Arnold, and Frances Ilg. *The Child from Five to Ten.* New York. Harper and Brothers, 1946.

Hamilton, Gordon. *Psychotherapy in Child Guidance.* New York. Columbia University Press, 1947.

Kanner, Leo. *Child Psychiatry.* Third Ed. Springfield, Illinois. Charles C. Thomas, 1960.

Kanner, Leo. "Problems of Nosology and Psychodynamics of Early Infantile Autism." *American Journal of Orthopsychiatry,* July, 1949.

Klein, Melanie. *The Psychoanalysis of Children.* New York. Grove Press, 1960.

Lewis, Nolan D. C., and B. L. Pacella, editors. *Modern Trends in Child Psychiatry.* New York. International Universities Press, 1945.

Lippman, Hyman S. *Treatment of the Child in Emotional Conflict.* New York. Blakiston Div., McGraw-Hill Book Co., Inc., 1956.

Mahler, Margaret. "On Child Psychosis and Schizophrenia," in *The Psychoanalytic Study of the Child,* Vol. VII. New York. International Universities Press, 1952.

Pearson, Gerald H. J. *Emotional Disorders of Children.* New York. W. W. Norton & Company, 1949.

Pearson, Gerald H. J. *Psychoanalysis and the Education of the Child.* New York. W. W. Norton & Company, 1954.

Ribble, Margaret. *The Rights of Infants.* New York. Columbia University Press, 1943.

Shirley, H. F. *Psychiatry for the Pediatrician.* New York. The Commonwealth Fund, 1948.

Witmer, H. L., editor. *Psychiatric Interviews with Children.* New York. The Commonwealth Fund, 1946.

Psychoneurotic Disorders

Alvarez, W. C. *The Neuroses*. Philadelphia. W. B. Saunders Co., 1951.

Deutsch, Helene. *Psychoanalysis of the Neuroses*. London. Hogarth Press and the Institute of Psychoanalysis, 1933.

English, O. S., and Gerald H. J. Pearson. *Common Neuroses in Children and Adults*. New York. W. W. Norton & Company, 1937.

Fenichel, Otto. *The Psychoanalytic Theory of Neurosis*. New York. W. W. Norton & Company, 1945.

Freud, Sigmund. "Analysis of a Case of Hysteria," in *Collected Papers*, Ed. by Ernest Jones, 5 vols., New York. Basic Books, 1959.

Freud, Sigmund. "From the History of an Infantile Neurosis," in *Collected Papers*, Ed. by Ernest Jones, 5 vols., New York. Basic Books, 1959.

Freud, Sigmund. "Notes Upon a Case of Obsessional Neurosis," in *Collected Papers*, Ed. by Ernest Jones, 5 vols., New York. Basic Books, 1959.

Prince, Morton. *The Dissociation of a Personality*. London. Longmans, Green and Co., 1925.

Sakel, M. *The Pharmacological Shock Treatment of Schizophrenia*. New York. Nervous & Mental Diseases Publ. Co., 1938.

Whitaker, Carl A., and Thomas P. Malone. *The Roots of Psychotherapy*. New York. Blakiston, 1953.

Forensic Psychiatry

Alexander, Franz, and William Healy. *Roots of Crime*. New York. Alfred A. Knopf, 1935.

Alexander, Franz, and Hugo Staub. *The Criminal, the Judge and the Public*, Rev. Ed. New York, Free Press, 1957.

Cleckley, H. M. *The Mask of Sanity*. Third Ed. St. Louis. C. V. Mosby Co., 1955.

Glueck, S., and E. Glueck. *Five Hundred Criminal Careers*. New York. Alfred A. Knopf, 1930.

Glueck, S., and E. Glueck. *Unraveling Juvenile Delinquency*. Cambridge, Mass. Harvard University Press, 1950.

Group for the Advancement of Psychiatry. *Confidentiality and Privileged Communication in the Practice of Psychiatry.* Report No. 45. New York. 1960.

Guttmacher, M. S. *Sex Offenses: The Problem, Causes and Prevention.* New York. W. W. Norton & Company, 1951.

Guttmacher, M. S., and H. Weihofen. *Psychiatry and the Law.* New York. W. W. Norton & Company, 1952.

Healy, William. *The Individual Delinquent.* Boston. Little, Brown and Co., 1927.

Kinsey, Alfred, et al. *Sexual Behavior in the Human Female.* Philadelphia. W. B. Saunders Co., 1953.

Kinsey, Alfred, et al. *Sexual Behavior in the Human Male.* Philadelphia. W. B. Saunders Co., 1948.

Overholser, Winfred. *The Psychiatrist and the Law.* New York. Harcourt, Brace & Co., 1953.

Roche, Philip Q. "Sexual Deviations." *Federal Probation,* September, 1950.

Roche, Philip Q. *The Criminal Mind.* New York. Farrar, Straus & Cudahy, 1958.

Watson, Andrew S. "Family Law and Its Challenge for Psychiatry." *Journal of Family Law* 2:71–84, 1962.

Weihofen, Henry. *The Urge to Punish.* New York. Farrar, Straus & Cudahy, 1956.

Williams, Glanville. *The Sanctity of Life and the Criminal Law.* New York. Alfred A. Knopf, 1957.

Zilboorg, Gregory. *The Psychology of the Criminal Act and Punishment.* New York. Harcourt, Brace and Co., 1954.

Personality Disorders

Aichhorn, August. *Wayward Youth.* New York. Viking Press, 1935.

Alexander, Franz. "The Neurotic Character." *International Journal of Psychoanalysis,* July, 1930.

Alexander, Franz, and William Healy. *Roots of Crime.* New York. Alfred A. Knopf, 1935.

Cleckley, H. M. *The Mask of Sanity.* St. Louis. C. V. Mosby Co., 1941.

Flugel, J. C. *Man, Morals and Society*. New York. International Universities Press, 1946.

Friedlander, Kate. *The Psychoanalytic Approach to Juvenile Delinquency*. New York. International Universities Press, 1947.

Group for the Advancement of Psychiatry. *Psychiatrically Deviated Sex Offenders*. Report No. 9. Topeka, 1949.

Guttmacher, M. S. *Sex Offenses: The Problem, Causes and Prevention*. New York. W. W. Norton & Company, 1951.

Guttmacher, M. S., and Henry Weihofen. *Psychiatry and the Law*. New York, W. W. Norton & Company, 1952.

Kinsey, Alfred, et al. *Sexual Behavior in the Human Female*. Philadelphia. W. B. Saunders Co., 1953.

Kinsey, Alfred, et al. *Sexual Behavior in the Human Male*. Philadelphia. W. B. Saunders Co., 1948.

Reich, Wilhelm. *Character Analysis*. New York. Orgone Press, 1949.

Roche, Philip Q. "Sexual Deviations." *Federal Probation,* September, 1950.

Saul, Leon J. *Emotional Maturity*. Philadelphia. J. B. Lippincott Co., 1947.

Psychophysiologic Disorders

Alexander, Franz. *Psychosomatic Medicine*. New York. W. W. Norton & Company, 1950.

Alexander, Franz, Thomas French, et al. *Studies in Psychosomatic Medicine*. New York. Ronald Press, 1948.

Derner, G. F. *Aspects of the Psychology of Tuberculosis*. New York. Paul B. Hoeber, Inc., 1953.

Deutsch, Felix, editor. *The Psychosomatic Concept in Psychoanalysis*. New York. International Universities Press, 1953.

Dunbar, Flanders. *Psychosomatic Diagnosis*. New York. Paul B. Hoeber, Inc., 1948.

Grinker, Roy R. *Psychosomatic Research*. New York. W. W. Norton & Company, 1953.

Grinker, Roy R., and J. P. Spiegel. *Men Under Stress*. Philadelphia. Blakiston Co., 1945.

Halliday, J. I. *Psychosocial Medicine.* New York. W. W. Norton & Company, 1948.

Hinsie, Leland. *The Person in the Body.* New York. W. W. Norton & Company, 1945.

Saul, Leon J. *Bases of Human Behavior.* Philadelphia. J. B. Lippincott Co., 1951.

Weiss, Edward. *Emotional Factors in Cardiovascular Disease.* Springfield, Illinois. Charles C. Thomas, 1951.

Weiss, Edward, and O. S. English. *Psychosomatic Medicine,* Third Ed. Philadelphia. W. B. Saunders Co., 1957.

Witthower, E., and Russell B. *Emotional Factors in Skin Disease.* New York. Paul B. Hoeber, Inc., 1953.

Wolf, Stewart, and Harold G. Wolff. *Headaches.* Boston. Little, Brown and Co., 1953.

Wolff, Harold G. *Headache and Other Head Pain.* New York. Oxford University Press, 1948.

Wolff, Harold G., et al. *Stress and Disease.* Springfield, Illinois. Charles C. Thomas, 1953.

Functional Psychotic Disorders

Abraham, Karl. *Selected Papers on Psychoanalysis.* 2 vols. Basic Books, 1953 and 1955.

Bleuler, Eugen. *Textbook of Psychiatry.* Translated by A. A. Brill. New York. The Macmillan ·Co., 1924 (Dover Publications reissue, 1951).

Bradley, Charles. *Schizophrenia in Childhood.* New York. The Macmillan Co., 1941.

Despert, J. Louise. "Some Considerations Relating to the Genesis of Autistic Behavior in Children." *American Journal of Orthopsychiatry,* April, 1951.

Freud, Sigmund. "A Case of Paranoia," in *Collected Papers,* Vol. III. London. Hogarth Press and the Institute of Psychoanalysis, 1949.

Freud, Sigmund. "Mourning and Melancholia," in *Collected Papers,* Ed. by Ernest Jones, 5 vols. New York. Basic Books, 1959.

Fromm-Reichmann, Frieda. *Principles of Intensive Psychotherapy.* Chicago. University of Chicago Press, 1950.

Greenacre, Phyllis, editor. *Affective Disorders.* New York. International Universities Press, 1953.

Hinsie, L. E. "Schizophrenias," in *Psychoanalysis Today.* Edited by Sandor Lorand. New York. International Universities Press, 1944.

Hoskins, Roy G. *The Biology of Schizophrenia.* New York. W. W. Norton & Company, 1946.

Kallmann, F. J. *Heredity in Health and Mental Disorder.* New York. W. W. Norton & Company, 1953.

Kanner, Leo. "Autistic Disturbances of Affective Contact." *The Nervous Child,* April, 1943.

Kanner, Leo. "Early Infantile Autism." *Journal of Pediatrics,* September, 1944.

Kasanin, J. *Language and Thought in Schizophrenia.* Berkeley. University of California Press, 1944.

Lewin, Bertram. *The Psychoanalysis of Elation.* New York. W. W. Norton & Company, 1950.

Lewis, N. D. C. *Research in Dementia Praecox.* National Committee for Mental Hygiene. Copyright, 1936, by the Supreme Council of the Thirty-third Degree Scottish Rite Masons of the Northern Jurisdiction, U.S.A.

Mahler, Margaret. "Clinical Studies in Benign and Malignant Cases of Childhood Psychosis (Schizophrenia-Like)." *American Journal of Orthopsychiatry,* April, 1949.

Rosen, John N. "The Treatment of Schizophrenic Psychosis by Direct Analytic Therapy." *Psychiatric Quarterly,* January, 1947.

Schilder, Paul. "Neuroses and Psychoses," in *Psychoanalysis Today.* Edited by Sandor Lorand. New York. International Universities Press, 1944.

Waelder, Robert. "The Structure of Paranoid Ideas, A Critical Survey of Various Theories." *International Journal of Psychoanalysis,* Vol. XXXII, Part 3, 1951.

Zilboorg, Gregory. "Manic Depressive Psychoses," in *Psychoanalysis Today.* Edited by Sandor Lorand. New York. International Universities Press, 1944.

Organic Brain Disorders

Alexander, Leo. *Treatment of Mental Disorders*. Philadelphia. W. B. Saunders Co., 1953.

Allen, E. B., and C. T. Prout. "Alcoholism," in *Progress in Neurology and Psychiatry*, Vol. VIII. New York. Grune and Stratton, 1953.

Bender, Lauretta. "Organic Brain Conditions Producing Behavior Disturbances," in *Modern Trends in Child Psychiatry*. Edited by N. D. C. Lewis and B. L. Pacella. New York. International Universities Press, 1945.

Cattell, James. "The Dynamics of Post-Topectomy Psychotherapy in Patients with Pseudoneurotic Schizophrenia." *American Journal of Psychiatry*, December, 1952.

Child, G. P., et al. "Therapeutic Results and Clinical Manifestations Following the Use of Tetraethylthiuram Disulfide (Antabuse)." *American Journal of Psychiatry*, April, 1951.

Dattner, Bernhard. *Penicillin in Neurosyphilis*. New York. Grune and Stratton, 1949.

Frank, J. "Clinical Survey and Results of 200 Cases of Prefrontal Leucotomy." *Journal of Mental Science*, July, 1946.

Himwich, H. E. *Brain Metabolism and Cerebral Disorders*. Baltimore. Williams and Wilkins, 1951.

Hoch, P. H., and R. P. Knight. *Epilepsy; Psychiatric Aspects of Convulsive Disorders*. New York. Grune and Stratton, 1947.

Kaplan, O. J. *Mental Diseases in Later Life*. Second Ed. Stanford. Stanford University Press, 1956.

Lennox, W. J. *Science and Seizures*. New York. Harper and Brothers, 1941.

Lennox, W. J. and Charles Markham. "The Sociopsychological Treatment of Epilepsy." *Journal of the American Medical Association*, August, 1953.

Lindemann, E., and L. D. Clarke. "Modifications in Ego Structure and Personality Reactions under the Influence of the Effects of Drugs." *American Journal of Psychiatry*, February, 1952.

Linden, Maurice E., and Douglas Courtney. "The Human Life Cycle and Its Interruption." *American Journal of Psychiatry*, June, 1953.

Menninger, William. *Juvenile Paresis*. Baltimore. Williams and Wilkins, 1936.

Putnam, T. J. *Convulsive Seizures*. Second Ed. Philadelphia, J. B. Lippincott Co., 1945.

Stieglitz, E. J. *Geriatric Medicine*. Philadelphia. W. B. Saunders Co., 1949.

Strecker, Edward, and F. T. Chambers. *Alcohol: One Man's Meat*. New York. The Macmillan Co., 1938.

William, W. "The Society of Alcoholics Anonymous." *American Journal of Psychiatry,* November, 1949.

Psychology and Mental Retardation

Benda, C. E. *Developmental Disorders of Mentation and Cerebral Palsies*. New York. Grune and Stratton, 1952.

Bender, Lauretta. *The Visual Motor Gestalt Test and Its Clinical Use*. New York. American Orthopsychiatric Association, 1938.

Bowman, Peter, and Hans Mautner, Eds. *Mental Retardation*. New York, Grune and Stratton, 1960.

Cattell, Psyche. *The Measurement of Intelligence of Infants and Young Children*. New York. Psychological Corporation, 1940.

Gesell, Arnold. *The First Five Years of Life*. New York. Harper and Brothers, 1940.

Gesell, Arnold, and Frances Ilg. *The Child from Five to Ten*. New York. Harper and Brothers, 1946.

Kanner, Leo. *A Miniature Textbook of Feeblemindedness*. New York. Child Care Publications, 1949.

Klopfer, B., and D. Kelley. *The Rorschach Technique*. New York. World Book Co., 1942.

Masland, R. L., S. B. Sarason, and T. Gladwin. *Mental Subnormality*. New York. Basic Books, 1958.

Merrill, Maud, and Lewis Terman. *Measuring Intelligence*. Boston. Houghton Mifflin Co., 1937.

President's Panel on Mental Retardation. *A Proposed Program for National Action to Combat Mental Retardation*. Washington, D.C. U.S. Government Printing Office. October 1962.

Rapaport, David, M. Gill, and R. Schafer. *Diagnostic Psychological Testing: The Theory, Statistical Evaluations, and Diagnostic Application of a Battery of Tests,* Vols. I and II. Chicago. Yearbook Publishers, Inc., 1946.

Rorschach, Hermann. *Psychodiagnostics.* Fifth Ed. New York. Grune and Stratton, 1951.

Tomkins, Silvan. *Thematic Apperception Test; Theory and Technique of Interpretation.* New York. Grune and Stratton, 1947.

Tredgold, A. F., and Kenneth Soddy. *A Textbook of Mental Deficiency (Amentia).* Tenth Ed. Baltimore. Williams and Wilkins (in preparation).

Wechsler, David. *Measurement and Appraisal of Adult Intelligence.* Fourth Ed. Baltimore. Williams and Wilkins, 1958.

Textbooks of Neurology

Brock, Samuel. *The Basis of Clinical Neurology.* Fourth Ed. Baltimore. William Wood and Co. (in preparation).

Buchanan, A. R. *Functional Neuroanatomy.* Fourth Ed. Philadelphia. Lea and Febiger, 1961.

Fulton, John. *Physiology of the Nervous System.* London. Third Ed. Oxford Medical Publications, 1949.

Grinker, Roy R., and Paul C. Bucy. *Neurology.* Fifth Ed. Springfield, Illinois. Charles C. Thomas, 1960.

Jelliffe, S. E., and W. A. White. *Diseases of the Nervous System.* Philadelphia. Lea and Febiger, 1935.

Nielsen, J. M. *A Textbook of Clinical Neurology.* New York. Paul B. Hoeber, Inc., 1941.

Wechsler, I. W. *A Textbook of Clinical Neurology.* Fifth Ed. Philadelphia. W .B. Saunders Co., 1943.

Wilson, S. A. *Neurology.* 2 vols. Baltimore. Williams and Wilkins, 1940.

Psychoanalysis

Abraham, Karl. *Selected Papers on Psychoanalysis.* Vols. I and II. Basic Books, 1953 and 1955.

Alexander, Franz. *Fundamentals of Psychoanalysis.* New York. W. W. Norton & Company, 1948.

Alexander, Franz. *Psychoanalysis of the Total Personality.* New York. Nervous and Mental Disease Publishing Co., 1930.

Fenichel, Otto. *Outline of Clinical Psychoanalysis.* New York. W. W. Norton & Company, 1934.

Ferenczi, Sandor. *Further Contributions to the Theory and Technique of Psychoanalysis.* London. Hogarth Press, 1950.

Freud, Anna. *The Ego and the Mechanisms of Defense.* New York. International Universities Press, 1946.

Freud, Sigmund. *The Standard Edition of the Complete Psychological Works of Sigmund Freud.* 24 vols. New York. The Macmillan Co.

Freud, Sigmund. *Beyond the Pleasure Principle.* New York. Liveright, 1950.

Freud, Sigmund. *Collected Papers.* 5 vols. Ed. by Ernest Jones. New York. Basic Books, 1959.

Freud, Sigmund. *The Ego and the Id.* New York. W. W. Norton & Company, 1961.

Freud, Sigmund. *A General Introduction to Psychoanalysis.* New York. Liveright, 1935.

Freud, Sigmund. *Group Psychology and the Analysis of the Ego.* London. Hogarth Press and the Institute of Psychoanalysis, 1950.

Freud, Sigmund. *New Introductory Lectures on Psychoanalysis.* New York. W. W. Norton & Company, 1933.

Freud, Sigmund. *An Outline of Psychoanalysis.* New York. W. W. Norton & Company, 1949.

Freud, Sigmund. *The Problem of Anxiety.* New York. W. W. Norton & Company, 1936.

Hendricks, Ives. *Facts and Theories of Psychoanalysis.* Third Rev. Ed. New York. Alfred A. Knopf, 1958.

Jones, Ernest. *Papers on Psychoanalysis.* Boston. Beacon Press, 1961.

Jones, Ernest. *Psychoanalysis of the Total Personality.* New York. Nervous and Mental Disease Publishing Co., 1930.

Kubie, Lawrence. *Practical Aspects of Psychoanalysis.* New York. Alfred A. Knopf, 1936.

Lorand, Sandor, editor. *Psychoanalysis Today.* New York. International Universities Press, 1944.

Menninger, Karl. *Theory of Psychoanalytic Technique.* New York. Basic Books. 1958.

Textbooks of Psychiatry

Arieti, Silvano, editor. *American Handbook of Psychiatry,* Vols. I and II. New York. Basic Books Inc. 1959.

Bleuler, Eugen. *Textbook of Psychiatry.* Translated by A. A. Brill. New York. The Macmillan Co., 1924 (Dover Publications reissue, 1951).

Engel, George. *Psychological Development in Health and Disease.* Philadelphia. W. B. Saunders, 1962.

Ewalt, Jack R., and Dana L. Farnsworth. *Textbook of Psychiatry.* New York. Blakiston Div. of McGraw-Hill Book Co., 1963.

Henderson, David, and R. D. Gillespie. *A Textbook of Psychiatry.* Ninth Ed. New York. Oxford University Press, 1962.

Hinsie, Leland, and Jacob Shatzky. *Psychiatric Dictionary.* New York. Oxford University Press, 1940.

Masserman, Jules. *Principles of Dynamic Psychiatry.* Second Ed. Philadelphia. W. B. Saunders Co., 1961.

Menninger, Karl. *The Human Mind.* New York. Alfred A. Knopf, 1947.

Noyes, Arthur. *Modern Clinical Psychiatry.* Fourth Ed. Philadelphia. W. B. Saunders Co., 1963.

Therapy

Ackerman, Nathan W. *The Psychodynamics of Family Life.* New York. Basic Books, 1958.

Alexander, Franz. *Fundamentals of Psychoanalysis.* New York. W. W. Norton & Company, 1948.

Alexander, Franz, and Thomas French. *Psychoanalytic Therapy.* New York. Ronald Press, 1946.

Alexander, Franz, and Helen Ross. *Dynamic Psychiatry*. Chicago. University of Chicago Press, 1952.

Alexander, Leo. *Treatment of Mental Disorders*. Philadelphia. W. B. Saunders Co., 1953.

Bell, J. E. "Recent Advances in Family Group Therapy." *Journal of Child Psychology and Psychiatry*, 3:1–15, 1962.

Boszormenyi-Nagy, I. "The Concept of Schizophrenia from the Perspective of Family Treatment." *Family Process*, 1:304–318, 1962.

Brenman, Margaret, and Merton Gill. *Hypnotherapy*. New York. Josiah Macy Foundation, 1944.

Brenman, Margaret, and Merton Gill. *Hypnotherapy, A Survey of the Literature*. New York. International Universities Press, 1947.

Bychowski, Gustav. *Psychotherapy of the Psychoses*. New York. Grune and Stratton, 1952.

Deutsch, Helene. *Psychoanalysis of the Neuroses*. London. Hogarth Press, 1951.

Diethelm, Oscar. *Treatment in Psychiatry*. Second Ed. Springfield, Illinois. Charles C. Thomas, 1950.

Frank, Jerome D. *Persuasion and Healing*. Baltimore. Johns Hopkins Press, 1961.

Freud, Sigmund. "The Dynamics of the Transference," in *Collected Papers*. Vol. II. London. Hogarth Press and the Institute of Psychoanalysis, 1949.

Freud, Sigmund. *The Interpretation of Dreams*. Ed. by James Strachey. New York. Basic Books, 1955.

Fromm-Reichmann, Frieda. *Principles of Intensive Psychotherapy*. Chicago. University of Chicago Press, 1950.

Grinker, Roy R., and J. P. Spiegel. *Men Under Stress*. Philadelphia. Blakiston Co., 1945.

Haley, J. "Whither Family Therapy." *Family Process*, 1:69–100, 1962.

Knight, Robert. "Evaluation of Psychotherapeutic Techniques." *Bulletin of the Menninger Clinic*, July, 1952.

Levine, Maurice. *Psychotherapy in Medical Practice*. New York. The Macmillan Co., 1942.

Miller, E., et al. *The Neuroses in War*. London and New York. The Macmillan Co., 1940.

Muncie, Wendell. "Psychobiologic Therapy." *American Journal of Psychotherapy*, April, 1953.

Powdermaker, Florence, and Jerome Frank. "Group Psychotherapy with Neurotics." *American Journal of Psychiatry*, December, 1948.

"Psychiatric Treatment," in the *1951 Proceedings of the Association for Research in Nervous and Mental Disease*, Vol. XXXI. Baltimore. Williams and Wilkins, 1951.

Rosen, John N. *Direct Analysis*. New York. Grune and Stratton, 1953.

Saul, Leon J. *Bases of Human Behavior*. Philadelphia. J. B. Lippincott Co., 1951.

Schilder, Paul. *Psychotherapy*. Revised Ed. New York. W. W. Norton & Company, 1951.

Sharpe, Ella. *Dream Analysis*. London. Hogarth Press, 1949.

Slavson, S. R. *Analytic Group Psychotherapy with Children, Adolescents and Adults*. New York. Columbia University Press, 1950.

Slavson, S. R. *An Introduction to Group Therapy*. New York. The Commonwealth Fund, 1954.

Towne, R. D., S. L. Messinger, and H. Sampson. "Schizophrenia and the Marital Family: Accommodations to Symbiosis." *Family Process*, 1:304–318, 1962.

Waelder, Robert. *Basic Theory of Psychoanalysis*. New York. International Universities Press, 1960.

Witmer, H. L., editor. *Teaching Psychotherapeutic Medicine*. New York. The Commonwealth Fund, 1947.

Psychiatry and Religion

Erikson, Erik. *Young Man Luther*. New York. W. W. Norton & Company, 1958.

Flugel, J. C. *Man, Morals and Society*. New York. International Universities Press, 1957.

Freud, Sigmund. *Civilization and Its Discontents*. New York. W. W. Norton & Company, 1962.

Freud, Sigmund. *Moses and Monotheism*. New York. Vintage Books, 1955.

Fromm, Erich. *Man for Himself*. New York. Rinehart & Co., 1947.

Fromm, Erich. *Psychoanalysis and Religion*. New Haven. Yale University Press, 1950.

May, Rollo. *Man's Search for Himself*. New York. W. W. Norton & Company, 1953.

Nuttin, Joseph. *Psychoanalysis and Personality*. Translated by George Lamb. New York. Sheed and Ward, 1953.

Otto, Max. *Science and the Moral Life*. New York. Mentor Books. New American Library, 1949.

Pfister, Oscar. *Christianity and Fear*. Translated by W. H. Johnston. New York. The Macmillan Co., 1949.

Stace, W. T. *Religion and the Modern Mind*. Philadelphia. J. B. Lippincott Co., 1960.

Weatherhead, Leslie D. *Psychology, Religion and Healing*. Nashville, Abingdon-Cokesbury Press, 1951.

Bibliotherapy

Adams, Clifford R. *Preparing for Marriage*. First Ed. New York. E. P. Dutton and Company, 1951.

Adams, Clifford R., and Vance O. Packard, *How to Pick a Mate*. First Ed. New York. E. P. Dutton and Company, 1946.

Baruch, Dorothy Walter. *New Ways in Discipline*. New York. McGraw-Hill Book Co., 1949.

Binger, Carl. *More About Psychiatry*. Chicago. University of Chicago Press, 1949.

Butterfield, Oliver M. *Sex Life in Marriage*. New York. Emerson Books, Inc., 1947.

Child Study Association of America. *A Reader for Parents*. W. W. Norton & Company, 1963.

Dunbar, F. *Mind and Body*. New York. Random House, 1955.

English, O. S., and Gerald H. J. Pearson. *Emotional Problems of Living*. Third Ed., New York. W. W. Norton & Company, 1963.

English, O. S., and C. J. Foster. *Fathers are Parents Too*. New York. G. P. Putmans Sons, 1951.

Farnham, Marynia F. *The Adolescent*. New York. Harper and Brothers, 1951.

Fishbein, M., and E. W. Burgess. *Successful Marriage*. Rev. Ed. New York. Doubleday, 1955.

Frazer, J. G. *The Golden Bough*. Third Ed. 13 vols. New York. St. Martins Press, 1955.

Fromm, Erich. *Psychoanalysis and Religion*. New Haven. Yale University Press, 1950.

Himes, James F. *Understanding Your Child*. New York. Prentice-Hall, 1952.

Horney, Karen. *Self-Analysis*. New York. W. W. Norton & Company, 1942.

Kinsey, Alfred, et al. *Sexual Behavior in the Human Female*. Philadelphia. W. B. Saunders Co., 1953.

Kinsey, Alfred, et al. *Sexual Behavior in the Human Male*. Philadelphia. W. B. Saunders Co., 1948.

Lawton, George. *Aging Successfully*. New York. Columbia University Press, 1946.

Levy, John and Ruth Munroe. *The Happy Family*. New York. Alfred A. Knopf, 1938.

Liebman, Joshua L. *Peace of Mind*. New York. Simon and Schuster, 1946.

May, Rollo. *Man's Search for Himself*. New York. W. W. Norton & Company, 1953.

Mead, M. *Male and Female*. New York. William Morrow and Co., 1944.

Menninger, K. A. *Love Against Hate*. New York. Harcourt, Brace & Co., 1959.

Menninger, K. A. *Man Against Himself*. New York. Harcourt, Brace & Co., 1956.

Menninger, W. C., and M. Leaf. *You and Psychiatry*. New York. Charles Scribner's Sons, 1948.

Montagu, Ashley. *On Being Human*. New York. Henry Schuman, 1950.

Mudd, Emily, and Aron Krich, Eds. *Man and Wife*. W. W. Norton & Company, 1957.

Overstreet, Harry A. *The Mature Mind*. New York. W. W. Norton & Company, 1949.

Peale, Norman Vincent. *A Guide to Confident Living*. New York. Prentice-Hall, Inc., 1948.

Preston, George H. *Should I Retire?* New York. Rinehart & Co., 1952.

Ribble, Margaret. *The Rights of Infants*. New York. Columbia University Press, 1943.

Spock, Benjamin. *Pocket Book of Baby and Child Care*. New York. Pocket Books, Inc., 1945.

Strecker, E., and K. Appel. *Discovering Ourselves*. Second Ed. New York. The Macmillan Co., 1943.

Wolf, A. W. M. *The Parents' Manual*. New York. Simon and Schuster, 1941.

Chemotherapy

Fisher, Seymour, editor. *Child Research in Psychopharmacology*. Springfield, Illinois, Charles C. Thomas, 1959.

Flach, Frederic F., and Peter F. Regan. *Chemotherapy in Emotional Disorders*. New York. McGraw-Hill Book Co., Inc. 1960.

Ostow, Mortimer. *Drugs in Psychoanalysis and Psychotherapy*. New York. Basic Books, 1962.

Uhr, Leonard, and James G. Miller, editors. *Drugs and Behavior*. New York. John Wiley & Sons, Inc., 1960.

Remmon, E., S. Cohen, K. S. Ditman, and J. R. Frantz. *Psychochemotherapy*. Los Angeles. Western Medical Publications, 1962.

Mental Health and Community Psychiatry

Harvard Medical School and Psychiatric Service Massachusetts General Hospital. *Community Mental Health and Social Psychiatry: A Reference Guide*. Cambridge, Mass. Harvard University Press, 1962.

Joint Commission on Mental Illness and Health. *Action for Mental Health*. New York. Basic Books, 1961.

Leighton, A. N., J. A. Clausen, and R. N. Wilson, editors. *Explorations in Social Psychiatry*. New York. Basic Books, 1957.

Caplan, Gerald, editor. *Prevention of Mental Disorders in Children*. New York. Basic Books, 1961.

Caplan, Gerald. *An Approach to Community Mental Health*. New York. Grune and Stratton, 1961.

Monographs published by the Joint Commission on Mental Illness and Health:

#1. Jahoda, M. *Current Concepts of Positive Mental Health*. New York. Basic Books, 1958.

#2. Fein, Rashi. *Economics of Mental Illness*. New York. Basic Books, 1958.

#3. Albee, G. W. *Mental Health Manpower Trends*. New York. Basic Books, 1959.

#4. Gurin, G., J. Veroff, and S. Feld. *Americans View Their Mental Health. A Nationwide Interview Survey*. New York. Basic Books, 1960.

#5. Robinson, R., D. DeMarche, and M. Wagle. *Community Resources in Mental Health*. New York. Basic Books, 1960.

#6. Plunkett, R., and J. Gordon. *Epidemiology and Mental Illness*. New York. Basic Books, 1960.

#7. Allinsmith, W., and G. Goethals. *The Role of Schools in Mental Health*. New York. Basic Books, 1962.

#8. McCann, R. *The Churches and Mental Health*. New York. Basic Books, 1962.

#9. Schwartz, M., et al. *New Perspectives of Mental Patient Care*. (In preparation)

#10. Soskin, W. *Research Resources in Mental Health*. (In preparation)

Miscellaneous

Reports and Symposiums of the Group for the Advancement of Psychiatry. Volumes I through IV. New York. Group for the Advancement of Psychiatry Publications Office.

Index